Japanese Psychotherapies

Japanese Psychotherapies

Silence and Body-Mind Interconnectedness in Morita, Naikan and Dohsa-hou

Velizara Chervenkova

日本の心理療法における「間」の治癒力と心身相関―

森田療法・内観療法・動作法に着目して

チェルヴェンコヴァ ヴェリザラ

Springer

Velizara Chervenkova
Osaka University
Osaka
Japan

ISBN 978-981-10-3125-0 ISBN 978-981-10-3126-7 (eBook)
DOI 10.1007/978-981-10-3126-7

Library of Congress Control Number: 2016961326

Printed on acid-free paper

This Springer imprint is published by Springer Nature
The registered company is Springer Nature Singapore Pte Ltd.
The registered company address is: 152 Beach Road, #21-01/04 Gateway East, Singapore 189721, Singapore

To the loving memory of
my grandmother Velika and
my father Minko
this book I wholeheartedly dedicate

The Gifts of Silence

It is said that "silence is golden." This saying is especially apt in Japan, where much cultural emphasis is placed upon showing sensitivity toward others' unspoken feelings and thoughts, as well as toward the "atmosphere" of places and situations. This can make Japan a bewildering place for visitors from the West who are typically more comfortable with direct, verbal communication. This difference is also evident when comparing approaches to psychotherapy that have developed in Japan and the West, and the emphasis in the former upon silence.

In this book, Velizara Chervenkova discusses both the theoretical and practical aspects of three representative Japanese psychotherapies—Morita, Naikan, and Dohsa-hou—with attention to their emphasis upon the therapeutic power of silence on the one hand, and upon body–mind interconnectedness on the other.

Morita Therapy was developed by the psychiatrist Shōma Morita as a method for dealing especially with anxiety-based disorders. Morita's view on human nature, which shaped the goals of his therapy and its phases of treatment (both of which are described in the pages ahead), holds that at the root of fears and anxiety there lies a strong desire for life. It is our deluded mind that causes suffering. Morita's concepts are often congruent with philosophical notions from Zen Buddhism, such as *arugamama*—accepting things as they are, and *jun-na kokoro*—a pure heart that sees without judgment, both qualities that are attributed to one who has attained an enlightened state.

Naikan literally means "looking within." Naikan therapy was developed by Rev. Ishin Yoshimoto from a spiritual practice called *mishirabe*, which was practiced among followers of the Jodo Shin Buddhist sect in a rural district in Nara, Japan, where he was born. *Mishirabe* incorporated deep self-reflection along with strict physical restrictions, often bringing practitioners to the point where they faced their own death. What Yoshimoto realized through *mishirabe* was the degree to which his own life had been sustained by others—by all living creatures and ultimately by Nature—instead of through his own self-centered efforts. Based on his experience, Yoshimoto established the Naikan approach as a gentler method that was suitable for anyone, not only Buddhist practitioners, and that would help them experience a new self-understanding and motivation for positive change. Naikan therapy has been successfully adapted for use in prisons, detention centers, schools and business trainings, and has also been found to be efficacious in treating patients with a variety of mental difficulties.

Dohsa-hou, the youngest among the three psychotherapies, was developed by the psychologist Gosaku Naruse. Dohsa-hou literally means “a way to act out; a way to perform an action, behavior or bodily movement.” Its method utilizes a holistic process of motor action which draws upon the inner psychic activities of bodily movement. Initially, Naruse applied this method to children with cerebral palsy to improve their motor difficulty. Subsequently, it has been applied to patients with various disorders and disabilities such as autistic disorder, Down syndrome, mental retardation, hyperactivities, and schizophrenia, in order to stabilize their emotions and to improve their patterns of behavior and posture in daily life. Since the majority of targeted patients suffer from intellectual disabilities, nonverbal communication—giving preference to touch and eye contact, as well as facial expressions—has remained essential to the method, in which trainer and trainee collaborate to accomplish particular movement tasks. By focusing together within the same space-time reality upon the performance of a certain task, both parties attempt to understand each others’ intentions, preferences, and mentality.

In this excellent and informative book, Velizara Chervenkova explores each therapy in its own chapter, and ends each such chapter with a comparison between the respective therapy and a Western counterpart in a search for similarities or differences. She pairs Morita therapy with Metapsychiatry, Naikan with Freudian psychoanalysis, and Dohsa-hou with Body-Mind Psychotherapy. Such a comparison reveals cultural differences, yet helps the reader to see the unbiased truth about the mutual reality that people share.

Velizara Chervenkova makes three other key contributions as well. First, in the opening chapter she usefully explores various aspects of Japanese culture as a background for the development of the three psychotherapies, which helps to bring out crucially different assumptions that inform them vis-à-vis Western psychotherapies. Notably, she offers an account of silence as a feature of Japanese life, and then proceeds with an original interpretation of silence’s therapeutic potential. Second, she also illuminates how each therapy operates upon assumptions of body–mind unity, and describes how this important concept can be of help to both physical and mental health, as well as contributing to personal growth. Finally, she presents the results of three original studies that she has carried out utilizing these therapies, both in Japan and in her native country of Bulgaria. The first is a six-day Dohsa-hou camp in Japan, in which she served as the trainer of a young patient with hydrocephaly; the second reports the findings of a pilot clinical study using written Naikan therapy among drug- and alcohol-addicted clients of a rehabilitation day-care center in Bulgaria; and finally, she offers her personal experiences with Morita therapy over a two-week period of experiential hospitalization.

I think readers will be impressed to observe how particular culture-bound phenomena are interwoven with the development of distinct psychotherapeutic approaches whose basic tenets differ from and sometimes even contradict those commonly known in the West. At the same time, however, while the therapeutic power of silence and the assumption of mind-body interconnectedness that animate these therapies arose from particular expressions of Japanese culture, the successful adaptation of these psychotherapies to non-Japanese contexts suggests that these principles are applicable more widely. It may be that these three therapies point to resources that can be of value to all humankind. In illuminating them so clearly and compellingly, Velizara Chervenkova has done a major service, tuning Western ears to the powerful gifts of silence.

Tottori, Japan
On the cusp of cherry blossom season 2016

Mari Sengoku

A Few Words in the Silence

Giving birth to a text may be likened to giving birth to a child: both processes require time and follow patterns of organic growth and development. In creating a text, however, the author needs some sort of demiurgic faculties for they have to call out *ex nihilo* the words one by one and then put them in such an order so as the author's unique creation—the text—to see the light of day. The author is indeed the creator of the text and the text is their creation. But if we take a glimpse below the surface, we may recognize the author's heart as a distiller where everything they have experienced and all the people they have met on their way now ripen into the mellow wine of their text. For even the life of a hermit cannot isolate the author completely.

Such was the creation process of the present book. Starting seven years ago as a project about Naikan therapy, it evolved into, I believe, a full-fledged monograph about three Japanese psychotherapies. Over all these years the text grew organically before my eyes and now, when the birth pangs have subsided, I realize that I have never been alone with my text. I therefore wish to express my gratitude to all the people who have been and still are right next to me on this inspiring trip—a trip which has probably started unnoticed back in the late 1990s when, as an undergraduate student, I first learned about the Japanese psychotherapies and let them fascinate me.

First, I thank Osamu Imura, Professor of Clinical Psychology at Osaka University. I vividly remember one of the first times we met at Osaka University: it was a Dohsa-hou therapeutic session. When I entered the room, I saw Prof. Imura playing on the floor and laughing merrily with several children with disabilities. I immediately understood that I have met a gifted teacher and a person with a generous heart. Over these years, Prof. Imura spared no effort to support me in my academic life and provide valuable advice on my research. I hope that our fruitful collaboration will continue in the future.

I also thank Katsuhiro Oimatsu, Professor of Clinical Psychology at Osaka University, and Wolfgang Schwentker, Professor of Intellectual History and Social Thought at Osaka University. Even the shortest discussions with them made me feel grateful to be part of the academic world.

My gratitude goes further to Kyō Kobayashi and Mitsuho Ikeda, both professors at the Faculty of Human Sciences, Osaka University. They helped me understand that true knowledge first has a place in the heart. A great deal of the inspiration for writing this book I owe to them.

I also thank the associate and assistant professors of the Clinical Psychology Department at Osaka University over the period 2010–2016: Haruo Nomura, Jun Sasaki, Reiko Ōmae, Shie Kamijō, Shōko Sugao, and Haruo Fujino, as well as Dr. Naoko Wada, Dr. Takuma Matsumoto, Dr. Tomonori Adachi, Dr. Tsuyoshi Takeda, Dr. Yukio Obunai, Dr. Yuki Doi, Naho Yūki, and Yukitaka Takimoto for their kind support.

A number of people outside of the Osaka University, too, accompanied me wholeheartedly on my way. I thank Prof. Yoshihiko Miki and Junko Miki of Nara Naikan Training Center, under whose guidance I made my first steps in the fascinating world of Naikan therapy, including my personal experience in intensive Naikan. Later, my skills as a Naikan interviewer were tested under the strict but nurturing guidance of Mieko Hariki, Director of Osaka Naikan Training Center, and of the members of the monthly research meetings held at the center. I received enormous moral support also from Prof. Teruaki Maeshiro, Director of Yamato Naikan Training Center; Prof. Makoto Kusano and his wife, Mrs. Setsuko Kusano, from Hokuriku Mental Health Research Center; Dr. Shō'ichi Ihara of St. Martin Hospital in Kagawa prefecture; and Dr. Takahiro Takemoto, head of Ibusuki Takemoto Hospital in Kagoshima prefecture.

In the field of Dohsa-hou I was first initiated by Prof. Osamu Imura, but I would like to also acknowledge the invaluable support of Atsushi Konishi, Hideaki Naohara, Hiroaki Ueno, and Toshio Iwai—supervisors at the monthly Dohsa-hou seminars held at Osaka University; and of Dohsa-hou supervisors Hiro'o Inoue, Toshiyuki Miyoshi, Yoshiko Noguchi, and the late Masaki Mabuchi from the "Sunflower" Dohsa-hou Society in Ibaraki city, Osaka prefecture; Prof. Kenji Ishikura from Hyogo University of Teacher Education; and Dr. Bunko Kouno, a Dohsa-hou supervisor, clinical psychologist, and chief priest of the Fukuju-ji Zen Buddhist temple in Aichi prefecture.

My sincere thanks go further to Sei Tanaka, my Dohsa-hou trainee since the very beginning, and to his devoted mother—Mrs. Miki Tanaka—who kindly allowed me to use the pictures and the real name of her son in this book (Part IV and Appendix III). I also thank all the trainees and their parents/caregivers of the Dohsa-hou seminars and intensive camps I have attended over the years. They taught me much through their courage and their faith in life. Above all, thanks to them I would never again doubt that pure joy exists in this world.

My insights into Morita therapy, and also into the genuine beauty and depth of the Japanese psychotherapies and of Japanese culture in general, I owe to Dr. Shin'ichi Usa, Director of Sansei Hospital in Kyoto (which has since closed down), who kindly admitted me for experiential hospitalization. The moments we exchanged only a few words, but lots of profound silence over a cup of green tea will always remain moments of Eternity.

I thank further all the inpatients of Sansei Hospital at the time of my experiential hospitalization for their silent, yet invaluable support and for sharing two weeks of precious communal life; as well as the nursing staff, especially Mrs. Yoshie Imanishi and Mrs. Saeko Ichida, for their kind help.

Many thanks go also to Prof. Shigeyoshi Okamoto, Director of Kyoto Institute of Morita Therapy and part-time physician at Sansei Hospital from 1974 to 2014; Dr. Nobuo Kurokawa, Director of Kurokawa Clinic of Internal Medicine in Osaka; and Mr. Hiroshi Mandai, librarian at The Mental Health Okamoto Memorial Foundation in Osaka. They all supported wholeheartedly my research in the field of Morita therapy.

I thank also music therapist Mrs. Hiroko Katō and Dr. Mari Fujisawa, clinical psychologist at Toneyama Municipal Hospital in Osaka, where I was admitted to volunteer during the music therapy sessions with the patients of the severe neurological disorders ward. Over the two years of volunteering at the hospital, I was given the chance to communicate, more often nonverbally, with the patients, and to witness how in their slowly dying bodies their spirit was blossoming out more and more with humor, wisdom, and unconditional love. I will always remember those simple but great lessons of life.

My thanks go further to Dr. Elena Nikolova, Director of "Solidarity" day-care center for drug and alcohol addicts in Sofia, for her open-mindedness toward the novelty that Naikan therapy was to Bulgaria back in 2011–2012. I am grateful also to the center's staff for their assistance during the two studies that we carried out there, and, of course, to the study participants—allowing me to take a glimpse into their life stories and into the brave struggles with their own addictive behavior will always remain a precious gem for me. I pray that wherever the participants are now, they have more courage and will to live.

I want to wholeheartedly thank all my friends both in Japan and in Bulgaria, especially Dr. Iskra Velinova for her timely, wise, and heartfelt support; and Andrey Mezan, Kalina Bogdanova, and Megelina Dimitrova-Koleva—for simply being here. Listing all the other names might take another page and I will therefore refrain from doing it. I will only name my dear friends whom I met in Japan: Akemi Sakurai and her *Geetanjali* group for classical Indian dances, Asataka Matsuda, Ayasa Ishii, Boris Todorov, Chikako Yamaji, Eline Sikkema, Father David and Olga Mizuguchi from the Osaka Orthodox Church, Hani Al-Shareef, Hiromi Ōmori, Kazuhiko and Chikako Fujita, Keishirō Suzuki and his family, Kenya Hirose, Liliya Totevska, Mahdi Choyekh, Mari Higuchi, Mari Washio, Marina Demeshko, Mariyana Voynikova, Masayuki Ijiri, Michiko and Kiyoko Imai, Miroslav Matev, Mohan Pyari Maharjan, Noriko Iwata, Petko Slavov, Peter Dimitrov, Regina Yakimenko, Reinis Udris, Sachiko Nanri, Samia Haseeb Khan, Satoyo Takisawa, Sophie Bocklandt, Stefan Hadjiev, Stefan Trifonov, Stoyan Ivanov, Takako Hayashi and all the members of the "Let's Talk in Japanese" volunteer group at Suita International Friendship Association, Tenko Ima and her *Kiraza* Butoh dance group, Tihomir Manev, Tomoko Yoshino, Toshihiro Suzuki, Yani Karavasilev, Yanko Popov, Yūko Miyoshi, and Zornitsa Cholakova-Uratani. I feel blessed to have met them here and to have shared the weal and woe of my life in Japan with them.

I am deeply indebted to Rev. Mari Sengoku, Ph.D., Director of *Shinshin-Mezame* Naikan Center in Tottori; Dr. David K. Reynolds, founder of the Constructive Living approach; and Paula Arai, Professor of Comparative Religion at Louisiana State University, for their unconditional help and encouragement on the publication of the present book. My sincere thanks go further to Mrs. Jayanthie Krishnan and Mr. Vishal Daryanomel, editors at Springer Nature Singapore, and to Mrs. Hema Suresh and Mr. Mohammed Ali from Scientific Publishing Services (P) Ltd., for their kind and timely guidance through the editorial process of the present book. My sincere gratitude goes also to my devoted friend, Dr. Irina Kyulanova, for sparing her time on the precise proofreading of the entire text and providing valuable advice. Had there not been her enormous and heartfelt help, I would not have been able to accomplish this book.

Last but not least, my deepest gratitude goes to my mother Todorka and my brother Sotir for their constant moral support. I thank them also for sharing unforgettable moments while enjoying the beauty of the Land of the Rising Sun.

I also reserve a great deal of my gratitude for my beloved Emil—sharing a mutual ardour for Japan and its culture was just the beginning of our trip. Without him, my academic life in Japan would not be as fruitful and inspiring. Although from the other side of the globe, Emil was steadfastly here with me throughout all these years to advise and encourage.

Finally, rather than from books, I learned more about Japan while I was traveling throughout its enchanting land in contemplation of the beautiful contrast between the green paddy fields and the blue roofs of the traditional houses; of its mystic mountains and unfathomable seas; its cities and villages—ever ancient and modern; and the faces of its people—sometimes cheerful and bright, sometimes gloomy and melancholic, but always genuine the way they are: *Japanese*.

To you all, I bow and give you my thanks from the depths of my heart.

Osaka, Japan
March 2016

Velizara Chervenkova

Contents

About the Author

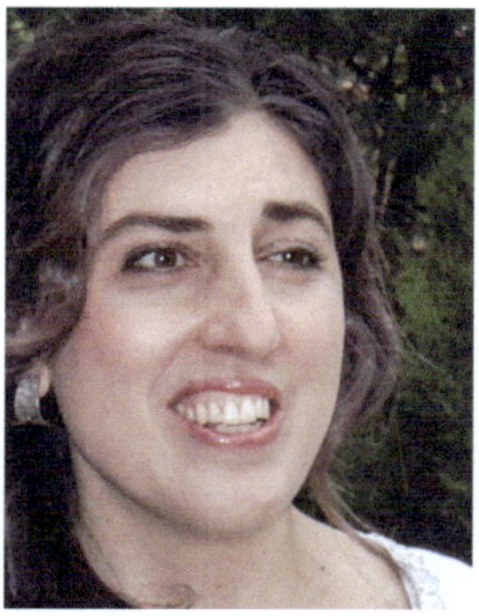

Velizara Chervenkova was born in October 1980 in Sofia, Bulgaria. She graduated from a Japanese- and English-language school in 1998 in her hometown. Four years later, she obtained bachelor degrees in Psychology and in Japanese Studies from the Sofia University, Bulgaria. Between 2002 and 2007 she obtained master degrees in Clinical and Counseling Psychology, and in Indology, also from the Sofia University. Over the years of her university education, she underwent trainings and individual psychotherapy with the C. G. Jung Bulgarian Society of Analytical Psychology. In parallel, she worked as a Japanese language teaching assistant at her alma mater, and as a Japanese- and English-language translator and journalist at the local branch of Factiva, a Dow Jones company.

In 2010 Velizara Chervenkova was accepted in Osaka University as a Japanese government scholarship student where in 2014 she finished a doctoral course in Clinical and Counseling Psychology. Her research and practical training are focused on the Japanese psychotherapies Morita, Naikan, and Dohsa-hou—especially the way they consider issues of body–mind interconnectedness—and on the opportunities for the further dissemination of these approaches outside of Japan.

Velizara Chervenkova has publications on the Japanese psychotherapies in both Japanese and international journals, and has translated from Japanese *Journey to Your Heart—Workbook for Practicing Written Naikan* (Nara Naikan Training Center, 2015). She is a regular member of the Association of Japanese Clinical Psychology, The Japan Naikan Association, and the Japanese Association of Rehabilitation Psychology; the latter handed to her in 2014 a Dohsa-hou trainer certificate.

Velizara Chervenkova is currently working as a specially appointed Assistant Professor in the Department of Clinical Psychology at Osaka University, where she is in charge of a project on the international popularization of Dohsa-hou therapy. As part of this project, she has compiled two non-sale books about Dohsa-hou: *Introduction to Rehabilitation Psychology—Theory and Application* (Osaka University, 2015; in Bulgarian) and *Introduction to Dohsa-hou—An Integrated Japanese Body-Mind Therapy* (Osaka University, 2016; co-authored, in English).

Part I
On the Threshold

Chapter 1
Why Japanese Psychotherapies?

Over the last decades, the interest toward Eastern culture, religion, and philosophy has grown significantly. This interest includes issues of general well-being, but also such spanning to the fields of specialized mental and physical healthcare. One of the recent examples in the specialized field is the so-called third wave in cognitive-behavioral therapy based on the concept of *mindfulness*—the seventh element of the Noble Eightfold Path across Buddhism. In this example, a centuries-old convention born within Eastern cultural and religious context influences the Western thought, which tries to dress it up in a scientific gown and apply it within a clinical setting. On the other hand, the West appears reluctant to adopt Eastern therapeutic approaches which have already been approved scientifically in their native countries. This tendency is especially valid for the original Japanese psychotherapies—the main subject of the present book. As the Japanese essayist Shū'ichi Kato points out, Japanese scholars readily research and adopt Western scientific approaches, but the opposite is rarely the case (Kato, as cited in Miki and Kuroki 1998: 5). Although Japanese culture has fascinated and influenced a great number of scientists, writers, and artists of the West, the country's psychotherapeutic approaches have remained confined to their homeland and some Asian neighbors; to the best of our knowledge, the non-Asian countries to which these approaches have been introduced and applied in a consistent way are rather few.

There are, we suggest, two main reasons for this *status quo*. First, because of certain cultural peculiarities, the Japanese psychotherapies remain somewhat veiled in mystery behind which their universal therapeutic potential is difficult to comprehend. Hence, their validity as psychotherapies in the Western sense of the word is often questioned, if not simply ignored. Perhaps for these reasons, some Western scholars harshly dispute even the use of the term "psychotherapy" when referring to the Japanese approaches in question. Such statements are based on the argument that assessment criteria and well-ordered theory of consciousness are *sine qua non*

V. Chervenkova, *Japanese Psychotherapies*,
DOI 10.1007/978-981-10-3126-7_1

for any approach to be classified as psychotherapy; that these methods are not intended to be practiced as psychodynamic ones, for which reason they should be labeled "Japanese-derived systems of therapy" or simply "therapies".[1] Other scholars claim that "to label a particular Japanese practice using the English word "psychotherapy" is to risk inaccurately circumscribing it through inappropriate connotations—in terms of what is implied about its origins, its purposes, and its likely meaning to participants. This is most clearly the case with Morita and Naikan therapies, for neither of which either "psychotherapy" or "religious practice" would be an entirely satisfactory tag" (Harding et al. 2015: 8). However, being too careful not to inaccurately circumscribe these approaches is yet another pitfall—that of naming them in ambiguous ways such as "practice," "meditation," or the previously mentioned "therapy," which may signify any other kind of original Japanese treatment—for example, approaches to health as completely irrelevant to the present topic as *shiatsu* massage therapy. In our case, such denotations threaten to make even the title of the present book ambiguous. Although in its origin "psychotherapy" is not an Eastern paradigm and it is often associated with the "talking cure" of the West, "the time now seems ripe for genuine synthesis of the great achievements of the Eastern and Western healing traditions" (Sheikh et al. 1996: xxi). Therefore, such a debate on terminology is far from constructive and, what is more, it threatens to aggravate unnecessarily the East–West gap. Considering this, we term the three Japanese approaches that are the subject of this book—Morita, Nakan, and Dohsa-hou—"psychotherapies" referring exclusively (i) to the Japanese term *shinri-ryōhō* (心理療法), which literally means "psychotherapy" and which is widely used by the contemporary Japanese specialists when describing these approaches[2], and (ii) to the fact that, as we explain throughout the book, these approaches are aimed at transforming the mindset of their clients and this aim implies psychotherapeutic endeavors *per se*, no matter the cultural context; the

[1]This is a summary of comments that the author received in the past from anonymous Western reviewers. For further details on the issue, see Sheikh et al. (1996: xx-xxii).

[2]For example, Miki and Kuroki (1998), Nagayama et al. (2006: 3–5), and a recently published work by Iwao Akita, *Japanese Psychotherapies* (2014), to name only a few. Also, *Flowing Bridges, Quiet Waters—Japanese Psychotherapies, Morita and Nakan* (1989) by David K. Reynolds, "Japanese Forms of Psychotherapy: Naikan Therapy and Morita Therapy" (Tanaka-Matsumi in Gielen et al. 2004: 277–291), and "Unique Psychotherapies Developed in Asia" (Tseng et al. in Chang 2012: 414–431).

The term *shinri-ryōhō* was first introduced by the Buddhist philosopher Enryō Inoue in his book of the same title (1904) to signify all non-medical approaches to healing, for example, hypnosis. *Shinri-ryōhō* came extensively into use after the influential Japanese psychiatrist Tsunerō Imura (1906–1981), disciple of Shōma Morita and Professor at Nihon University, published a book of the same title in 1952. Imura suggested that the English word "psychotherapy" should be rendered into Japanese by *shinri-ryōhō* because the prewar term for "psychotherapy"—*seishin-ryōhō*(精神療法)—was easy to mistake for non-scientific approaches, magic included. In postwar Japan, such connotations of *seishin-ryōhō* faded away; today, when having in mind "psychiotherapy," Japanese psychologists tend to use more often *shinri-ryōhō*, whereas physicians and psychiatrists—*seishin-ryōhō* (Koizumi 2004:41–42). The Japanese transliteration "saikoserapī"(サイコセラピー) is also used sometimes as a more neutral term.

outcomes of these endeavors are supported through numerous evidence-based research. In the end, the fact that the Japanese approaches do not fit completely into the domain of the extant Western psychotherapies does not mean that they cannot offer efficacious psychotherapeutic models. On the contrary, as Miki and Kuroki aptly point out, the Japanese psychotherapies can provide important notions that their Western counterparts lack (Miki and Kuroki 1998: 7), broadening this way the range of healing paradigms across cultures and enriching the psychotherapeutic domain with models that differ from, or sometimes even contradict, the existent ones, but are no less efficacious than them.

Second, despite a recent increase in the English-language literature on the subject, there are still some gaps that need filling. The lack of sources other than Japanese-language ones—especially about Naikan therapy and Dohsa-hou therapy—becomes an insurmountable impediment to gaining access to the precious knowledge that the Japanese psychotherapies offer. The present book therefore shoulders the task to remedy—to the best of our abilities—this gap and present in a streamlined manner a general historical overview and an outline of the main components, both theoretical and practical, of three representative Japanese psychotherapies—Morita, Naikan, and Dohsa-hou. The term "representative" we use in the sense that these therapies have originated in Japan and bear certain cultural peculiarities, but not because they should be distinguished as deserving more attention than other Japanese therapeutic methods. According to Miki and Kuroki, there are several psychotherapeutic approaches we could term "Japanese." Besides the three mentioned above, these further include, for example, pot image therapy (壺イメージ療法) where the client is encouraged to imagine a vessel, "fill" its interiors with images, then "cover" it and distance themselves from it; and *haiku* therapy (俳句療法) where composing the traditional Japanese verses is believed to possess a therapeutic potential (Miki and Kuroki 1998).[3]

Despite the fact that the oldest among these approaches, Morita therapy, has gained significant international popularity over the years, which one of them is most recognizable and systematically applied outside of Japan is difficult to estimate. We decided to present exactly these three psychotherapies—Morita, Naikan, and Dohsa-hou—in the chronological order of their development, because they offer an opportunity for tracing how their cultural features converge in two focal points, namely the *therapeutic power of silence* and the *body–mind interconnectedness*. We suggest that these two points concern issues common to all humans and their psycho-physical well-being and personal growth, and as such these points have the potential to acknowledge the three Japanese approaches as *psychotherapies*.

---

[3]Another form of original Japanese therapy that deserves attention—forest therapy (*shinrin-ryōhō* – 森林療法)—is also being promoted in the country but, within our knowledge, not extensively enough outside of it. For further details, see the works of Tanaka (2009) and Morimoto et al. (2006), the second of which focuses on the so-called forest medicine.

References

Akita, Iwao (ed.): Japanese Psychotherapies—A Thought Compendium, Shinyosha, 2014 (in Japanese)

Chang, Edward C. (ed.): Handbook of Adult Psychopathology in Asians—Theory, Diagnosis, and Treatment, Oxford University Press, 2012

Gielen, Uwe P., J. M. Fish, J. G. Draguns (ed.): Handbook of Culture, Therapy, and Healing, Routledge, 2004

Harding, Christopher, F. Iwaki, S. Yoshinaga (ed.): Religion and Psychotherapy in Modern Japan, Routledge, 2015

Koizumi, Shin'ichi: *Shinri-ryōhō* and *Seishin-ryōhō* in Prewar Japan, in "Introduction and Adoption of Clinical Psychology in Japan"—The 68th Congress of the Japanese Psychological Association, retrieved from http://www.ritsumeihuman.com/uploads/publications/97/9_35.pdf, Ritsumeikan University, 2004 (in Japanese)

Miki, Yoshihiko, K. Kuroki (co-ed.): Japanese Psychotherapies—Essence and Practice, Tokishobo, 1998 (in Japanese)

Morimoto, Kanehisa, Y. Miyazaki, H. Hirano (ed.): Forest Medicine, Asakura Publishing, 2006 (in Japanese)

Nagayama, Kei'ichi, Y. Shimizu: Naikan Method—Theory and Practical Structure, Nippon Hyoron Sha, 2006 (in Japanese)

Reynolds, David K.: Flowing Bridges, Quiet Waters—Japanese Psychotherapies, Morita and Naikan, State University of New York Press, 1989

Sheikh, Anees A., K.S. Sheikh, J. Achterberg (ed.): Healing East and West—Ancient Wisdom and Modern Psychology, Wiley & Sons Inc, 1996

Tanaka, Atsuo: Walking the Forests—An Invitation to Forest Therapy, Akatsuki Printing Inc, 2009 (in Japanese)

Chapter 2
Structure and Content of the Book

The present book is based on a general-to-particular approach. Seemingly, its starting point is not related directly to psychology and psychotherapy, but it has to be discussed so that a more profound understanding about the three psychotherapies can be gained. In other words, we need to specify what "Japanese" means, what makes the psychotherapies in question different from others we know and why we need to label them "Japanese."

To this end, after explaining in **Part I** the importance of the core topic of the present book—the Japanese psychotherapies—in **Part II** we briefly discuss Japan's geographical and national characteristics, and historical circumstances that likely relate to the peculiarities of the Japanese mentality. All these characteristics and circumstances serve as a background, although not an absolute one, for the development of the three psychotherapeutic methods. If we fail to consider the methods against such a background, we risk losing sight of the forest for the trees and thus draw too narrow and culturally biased conclusions, which erroneously explain phenomena that are not completely familiar to the Western psychological science. Although Part II speculates upon key cultural concepts such as *Dō*, *ma*, and *gen-fūkei*, it does not aspire to meet any scientific ends in the field of Cultural Studies, Anthropology, and Japanology; such speculation only serves as a likely gateway to the book's core topic—the Japanese psychotherapies. However, before embarking on a detailed study of the main subject, we need to take a step back and attempt to see the full picture of the culture where these psychotherapies were born—a culture that is multilayered rather than multifaceted or mosaic; hence the need of a general-to-particular approach.

Based on the author's interpretation of silence as a distinctive Japanese cultural phenomenon related to the characteristics of the country's landscape, Part II further discusses what the therapeutic effect of silence is and how it is harnessed in service of both physical and mental health and personal growth. In Japan, these are tantamount to attaining balance between body and mind, and this process is exclusively conducted in seclusion and silence.

V. Chervenkova, *Japanese Psychotherapies*,
DOI 10.1007/978-981-10-3126-7_2

Part III presents the theoretical interpretation of the three psychotherapies, partly based on the author's personal experience with them. First, we introduce Morita therapy as the oldest one, which is rather popular outside of Japan and which partly adopts Western psychological thought in its tenets. Presenting in brief its founder Shōma Morita's life is also important for gaining more profound understanding of the method's key therapeutic components.

Then we introduce Naikan therapy, which can be considered a unique phenomenon in the world of mental healthcare for it was born out of an indigenous religious practice and established by a Buddhist priest, Rev. Ishin Yoshimoto. For this reason, the readers will notice that the chapter on the development and theory of the Naikan therapy is almost twice the volume of the chapters presenting the other two therapies. It is so because we need to explain how exactly this practice has evolved into a psychotherapy, emphasizing the founder's biography as well.[1]

Finally, we introduce the youngest among the three psychotherapies—Dohsa-hou—which, similarly to Morita therapy, was conceived under the influence of Western psychological thought, primarily hypnotherapy and autogenic training, by academic scholar Gosaku Naruse; but it eventually evolved into an approach with distinctive Japanese features. These we explain in detail.

Each of the chapters closes with a brief comparison between the respective therapy and a Western counterpart in a search for similarities or differences: Morita therapy and Metapsychiatry; Naikan therapy and Freudian psychoanalysis; and Dohsa-hou and Body–Mind Psychotherapy. Although many aspects cannot be readily transferred between the respective approaches, we decided to make such comparisons in order to prove that approaches on well-being in different cultures have not been developed entirely separately from each other and that the development of the Japanese psychotherapies is part of the global tendencies. On the other hand, these comparisons may help readers better comprehend the specific Japanese nature of the approaches in question.

The next **Part IV** presents the results of three studies the author carried out in Japan and in Bulgaria. The first chapter of this part discusses the results of a six-day summer Dohsa-hou camp in Japan, in which the author participated as trainer of a 6-year-old boy suffering from hydrocephaly. The tasks during the camp and the outcomes are described in detail as evidence for the trainee's improvement, both physical, in improved posture and bodily movements, and mental and social, with richer facial expression and enhanced communication skills.

The second study—that on Naikan therapy through writing—was aimed at drug- and alcohol-addicted clients of a rehabilitation day-care center in Bulgaria. A pilot study of Naikan therapy in the country, it comprised two phases: an introductory phase and a follow-up phase, which were implemented within 6 months. The positive outcomes shed light upon important issues related to the applicability of the

[1]It is worth mentioning that the founders of both Morita and Naikan therapies had childhood encounters with death. These encounters, as explained in detail in the respective chapters, influenced both their personal lives and the origin of the psychotherapeutic approaches they developed.

Japanese therapies to foreign clients, as well as to the high rehabilitative potential of Naikan therapy in the field of addictions.

The final chapter of Part IV depicts the author's personal experiences in Morita therapy over a two-week experiential hospitalization in the now former Sansei Hospital in Kyoto. This chapter moves away from the objective tone of scientific prose to a more autobiographical mode of writing, which we believe lends it authenticity and more faithfully represents the very nature of Morita therapy with its emphasis on creativity and the concept of true human nature. Additionally, this text may serve as a snapshot of the last months of Sansei Hospital not long before it was closed down and demolished for financial and other reasons. We also believe that such mode of writing that voices the experience and work of a non-Japanese researcher may elucidate further the applicability of these psychotherapies in broader context, i.e., outside of Japan and to non-Japanese clients.

The closing part, **Part V**, presents a general conclusion on the three psychotherapies and summarizes some of their most distinctive features—for example, lack of interest in verbal communication and emphasis on the concept of the natural body–mind unity.

In the end, in three **Appendixes** we present pictures related to the history, development, and present condition of each of the three psychotherapies. For the readers' convenience, the book closes with a brief **Glossary** of those Japanese terms that appear in the text more than once. To those familiar with the Japanese script, in a separate **Reference List** we list the original titles of all Japanese-language sources that this book refers to.

*

It would be presumptuous to attempt to compress between the covers of a single book centuries of human experience and wisdom distilled in the form of these three psychotherapies. As the readers will recognize, this is an enormous subject and it therefore would be exaggerated also to claim that one researcher may be so well grounded in all three of them as to be able to discuss them down to the minutest details. Therefore, all we do is to offer a guide for those who look for a relatively quick tour of the Japanese psychotherapies and perhaps a few signposts for those planning a more extended trip.

To this end, the present book explores mainly the three approaches and the cultural background within which they originated, and to which, we suggest, they owe the specificities of their therapeutic structure and functions. Also, it presents the orthodox versions of the methods the way they were originally established and applied by their founders. Much less attention is given to the general context of the psychotherapy in Japan, how the three psychotherapies are positioned within it now, how they have transformed over the years, and how they are applied nowadays, not because these topics are less important, but because there is not enough space to do them justice. For this reason, there are certain generalizations that may appear too schematized or even inadequate to the contemporary psychotherapeutic milieu.

Moreover, the readers may probably come across some biased statements that inevitably stereotype Japanese culture or overstate its enigmatic nature. Japanese culture and society are changing and so are the psychotherapies in question: in contemporary Japan, different practitioners have different ways of applying the methods and many of them introduce new possibilities to the orthodox versions. Also, it is important to draw attention to the fact that psychological and psychiatric issues in the country are dealt with mainly using Western medical models and that treatments predominantly rely on medication. On top of that, the Japanese psychotherapies are rarely subjects of the Clinical Psychology curricula in the Japanese universities—a situation which Iwao Akita, Professor at Kyoto Bunkyo University, defines as abnormal (Akita 2014: ii). However, discussing all these issues could be the subject of another work. To emphasize some aspects of Japanese culture and society at the expense of others was therefore the necessary evil in order to keep the book's initial concept intact.

Also, the discerning readers will probably notice that not all existing English-language literature on the three approaches was necessarily referred to. Omitting them should not be considered deliberate negligence, but only the result of the natural development of the text: in order to fulfill its aim of outlining the original structure of the three psychotherapies and their development, the present book refers predominantly to original Japanese sources and also to the author's private communication with Japanese specialists who practice in the respective fields, some of them direct disciples of the founders of these therapies. To echo or largely summarize what has already been done in the existent English-language literature is outside of the purpose of this book, both in terms of content and structure. Rather, the book focuses on introducing what, to the best of our knowledge, is not yet available in English. In so doing, we believe that the present book will contribute to broadening and systematizing the yet partial knowledge about the three psychotherapies outside of Japan and among non-Japanese readers and researches. Despite some apparent idiosyncrasies in emphasis and coverage, we also believe that this work is a starting point for a more comprehensive study of the fascinating world of the Japanese psychotherapies rather than a final destination.

*

When introducing Japanese names, we adhere to the Western tradition of placing the personal name first, followed by the surname. This rule we break only on occasions when the individual is already known in the West by their surname placed first—for example, Nishida Kitarō. The Japanese terms we transliterate through the Hepburn romanization system, as we do with the personal names, and present them in Italics; the original Japanese words are parenthesized when the term is introduced for the first time. Exceptions to this romanization system are made in the reference lists for some of the names of Japanese authors and publishing companies—we abide by the transliteration they themselves use for their names. Also, when a Japanese-language source is cited within the text, its author is presented by their family name written in Roman letters only. The author's full name and the source cited are available in the detailed reference list that follow the respective chapter. However, since many of the citations in the text are translated by the author from

Japanese-language sources, we do not put quotations marks as the common rule suggests. Instead, we specify the sources precisely, including (i) the author's family name, (ii) the year the source was published, and (iii) the number of the page where the quotation was taken from—for example, (Yoshimoto 1977: 12).

Unless otherwise stated, all the pictures in the present book were taken by the author in the period from July 2010 to March 2016. They all are used with due permission.

The Dohsa-hou illustrations in Appendix III were kindly done by Shōko Sugao, Assistant Professor in the Department of Clinical Psychology at Osaka University. The illustrations for the first pages of each of the three appendixes were done by the author. These illustrations represent the Japanese "three friends of winter"—*shō-chiku-bai* (松竹梅)—pine, bamboo, and plum blossom, which are praised for their natural abilities to survive harsh environments intact due to their steadfastness, flexibility and resilience, respectively. We find each of these qualities to respectively symbolize the very essence of each of the three Japanese psychotherapeutic approaches—Naikan, Dohsa-hou, and Morita therapy.

Reference

Akita, Iwao (ed.): Japanese Psychotherapies—A Thought Compendium, Shinyosha, 2014 (in Japanese)

Part II
Japan—A Land on the Edge of the World

Often metaphorically referred to as "The Land of the Rising Sun," "The Paradise of Far East," or the less popular but intimate to natives "The Land of Rich Reed Plains and Fresh Rice Ears" (Watsuji 1961: 20) and "The Bountiful Land of Ripening Grain" (Fukuoka, as cited in McLuhan 1994: 150), the islands that make up the country of Japan have for centuries held a fascination for Westerners that has been both exotic and mysterious. For much of its history Japan has been far off the map of the world and even nowadays, in the era of bullet trains and glass skyscrapers, those who look beneath the surface of things can see that, as the Japanese scholar Kakuzō Okakura noticed back in 1905, "in spite of her modern garb, the heart of Old Japan is still beating strongly" (Okakura 1905: 191–192); and this heart is zealously keeping its inmost secrets veiled in mystery.

A turning point in Japan's historical development, the 19th-century Meiji Restoration marked the end of the feudal isolation and the country's subsequent "opening" to the Western world: Japan was "no longer the hermit of the East, but the most Western of the nations of the West" (Sladen, as cited in Lehmann 1978: 20). However, there were Japanese people "significant both in number and influence, who felt very strongly that under no circumstances should Japan be allowed to modernize; they saw Japan as a pre-industrial earthly paradise which should be preserved from the evils of modernity" (Lehmann 1978:14). These evils likely involved the technological advancements that the West so lavishly introduced, but much more ideas and beliefs that threatened to defile the primordial purity of the Japanese soul. Nevertheless, Japan chose modernization, thus turning within the span of a century into one of the world's most scientifically, technologically, and industrially advanced countries.

Even though contemporary Japanese culture may resemble that of the West, remarkably, it has managed to retain the pulsation of the past and preserve manners and social principles so distinctly different from that of other modern nations. We should not forget that "Japan is the only industrialized country in the world with its own primitive religion still intact" (Rapoport 1989:16) and that its traditional attitudes are "not merely traits to be overcome but also assets in the building of the new Japan" (Duus 1976: 10), "making present-day Japan both modern and uniquely Japanese" (Duus 1976: 9). It is the so-called "uniquely Japanese" that often puzzles anyone who embarks on studying the Japanese nation and culture: the moment one phenomenon is "tamed" and put into words, a deeper mystery emerges to provide a different and more comprehensive perspective to the whole picture. As such, this "uniquely Japanese" is difficult to be captured in clear-cut definitions and some authors even consider it a myth that reflects a nationalist ideology (Dale 2012), but still there are many—from mere tourists to long-time devoted researchers—who unanimously agree on its existence.

As mentioned in Chap. 2, in this book we refer to Japanese culture as a *multi-layered* one where different and even contrasting layers are superimposed on one another to create the "uniquely Japanese." "Although history continually undergoes change," the Japanese philosopher Yasuo Yuasa notes, "all that is newly introduced to Japan does not obviate things of the old, but rather, places itself upon the latter. In other words, things of old, like the annual layers of a tree, continue to exist and work in the center" (Yuasa in Carter 2001: xiv). It is the multilayered structure of Japanese culture that is likely to provide clues for an in-depth research of the core topic of the present book—the three Japanese psychotherapies Morita, Naikan, and Dohsa-hou. That is why, as readers will probably notice for themselves, in some of the chapters it is difficult to draw clear-cut boundaries between psychology on the one hand, and culture and religion on the other. This, however, appears to be the major advantage when researching the Japanese psychotherapies for it gives clues on their truly Japanese "soul," which distinguishes them from other approaches we are familiar with.

For all of these reasons, as mentioned in Chap. 2, before embarking on the core subject, we will set off for the world of the "uniquely Japanese," starting from the country's geographical and historical specificities, traditional attitudes, and mentality of its people. All of these, we suggest, form the background that the three psychotherapies have sprung from. Ignoring these cultural layers would be nearly tantamount to reducing the Japanese psychotherapies to yet another bunch of exotic techniques for body–mind wellness. In so doing, we may easily miss the chance to gain intimate knowledge of the centuries-old spiritual legacy of the Japanese people and, more dangerously, of the therapeutic potential of the approaches themselves.

Chapter 3
Traveling in Silence—An Attempt for Cultural–Anthropological Reading of the Japanese *Kokoro**

Magical indeed is the charm of this land, as of a land haunted by gods; so lovely the spectral delicacy of colors, so lovely the forms of its hills blending with the forms of its clouds, so lovely, above all, those long trailings and bandings of its mists which make its altitudes appear to hang in the air. A land where sky and earth so strangely intermingle that what is reality may not be distinguished from what is illusion, that all seems a mirage about to vanish.

Lafcadio Hearn ("Sayonara!")

3.1 "He Who Greets the Effulgent Dawn … "

The very first fact regarding the presence of Japan on the world map is that it is an island country—an archipelago of four main islands and thousands of smaller ones off the Asiatic continent. Geographical similarities between Japan and other island countries—for example, UK in Europe—certainly cannot go unnoticed. However, considering the country's physical isolation from the rest of the world, both from the Asian mainland on the west and the Americas on the east, Japan has almost never been involved in continental Asian affairs nor has it ever "experienced military invasions until 1945" (Lehmann 1978: 21). Even the two significant waves of

*In this case we prefer to stick to the Japanese word for "heart; mind"—*kokoro* (心)—referring to the Japanese-born American anthropologist Takie Sugiyama Lebra's interpretation of the self in Japanese culture. According to Lebra, the infinitely variable selves could be organized into three dimensions, namely "the interactional self," "the inner self," and "the boundless self," each of them linked up or flowing into another. "At the center of the inner self," Lebra suggests, "is the *kokoro* which stands for heart, sentiment, spirit, will, or mind. While the outer self is socially circumscribed, the *kokoro* can be free and spontaneous, and even asocial. Further, the *kokoro* claims moral superiority over the outer self in that it is a reservoir of truthfulness and purity, uncontaminated by circumspections and contrivances to which the outer self is subject. This association of the *kokoro* (or inner self) with truthfulness gives rise to the paradoxical notion that the "real" truth is inexpressible. Thus words and speech as means of expression are often regarded as potentially deceptive and false, and silence as indicative of the true *kokoro*" (Lebra in Rosenberger 1992: 112). Hence our decision to use the original Japanese word untranslated.

V. Chervenkova, *Japanese Psychotherapies*,
DOI 10.1007/978-981-10-3126-7_3

cultural influence—that from China over the 5–8th century and from Western Europe, mainly Portugal and the Netherlands, in the 16th century—were not enough to prevent the country from "taking a vow of silence" from the early 17th century onward.

Born from the sea on the earthquake-prone Pacific Rim's Ring of Fire, the thin and narrow body of Japan stretches from north to south crowned with lofty volcanic mountains; full rivers cut through its picturesque landscape to water the paddy fields scattered in a patchwork manner across the narrow lowlands. The characteristics of the country's geographical position—an archipelago with four distinct seasons that encompass extremities varying from icy cold winter in the north, in Hokkaido, to eternal summer in the south, in Okinawa—are further enriched by opposites found in the east-western dimension: Japan's "western shores are washed by heavy seas, being exposed to the strong and cold north-westerly winds coming from the Siberian plains" (Nitobe 1912: 37). In contrast, its eastern shores, also known as Outer Japan, are milder in climate, have more bright days, and are abound in gulfs and bays, harbors and ports (ibid.). However, "the seas about Japan were never a means of communication but were first and foremost the fields from which the Japanese obtained his food. Until modern times, they served not so much as a means of communication but as a barrier to separate an island kingdom from a continent" (Watsuji 1961: 65). It appears as if "Japan turns her back upon the sea which separates her from mainland Asia" (Nitobe 1912: 37), while gladly facing the Pacific Ocean and the morning sun. Yet another fact about Japan is that, indeed, it is the Land of the Rising Sun as its people have long believed that they were the first on Earth to greet the dawn of day.

While attempting to refrain from drawing too much environmentally and geographically determined conclusions about the Japanese mentality, we cannot ignore some objective factors, which could be supposed to have affected it: the Japanese are born and bred on a narrow island within sight of mountains all surrounded by seas from whose depths the life-giving Sun rises every morning. Needless to specify, this is not the common vista for all the denizens of the archipelago; but if we search a generalized outline of the "uniquely Japanese" physical landscape, of "*the* first landscape, the arche-landscape—*gen-fūkei* (原風景)—which is in the heart of every Japanese" (Berque 1997: 176), this is probably among the most figurative ones[1].

[1]"The term "arche-landscape" (*gen-fūkei*) frequently appears in conjunction with *furusato* (故郷). What the word refers to is the first landscape that a person experiences, which remains in the deepest recesses of his or her memory as a photographic image" (Morrison 2013: 12). *Furusato* then is "the most primary, deeply rooted image in the Japanese psyche" (Morrison 2013: 13), which could refer to, for example, the thatched roofs of the farming village houses or to the streets of a small castle town at sunset. Ordinary people often percevie "*furusato* as a mother, and it fulfills their longing to return to the womb. For them, it is not so much the spirit of the home that takes the substance; what consumes them is the sentiment of returning to the mothering of the village, to be enveloped by the home-as-womb" (Matsunaga, as cited in Berque 1997: 179).

However, for the purposes of the present work we need something more comprehensive than *gen-fūkei*. Considering landscape "a visual scroll which provides insights into the nature of a people" (Mather et al. 1998: 1), we introduce the concept of the inner landscape—psychoscape—and term it *shin-fūkei* (心風景). *Shin-fūkei* transcends the memories and nostalgic sentiments about one's native place, to expand to the primordial interconnectedness between the whole nation and the peculiarities of the physical landscape and climate that the nation has been exposed to since the very beginning of its history. This nation–landscape/climate connection is fed by a constant interplay between (i) people's respond to the surrounding environment and (ii) the imprints that the environment leaves on people's psyche from one generation to the next. These imprints are bound up not only with "the principle of landscape evocation" (Berque 1997: 19) as reflected, for example, in the Japanese season words *kigo* (季語), but, on a deeper plane, they shape the nation's mentality and sensibility in accordance with a web of symbols—for example, opposites such as high–low or vast–narrow, as well as the archetypal symbolism of water (rivers; seas) or fire (volcanoes).

Considering the already mentioned characteristics of the Japanese physical landscape, we suggest that the Japanese psychoscape, *shin-fūkei*, is then outlined by the horizontal dimension of the sea and the vertical dimension of the mountains; at their cross-point, the man witnesses the miracle of regenesis as symbolized by the sunrise with every new day. "He who greets the effulgent dawn," Nitobe summarizes, "is therewith content and cares not for its further course, but rather turns in wonderment to the source whence it came, hence his religion is the cult of the past. The matin disposes man to contemplation" (Nitobe 1912: 12). Similarly to their land which figuratively turns its back to the human realm—the vast Asiatic continent to the west—the Japanese do so for the sake of Nature and for gaining an insight into her divine order. In addition to the "agricultural society's need to know when to plant, cultivate, and harvest its crops" (Gakken 2002: 31), such a distance has likely "sharpened the Japanese sensitivity to seasonal changes, heightening their awareness of the minutiae of nature—the wind in the pines and the singing of the insects—and giving rise to a wide variety of arts and customs embodying this sensitivity" (ibid.). "Even today, there is a widespread belief that the Japanese have an inherent affinity with nature and that this affinity is one of the major characteristics of Japanese culture" (Shirane 2013: 5).

This physical distance from the rest of the world together with the peculiarities of the insular landscape likely account for "two important psychological consequences: the sense of isolation and of discontinuity" (Nitobe 1912: 43). First, despite all the modern means of communication and transportation, there seems an ancient layer of the Japanese *kokoro* is still alive. This layer allows "half the convex world to intrude between Japan and the rest of the world" (ibid.) and likely makes its denizens "frontier people" (Uchida 2009). It is exactly this sense of isolation that allows the Japanese to easily enter a preverbal state of mind where boundaries between the individual and Nature are rarely present or, at least, are ambiguous. In other words, compared to other nations, the Japanese appear to be able to easily "immerse" themselves in the phenomenal world of Nature. A man sitting in their mountain hut, the Japanese philosopher Daisetz Teitarō Suzuki notes, "is in no way different from the birds singing, the insects buzzing, the leaves swaying, and the waters murmuring—nor even from Mount Fuji, looming up on the other side of the bay. Here is a complete merging of Nature and man" (Suzuki 1959: 336).

Second, the sense of discontinuity likely ensues from a tension between inner polarities that are not alien to other ethnicities, but which in the Japanese *kokoro* are brought to an extreme. In his theory of the Japanese landscape, the Meiji era geographer and thinker Shigetaka Shiga suggests that the essence of the Japanese landscape is in its (i) elegance, represented by the Japanese autumn scenery; (ii) beauty, as seen in the spring scenery; and (iii) the magnificence of the volcanoes, typhoons, and rough sea waves. The third specificity contrasts with the first two and embodies the rough dynamism of the natural forces behind the native beauty and grace (Nakano and Ohkubo 2015: 93–94). Indeed, "living on an island exposed at every point to the sea, the Japanese realized that they could not retreat into a vast continental interior, like the Chinese, to escape a seaborne threat" (Duus 1976: 24), which rendered the Japanese cultural identity "a strong sense of vulnerability" (ibid.). This vulnerability, as represented by the first two sceneries that Shiga suggests, always goes hand in hand with the untamed "volcanic" force that fuels the inner dynamism of the Japanese *kokoro*. There, in its depths, the bounty and beauty of the Japanese nature, philosopher Takashi Uozumi points out, evokes gratitude, whereas its rough forces as manifested in typhoons, volcanoes, and earthquakes awe people into silence (Uozumi 2016: 18).

Alternative interpretations, as these suggested by the Japanese writer Nyozekan Hasegawa, claim that the Japanese landscape contrasts the continental one in the sense that it knows no extremes, "but tends to the moderate, the delicate, the minute, and the approachable" (Hasegawa 1983: 10). This specificity likely accounts for a "national dislike of extremes", Hasegawa concludes (Hasegawa 1983: 11). Indeed, "the extreme spaciousness of feeling" (ibid.) typical for the continental landscape cannot be found in Japan. Our assumption, however, is that the Japanese attitude toward extremes is different as it derives from another type of extremes—those peculiar to a narrow and mountainous island country, and also to the extremes described by Shiga. These natural contrasts differ from the continental ones that Hasegawa refers to, such as, for example, "the great conglomerations of mountains and water" (ibid.) and vast plains of the Chinese landscape. In Japan, the symbolical oppositions found in the continent—*vertical* (mountains) versus *horizontal* (plains)—expands to *high* (mountains) versus *vast, but also deep* (seas). And because, on the other hand, we cannot but agree with Hasegawa that "a people which has been exposed to such things for thousands of years naturally comes to have a special character very different from that of peoples used to different environments" (Hasegawa 1983: 10–11), we assume that the Japanese attitude toward extremities is an *unconscious intention for reconciling them* rather than a mere dislike and avoidance—the intention for reconciliation represents an incessant movement toward a point of balance, whereas a mere dislike and avoidance are rather static, with less of inner dynamics.

If we accept this speculation, we will then understand that "insular" is by no means tantamount to narrowness of vision. On the contrary, the capacity of the

Japanese *kokoro* to encompass extremities reveals a profound view that life "cannot be formulated in a single idea, because reality is more complex than any logic and at the same time so much more simple" (Hoffmann 1986:29). Returning to the two key psychological consequences engendered by the island landscape—the sense of isolation and that of discontinuity—we can now see how they flesh out the Japanese psychoscape (*shin-fūkei*) as a point where the depths of the seas and the heights of the mountains meet; a point symbolically represented by the image of the rising sun, into which the chasm between the polarities is bridged over and the otherwise unbearable tension between them is eased. It is probable that the quest for balancing these polarities in the Japanese *kokoro*, in the, as the Japanese psychiatrist Bin Kimura defines it, spasmodic Japanese character (Kimura 1972: 125) and the "north-south structure" of Japanese culture (Nakanishi 2008: 6), have made the denizens of this island intuitively resort to contemplation and silence: close contemplation of the ordered state of Nature; and silence, which is approached not as a deliberate refusal to communicate, but as an opportunity for enhancing one's ability to "listen" to this order and internalize it. Indeed, as the Swiss philosopher Max Picard emphasizes, "man is better able to endure things hostile to his own nature, things that use him up, if he has the silent substance within" (Picard 2002: 67).

For this reason, we should discuss also the specific attitude the Japanese take toward words and language as generally opposed to the phenomenon of silence. The Japanese are famous for their passive verbal behavior, and for their language abound with passive expressions and non-attributive sentences. According to the Japanese linguist Yasushi Haga, if we do not count the traditional Japanese belief in the power of words—*kotodama* (言霊)[2]—such a behavior could be explained with distrust in the practical aspects of language as a means of self-expression and communication *per se*; hence the belief that where no words are present, there truth is (Haga 2004: 260). As previously explained, "Japan is a homogeneous island that had not experienced colonization or invasion" (Oyamatsu 2013: 7). Probably because of this it "did not need to develop linguistic communication extensively throughout its history" (ibid.). The implicit silence-orientated communication of the Japanese, together with the ambiguity of their speech[3], makes many "foreigners criticize the Japanese because

[2]There are records that the ancient Japanese called their land "The Country that Thrives by Virtue of *Kotodama*"(「言霊の幸わう国」) (Takahashi 2014: 130). In ancient Japan, *kotodama* signified the magical power that dwells in words and could bring about different events in the physical world—propitious or ominous. As Lebra points out, "in contrast to transcendentalized biblical "Word", which is associated with logos, rationality, and the mind, *kotodama* was magically empowered" (Lebra 2004: 185) and "language itself was imbued with an autonomous power of truth that transcended semantic nuances" (Kurita 1987: 45). That is why the Japanese are very careful in their choice of words (Yoshida 2015: 126). On the other hand, spoken language in Japan is rarely considered an effective means for communication; rather, "the Japanese inner self, apart from *kotodama*, is tied to spiritual serenity, integrity, sincerity, and silence" (Lebra 2004: 185).

[3]For example, phrases such as "That is right" do not necessarily imply consent. The receiver therefore needs to "astutely monitor the context and non-verbal manifestations to determine the intended meaning" (McDaniel 1993:4).

what they are thinking is imperceptible" (Minami 1971: 178) and because their appreciation of taciturnity is certainly odd. In the end, the Japanese are unfathomable. However, "this criticism results from a superficial view" (ibid.) not uncommon among people of the Western societies for whom gap filling is the norm in conversation, and verbal "silences" are often regarded as negative and undesirable phenomena. By contrast, the Japanese seem to trust much more quasi- and nonverbal communication—for them "tasting" the atmosphere and "listening" to the pregnant silence between words are more reliable means of communication. The true meaning of words can be found only in the silence in-between, in the atmosphere that people create simply by being together in this unique space-time—an atmosphere which can be referred to the Japanese Jungian psychologist Hayao Kawai's concept of the empty-centered structure—*chūkū-kōzō* (中空構造)—as a principle deeply innate to Japanese mentality (Kawai 1999)[4].

Additionally, by according more importance than Western societies to nonverbal communication, Haga suggests, the Japanese reveal the concave-shaped nature of their culture as opposed to the continental convex-shaped cultures: in Japanese culture communication is governed by an emphasis on the identification with the other person's mind and presence, rather than on what is or should be actually verbalized (Haga 2004: 240). In so doing, Japanese culture "privileges perceptible reality (the presence of things); and, at the same time, it privileges the matrix field constituted by the milieu at the expense of personal consciousness: it glorifies the collective subject at the expense of the individual subject" (Berque 1997: 223). To keep this "glorification" intact, the Japanese have retained their centuries-old reverence toward silence knowing that silence "clears away the smoke screen of words that man has laid down between his mind and things" (Merton 1999: 82). For the Japanese—as if in complete agreement with Picard's view that "language becomes emaciated if it loses its connection with silence" (Picard 2002: 15)—silence is so much bound up to discourse and in-between pauses that it governs the issues of what is to be said and what is not to be said. To summarize, "what we hear sometimes are not the words, but the intention behind the words. The interval may bring a deeper communion than the words alone" (Miyamoto 1960: 201).

Considering all of the above, it is important to discuss also the emphasis that the Japanese put upon the concept of *ma* (間)—a polysemic word, which literally means "interval", "space", "room, chamber", and "between, in-between", but also "valid interval" or "meaningful pause" (Miyamoto 1960: 201); "relationship", "man-to-man" (Nagasawa 1967: 989); "interval between two musical tones or two lines used to emphasize them" (Kurita 2010: 85); "the crossover between light and darkness" (Oyamatsu 2013: 3), which has both temporal and spatial qualities within a static, yet internally dynamic structure (Fujita 1969: 68). *Ma* is further rendered ontological as a "place of Being—that positive void where Being can unfold"

[4]This principle can be observed even in the emotional patterning of Japanese infants: their mothers "tend to quietly rock the infants rather than provide vigorous physical stimulation" (Befu 1971: 153); mother–infant interaction "tends to be less active and less verbal and instead tends to have a soothing and quieting effect on the infant" (ibid.).

(Berque 1997: 206); it is "a field where "things" are being born and disappearing" (Oyamatsu 2013: 40), for which reason it bears a potential for development (Tada 1988:87) and a capacity to reveal "the acceptance and beauty of becoming; the process" (Oyamatsu 2013: 40). A "*productive* emptiness like the place prepared and purified to receive the gods, *yuniwa*" (Isozaki 2006: 100), *ma* is "the binding force of all things" (Oyamatsu 2013: 40) and "the space of intersubjectivity" (Berque 1997: 206). In psychotherapy, *ma* "stands for the relationship between the therapist and a patient" (Fujita 1986:225) or also for the notion that the patient is able to control themselves "by maintaining a proper distance" (ibid.) between themselves and the symptom. Considered also one of the most important mastery in every Japanese art (Nishiyama, as cited in Yasuda 1984: 55), last, but not least, *ma* can be used "to suggest what we know as silence" (Wilmer 2000: 119)[5].

Why is silence given such a cultural significance in Japan to an extent that it is intentionally cultivated through the concept of *ma*: aesthetically—in traditional music, visual and performing arts, the latter extensively employing "gestures and disciplined movements rather than sounds" (Dauenhauer 1980: 3), and socially—in speech and interpersonal relationships? Why the Japanese "originally exist in "betweenness" of *ma*, that is, in a relationship between person and person" (Yuasa in Carter 2001: xxvi)?[6].

Although often taken for a mere absence of noise or lack of speech, silence for the Japanese, more than any other ethnicities, appears to be "a positive, a complete world in itself" (Picard 2002: 17). This world "contains everything within itself" (ibid.) and is therefore an efficacious world, a world of "active performance" (Dauenhauer 1980: 3). Opening room for this world to manifest itself amidst the flow of daily life seems to be very important for the Japanese for it fills everything with its own wholesome nature. While put in silence, things are as if in a "period of incubation towards growth" (Miyamoto 1960: 201); silence "enables the becoming of human potentials and reinforces the possibility of growth and creativeness" (ibid.).

All these aspects of silence correspond to what Suzuki summarizes about the peoples of the East, especially the Japanese nation: its soul is directed inward so

---

[5]There are many Japanese phrases that use *ma*, for example *ma-ga-warui* (間が悪い), which means "inappropriate" or "awkward, embarrassed", but the literal meaning is "to experience bad *ma*"; or *ma-nuke* (間抜け), which means "fool, stupid", but the literal meaning is "to lose one's *ma*". *Ma-ni-au* (間に合う), on the contrary, means "to be on time" or "to be useful", with a literal meaning of "to meet *ma*". The character for *ma* consists of two poles(門), which means "gate", and the ideogram signifying "sun"(日)located at the gate, that is, "a gate with space to let the Sun shine through" (Henshall 1998: 26). This character is used also in the Japanese words for space and time — *kūkan* (空間) and *jikan* (時間)—implying that in Japanese culture concepts of time and space are not considered separately. For further details on this topic, see Isozaki (2006: 81–100).

[6]Takie Sugiyama Lebra discusses this phenomenon as "compulsion for silence" (Lebra 2004: 180). For further details on the cultural significance of silence in Japanese communication, see Lebra's paper of the same title (1987).

In Japanese, the word "human being"—*ningen*(人間)—consists of the characters for "person" and "*ma*", that is, one becomes a human being only in the in-betweenness/silence of two (or more) persons.

much that its external manifestations could easily be mistaken for indifference and negligence (Suzuki 1997: 58). It is not rare, indeed, for foreigners to liken the faces of the Japanese to blank masks. However, it is exactly this comparison that gives an important clue: for example, *Nō*-theater masks look completely expressionless, but when lit up in certain ways or seen from a certain angle, they can "laugh" or "cry", or "be angry", i.e., they can "express" various emotions. Therefore, as the Japanese art historian Masa'aki Kambara emphasizes, the lack of expression is not necessarily tantamount to lack of emotions. On the contrary, being expressionless, masks *encompass* all possible emotions (Kambara 2001: 85–86) and these "emotions can alternate with the unanticipated and abrupt intensity of a seasonal yet savage typhoon" (Watsuji 1961: 136). Again as Suzuki summarizes about the introverted character of Eastern people in contrast to extraverted Westerners, the exterior is wide, whereas the interior is deep (Suzuki 1997: 58). That is, the rich and polyvalent emotional world of the Japanese is somewhere behind the mask-like faces, in the depths of the interiors, while the surface remains apparently blank, only rarely to allow the depths to emerge.

Such a seeming lack of expressions suggests that all vital forces are withdrawn from the surface to fuel a delicate, yet active movement toward the innermost silent recesses of the heart where all antipodes are brought together into "a state where only being is valid" (Picard 2002: 20). This inward movement visibly manifests itself throughout Japanese culture—from gift wrapping to wrapping thoughts and intentions in polite language; bodies literally wrapped in multilayered garments, and even space—by the traditional Japanese gardens and buildings, where "there is some notion of "creasing" or layering of space to create an impression of depth and mystery. The Japanese architect Fumihiko Maki regards this creation of *oku* (depth) as a distinctive feature of Japanese architecture which he contrasts with the "center demarcation" of Western cultures" (Hendry 1995: 100).[7] In short, the Japanese *kokoro* moves incessantly inward and the general cultural pattern therefore corresponds, in one form or another, to the idea of seclusion and silence usually perceived as opposites of outwardness and expression, verbal one included.

At the same time, paradoxically, the Japanese are the same people "who greet the effulgent dawn" (Nitobe 1912: 12) and who have come "to believe in the sun-origin of their rulers and, finally, of the whole nation" (Singer 1997: 52). How can this paradox be explained? Again, in contrast to the peoples of the vast continental plains, the Japanese have remained unfamiliar with (or have unconsciously kept at bay) the characteristics of a full-blown manifestation—both in terms of

[7]While the space of the traditional Japanese living interior is only symbolically marked by sliding doors and walls made of paper, the exterior is clearly outlined (Berque 1994: 176) and the garden and its fence look as if wrapping up the house. At the same time, the interior space creates an impression of as if moving toward the recesses of the house – *tokonoma* (床の間)– the family altar. "Japan seems to have developed its land potential according to inward-looking dynamics. It has been intensive rather than extensive" (Berque 1997: 51) and the logic of "introverted development" has marked "the entire Japanese relationship to space" (ibid.). For additional references on this cultural tendency, see the Korean scholar O-Young Lee's concept of *chijimi* (縮み—"shrinkage")as a truly Japanese proclivity (1992).

national mentality and behavior, and as a distinctive cultural feature. "Nothing is more alien to their souls than pure radiance and the blazing light that forces clarity and distinctness on everything" (ibid.). Perhaps the earthquake-prone homeland of the Japanese has made them search unconsciously for a psychological prop not on the surface, but deep down in the center of the earth and this tendency is manifested in the shuffle gait typical for many of their traditional performing arts (Yamazaki 2011: 24–25). The Japanese religious and spiritual traditions, too, have always maintained the importance of a minimalist seed-like mode of existence for it is only in darkness, seclusion and silence where the process of growth and gradual transformation can naturally begin from within.

We can therefore conclude that in Japan silence has always been recognized as a nurturing, healing and life-affirming phenomenon to be sought after and emphasized through various forms of the nation's material and spiritual culture as an *unquestionable sign of inner integrity*. The ontological primacy of silence over eloquence and expressiveness has, after all, nothing to do with negation of the latter. Rather, it suggests a quest for integrity of what cannot be integrated, or at least not without an effort: exteriority and interiority, center and periphery, mountain heights and ocean depths. For it appears that for the Japanese what is expressed is already brought to the verge of dissipation and all vital forces are being drained out of it; whereas what remains inexplicit and is yet to be born out of the bosom of silence has all the possibilities and futures within it—like an effulgent dawn and a brand new day.

3.2 Pathways of the Mountains, Pathways of the Heart

Reading the previous section, one may hasten to conclude that the Japanese are involved in abstract speculations about universal and other-worldly issues. Discussing the psychoscape of the inhabitants of an island, which "is the legacy of primeval fire" (Nitobe 1912: 31) may, indeed, evoke such conclusions. Quite the contrary, however, the Japanese recognize "the phenomenal world itself as Absolute and reject the recognition of anything excisting over and above the phenomenal world" (Nakamura 1964: 350).

Although with the advent of Buddhism in the 6th century the Japanese came to think of metaphysical issues such as life after death, it did not prevent them from accepting Buddhism, too, as this-worldly. Actually, "it was the Japanese themselves that transformed Buddhism, which they accepted from the continent, into a religion centered upon this world" (Nakamura 1964: 362). Significant proof of that can be found in the arrival of the prominent Buddhist monks and thinkers Hōnen and Shinran in the 13th century, who brought even basic Buddhist doctrines "down to the earth," among the ordinary people, emphasizing that "even ordinary men would be able to become Buddhas, should they attain enlightenment in this world" (Nakamura 1964: 363).[8]

[8]This topic we discuss in the context of Naikan therapy and the Pure Land Buddhism (see Sect. 6.1).

Indeed, a great deal of practicality dwells in the Japanese *kokoro* and issues of abstract and metaphysical character are difficult to captivate it. Rather, the Japanese turn their attention to this world, to "the fluid, arresting character of observed events" (Nakamura 1964: 350). Probably as a result of that, the Japanese have developed sensibility toward the phenomenal world and Nature that no other nation could share to such an extent. This susceptibility has helped them recognize that behind Nature's diversity and seeming topsy-turvyness there is a hidden order, a pattern "which contains the nature of Nature" (Yanagi, as cited in McLuhan 1994: 119).

This sounds not too distant an echo of the ancient East Asian doctrine of Tao—the Way of the Universe: "Man models himself on Earth, Earth on Heaven, Heaven on the Way, and the Way on Nature" (Lao-tzu, as cited in McLuhan 1994: 18). Tao functions primarily "as an ethical and aesthetic guide to transforming the body-mind to be in accord with the activity of the universe" (Arai 2011: 31). The Japanese, however, have brought this paradigm, as they did with Buddhism, "down to the earth" and have weaved it into their daily life: from gestures and the cadence of a sentence to arranging flowers and pouring and receiving a cup of sake, even the minutest daily action should be performed in accordance with a predetermined pattern. While focusing their attention on the pattern, the Japanese seem to attain greater understanding of the Way—the whole from which the particular pattern has been extracted. That is how daily life is attached a value to an extent that there are no ordinary experiences anymore—even the mere utilities flow into a quiet stream of preternatural beauty, and life thus becomes intelligible, significant and, most of all, worth living.

Such an attitude toward life appears to be so deeply ingrained in the Japanese mentality that it formed a distinctive tradition (Kadowaki 1990: 5–6), which became the true manifestation of the consistency and intactness of Japanese culture (Uozumi 2016: 19): this is the concept of *Dō* (道—way, path, road)[9]. While in the Western languages words such as "way" or "road" are used either in their literal sense or as abstract metaphors for life, in Japan they also describe circumstances where one "must learn or polish a skill" (Yamakuse 2011: 59)[10]. This practical aspect of the concept of the Way, however, by no means detracts from its philosophical implications, i.e., the Japanese understanding that it is exactly through

[9]It is worth mentioning that the Japanese word for religion—*shūkyō* (宗教)—"is actually a term coined specifically to translate a Western concept. The most important terms that existed in Japan previously to denote something approximating religion were *hō* (法)(Buddhist truth, Buddhist law, usually including reference to the institutions propagating it and the objects used in the associated practices) and *Dō* (the path a practitioner should pursue)" (Alisal et al. 2007: xx). However, *Dō* came into extensive use with the 1868 Meiji Restoration so that the traditional Japanese practices could be clearly distinguished from the substantial Western cultural influences. Before that it was self-evident that every art—aesthetic or martial—is a way that practitioners advance on. *Dō* is therefore neither the beginning nor the end of the road, but the process of advancement and inner transformation itself (Kurita 2010: 135).

[10]For example, *michi-wo-kiwameru* (道を極める) means "pushing one's skills", but the literal meaning is "to take the road to its ultimate destination" (Yamakuse 2011: 59). According to Uozumi, *michi-wo-kiwameru* refers to the way of living of individuals who dedicate their whole life to practicing a certain art or activity (Uozumi 2016: 271).

concrete physical actions and behavioral patterns that one can attain self-transformation and develop proper attitude with regard to how one relates to others, Nature and even the Universe. This describes to great extent the essence of *Dō*, which encompasses such artistic "ways" as martial arts *aikidō* (合気道) and *judō*(柔道), calligraphy *shodō*(書道), flower arranging *kadō* (華道), and tea ceremony *chadō* (茶道). "None of these," the Canadian philosopher Robert E. Carter emphasizes, "is to be understood and undertaken merely as entertainment or distraction: they are all ways of self-development, leading to a transformation of who a person is" (Carter 2008: 3).

A characteristic common to all of these *Dō*-practices is that they require intense and diligent physical efforts, thus exemplifying the fundamental Japanese concept of body-mind unity: self-transformation is possible through concrete physical actions that follow a preset pattern within the framework of a particular art, e.g., *aikidō*, *chadō*, etc. These practices involve not only the practitioner's body, but the triunity of their body, mind and spirit; they urge the practitioner to "throw" themselves into the bosom of Nature (Kurita 2010: 138). Mastering one's skills in, for example, using a calligraphy brush, the Japanese sword, or tea ceremony utensils is based on the integration of body and mind, hence phrases such as "unity of mind and brush" and "if the mind is correct, the brush is correct" (Davey 2007: 8). Such an integration is essential for mastering any Japanese *Dō* for it allows practitioners to grasp "the ultimate nature of the whole of life by closely examining themselves through a singular activity of life: to arrive at the universal through studying the particular" (ibid.). In other words, to explore and understand "what it means to live our very lives as art" (Davey 2007: vi).

Probably because of this, verbal, analytical and intellectual approaches are not attached great value in the Japanese *Dō*-s—the actual physical practice is what counts and the degree of purity of one's direct experience is used as an unequivocal proof that one is "walking" the Way. Borrowing the Japanese philosopher Nishida Kitarō's concepts, it would mean that one has achieved a state of mind where "there is yet neither subject nor object, and knowledge and its object are completely united" (Nishida 1960: 1–2); a state where no words, thoughts or judgments threaten to blur the experience itself. Undoubtedly, mere action will not lead to insight, but it is considered the most helpful tool if one aims to restore the lost harmony between body and mind. Despite its seeming simplicity, such an approach hides a depth and complexity that takes decades to comprehend through firsthand experience.

Therefore, the true understanding in the Japanese *Dō*-s is never just a theory, but everyday practice until this specific state of consciousness and body-mind coordination is attained; until Nature is represented through the practitioner the way it is and "the divine potential that is to be found in the depths of each and every individual who cares to discover it" (Carter 2008: 4) comes to realization. "The *Dō* begins with body discipline, the ultimate goal being the body's spiritualization or enlightenment" (Lebra 2004: 192), because "strength comes only when one is completely relaxed and as much at one with nature as possible" (Gakken 2002: 31). Achieving such a state of naturalness may result in the cultivation of ethical, social, and spiritual virtues as well.

The idea of self-transformation and self-realization can also be found in another Japanese convention outside of the *Dō*-practices, which adopts much the same concrete and practical aspects: this is the convention of journeying and pilgrimaging.

The concept of journey, both literal and figurative, has permeated the minds of the Japanese and unambiguously manifested itself in "numerous literary works which attempt to depict the evanescence and frailty of life or to show flowing and changing using the travel convention" (Minami 1971: 60). Pilgrimage, in turn, despite the concrete religious context within which it is usually performed, may also refer to more neutral concepts such as those of spiritual seeking and inner transformation.[11]

The centuries-old pilgrimage convention in Japan is most frequently a quest for this-worldly favors—*gense-riyaku* (現世利益)—such as good health, successful marriage and childbirth, protection from natural disasters, etc., all of which are expected to be granted by transcendental powers (Nishiyama, as paraphrased in Alisal et al. 2007: xii). Despite the this-worldly nature of the favors, such a quest is nevertheless considered "spiritual" as far as the pilgrim makes a sacrifice in the form of time and energy spent. More importantly, any pilgrimage involves a great deal of, in the French ethnologist Arnold van Gennep's terms, liminal experiences for it requires one's courage and strength to disconnect oneself—both physically and mentally—from daily life and be ready to encounter the unknown. Seclusion from the familiar human world and traveling the silent roads of the mountain wilderness[12] promises to bestow the expected good health, wealth and happiness. However, on a deeper plane and quite the contrary, the journey should help the pilgrim grasp the transient nature of life and "teach" them to live without attaching to this-worldly matters, i.e., to transform themselves.[13]

---

[11]The popularization of the pilgrimage concept in Japan should be discussed in the context of the spread of Buddhism and even in the broader context of the spiritual journeys in the East Asian cultural sphere. This, however, is a vast subject and doing it justice is beyond the scope of the present work. What we aim for is simply sketching the convention itself the way it dwells in the Japanese *kokoro* and the fundamental components that form it as a distinctive cultural phenomenon.

[12]Sacred mountains, symbolizing the exaltation of Divinity, are to be found in every corner of the globe, but they appear especially abundant in Japan: "it has 354 major sacred mountains, not to mention countless minor ones. They are the lifeblood of Japan's spiritual and physical landscape" (McLuhan 1994: 118); also, "*Yamato*, the ancient name for Japan, shares a rich association with Japan's mountain world, say philologists. *Yama* (山) means "mountain". The name Yamato has been explained as "mountain door," "mountain tracks" and "mountain stop" (McLuhan 1994: 119). The Japanese mountaineer Akihiko Ota even likens the hallowed grounds of the Japanese mountains to four-dimensional mandalas (Ota 2016: 2).

The Japanese-American historian of religions Joseph Kitagawa distinguishes three types of pilgrimage in Japan: (i) pilgrimages to sacred mountains related to *sanrin-tōsō* (山林逃走)—rigorous ascetic trainings in the mountain; (ii) pilgrimages based on faith in certain divinities—for example, the Pilgrimage to the Thirty-tree Sanctuaries in Western Japan, *saigoku-sanjūsan-sho* (西国三十三所), which is based on devotion to Kannon, the goddess of mercy; and (iii) pilgrimages based on faith in charismatic persons—for example, the cult that developed around the memory of Kōbō Daishi, systematizer of the esoteric Buddhist school Shingon, and his birthplace in Shikoku (Kitagawa 1987: 127–136). The pilgrimage convention in Japan is therefore intimately related to the country's mountainous landscape.

[13]For further details on the concept of the sense of impermanance—*mujōkan* (無常観)—see Sect. 6.1.1.

Here again, as with the concept of *Dō*, we arrive at the idea of self-transformation through physical effort. As the Japanese theologian Kakichi Kadowaki emphasizes, journey means first of all "to walk with one's body" (Kadowaki 1990: 4) and body, through which the physical action of pilgrimage is realized, is therefore *sine qua non* for gaining the spiritual fruits of the journey. Reversing the sequence of the personal quest—namely, first attaining spiritual truth by some abstract and intellectual means and then practicing it—is unthinkable a process in Japanese culture. For the Japanese, diligent practice and direct experience of reality on a physical level become the gateway through which metaphysical understanding can be attained. Only through training and self-discipline—*shūyō* (修養)—"can man or woman gain the power to live fully and to "get the taste" of life" (Benedict 2005: 233). Training "enlarges life" (ibid.) and "polishes away "the rust of the body", thus making "a man a bright sharp sword" (Benedict 2005: 234). *Shūyō* thus becomes a metaphor for the profound understanding of what it means to be a human.

To recapitulate, there are two pillars upon which the convention of the Way in Japan is built. First, this is the importance of selflessness and nonattachment[14], as far as "tasting" life corresponds to the idea of pure experience—an experience through which the screen of the "observing self" between one's mind and the world falls aside. Paradoxically, however, both in the conventions of *Dō* and of pilgrimage, selflessness induces self-reliance for "it enables a man to meet any situation with exactly the right expenditure of effort, neither too much nor too little, and it gives him control of his otherwise wayward mind so neither physical danger from outside nor passion from within can dislodge him" (Benedict 2005: 241). In short, it educates in self-control.

The second pillar of the convention of the Way is the gradual inner transformation that results from selflessness and nonattachment. Through this transformation, seemingly unfavorable situations might be observed, reflected upon and accepted as "containing the seeds for improvement and enlightenment" (Alisal et al. 2007: 9). These two pillars appear to be what the tradition of the Way in Japanese culture—be it of the artist (*Dō*) or that of the pilgrim—is all about.

In this chapter we discussed two phenomena which can be lined up with the most representative manifestations of Japanese culture. These are the concept of silence and that of the Way, the latter seen both figuratively as a lifelong journey toward mastering a certain skill or art, and literally—as a journey or a pilgrimage to a sacred place. Our basic assumption is that these two phenomena go hand in hand and complement each other: walking the Way requires temporary withdrawal from daily life and is usually conducted in silence, whereas silence, as if in return to the pilgrims' diligent efforts, nurtures their soul with "its own holy uselessness" (Picard 2002: 19). Figuratively, silence is the vessel where the path (the individual pattern) unfolds naturally as part of the greater Way.

In the next chapter we explore how this symbolic image of a man traveling in silence is recreated within the context of the Japanese psychotherapies and what therapeutic function it has.

---

[14]The concept of selflessness—*muga* (無我)—we discuss in Sect. 6.1.2.

References

Alisal, Maria Rodriguez del, P. Ackermann, D.P. Martinez (ed.): Pilgrimages and Spiritual Quests in Japan, Routledge, 2007
Arai, Paula: Bringing Zen Home: The Healing Heart of Japanese Women's Rituals, University of Hawaii Press, 2011
Befu, Harumi: Japan: An Anthropological Introduction, Harper & Row Publishers, 1971
Benedict, Ruth: The Chrysanthemum and the Sword—Patterns of Japanese Culture, Houghton Mifflin Company, 2005
Berque, Augustin: Vivre L'Espace au Japon (transl. Makoto Miyahara), Chikuma Shobo, 1994 (in Japanese)
Berque, Augustin: Japan—Nature, Artifice and Japanese Culture (transl. Ros Schwartz), Pilkington Press, 1997
Carter, Robert E.: Encounter with Enlightenment: A Study of Japanese Ethics, State University of New York Press, 2001
Carter, Robert E.: The Japanese Arts and Self-Cultivation, State University of New York Press, 2008
Dale, Peter N.: The Myth of Japanese Uniqueness, Routledge, 2012
Dauenhauer, Bernard P.: Silence—The Phenomenon and Its Ontological Significance, Indiana University Press, 1980
Davey, Hugh E.: The Japanese Way of the Artist, Stone Bridge Press, 2007
Duus, Peter: The Rise of Modern Japan, Houghton Mifflin Company, 1976
Fujita, Chihiro: On the Meanings of *Fumon* (Disregard of Symptoms) in Morita Therapy, Journal of Psychotherapy, Vol.1 (1), Japanese Psychotherapy Association, 1969 (in Japanese)
Fujita, Chihiro: Morita Therapy—Psychotherapeutic System for Neurosis, Igaku-Shoin, 1986
Gakken Editorial Board: Japan As It Is—A Bilingual Guide (Fourth Edition), Gakken, 2002
Haga, Yasushi: Structure of the Japaneseness—Lectures on Theory of Linguistic Culture, Taishukan Publishing, 2004 (in Japanese)
Hasegawa, Nyozekan: The Japanese Character—A Cultural Profile (transl. John Bester), Kodansha International, 1983
Hendry, Joy: Wrapping Culture: Politeness, Presentation and Power in Japan and Other Societies, Clarendon Press, 1995
Henshall, Kenneth G.: A Guide to Remembering Japanese Characters, Tuttle Publishing, 1998
Hoffmann, Yoel (transl.): Japanese Death Poems Written by Zen Monks and Haiku Poets on the Verge of Death, Tuttle Publishing, 1986
Isozaki, Arata: Japan-ness in Architecture (transl. Sabu Kohso, ed. David B. Stewart), MIT Press, 2006
Kadowaki, Kakichi: Metaphysics of *Dō*—Basho, Dogen, and Jesus, Iwanami Shoten, 1990 (in Japanese)
Kambara, Masa'aki: Japanese Arts—Searching the Roots of the Aesthetic Sense, Keiso Shobo, 2001 (in Japanese)
Kawai, Hayao: Into the Depths of Japan—The Empty-Centered Structure, Chuokoron-sha, 1999 (in Japanese)
Kimura, Bin: Man-to-Man—Psychopathological Theory on Japan, Koubundou Publishers, 1972 (in Japanese)
Kitagawa, Joseph: On Understanding Japanese Religion, Princeton University Press, 1987
Kurita, Isamu: Japanese Identity, Shodensha, 1987
Kurita, Isamu: Keywords to Japanese Cutlure—Seven Indigenous Japanese Words, Shodensha, 2010 (in Japanese)

Lebra, Takie Sugiyama: The Cultural Significance of Silence in Japanese Communication, Multilingua, Vol. 6, Mouton Pulbishers, 1987
Lebra, Takie Sugiyama: The Japanese Self in Cultural Logic, University of Hawai'i Press, 2004
Lee, O-Young: The Compact Culture: The Japanese Tradition of "Smaller is Better" (originally published in Japanese as "Shrinkage-Minded Japanese"; transl. Robert N. Huey), Kodansha America Inc, 1992
Lehmann, Jean-Pierre: The Image of Japan: From Feudal Isolation to World Power 1850–1905, George Allen & Unwin, 1978
Mather, Cotton, P.P. Karan, S. Iijima: Japanese Landscapes—Where Land and Culture Merge, The University Press of Kentucky, 1998
McDaniel, Edwin R.: Japanese Nonverbal Communication: A Review and Critique of Literature, San Diego State University, 1993
McLuhan, Teri C.: The Way of the Earth—Encounters with Nature in Ancient and Contemporary Thought, Touchstone, 1994
Merton, Thomas: Thoughts in Solitude, Farrar, Straus and Giroux, 1999
Minami, Hiroshi: Psychology of the Japanese People (transl. Albert R. Ikoma), University of Tokyo Press, 1971
Miyamoto, Misako: Zen in Play Therapy, Psychologia—An International Journal of Psychology of the Orient, Vol.3 (4), Psychologia Society, 1960
Morrison, Lindsay R.: Home of the Heart: the Modern Origins of *Furusato*, ICU Comparative Culture, Vol. 45, International Christian University, 2013
Nagasawa, Kikuya (ed.): New Japanese Dictionary of Chinese Characters, Sanseido, 1967
Nakamura, Hajime: Ways of Thinking of Eastern Peoples—India, China, Tibet, Japan (ed. Philip P. Wiener), University of Hawaii Press, 1964
Nakanishi, Susumu: The Lost Things of the Japanese (part 2), Wedge Co, 2008 (in Japanese)
Nakano, Akira, T. Ohkubo: Twenty Five Masterpieces of the Japanese Cultural Theory—Toward Understanding the Japanese Identity, Asahi Shimbun Publications, 2015 (in Japanese)
Nishida, Kitarō: A Study of Good (transl. V.H. Viglielmo), Tokyo Printing Bureau, 1960
Nitobe, Inazo: The Japanese Nation—Its Land, Its People and Its Life, G.P. Putnam's Sons, 1912
Okakura, Kakuzo: The Awakening of Japan, The Century Co, 1905
Ota, Akihiko: Mountain Gods and Buddhas—An Interesting and Informative Talk on the Shinto and Buddhist Mountain Deities, Yamakei Shinsho, 2016 (in Japanese)
Oyamatsu, Keiko, *Ma*—The Presence of Absence, Gerrit Rietveld Academie, 2013
Picard, Max: The World of Silence, Eighth Day Press, 2002
Rapoport, Carla: Understanding How Japanese Works, in Fortune Magazine—Special Issue (Fall), Time Inc, 1989
Rosenberger, Nancy R. (ed.): Japanese Sense of Self, Cambridge University Press, 1992
Shirane, Haruo: Japan and the Culture of Four Seasons: Nature, Literature, and the Arts, Columbia University Press, 2013
Singer, Kurt: Mirror, Sword and Jewel—A Study of Japanese Characteristics, Japan Library, 1997
Suzuki, Daisetz T.: Zen and Japanese Culture, MJF Books, 1959
Suzuki, Daisetz T.: Eastern Point of View, Iwanami Shoten, 1997 (in Japanese)
Tada, Michitaro: Japanese Culture at Hand, Kodansha Gakujutsu Bunko, 1988 (in Japanese)
Takahashi, Kouji: Speaking Indigenous Japanese in a Beautiful Way—Understanding Each Other's Expressions of Harmony, Toho Publishing, 2014 (in Japanese)
Uchida, Tatsuru: Theory of Japan as a Periphery, Shinchosha Publishing, 2009 (in Japanese)
Uozumi, Takashi: Taking the Road to Its Utmost—History of Japanese Mentality, Foundation for the Promotion of the Open University of Japan, 2016 (in Japanese)
Watsuji, Tetsuro: Climate and Culture: A Philosophical Study (transl. Geoffrey Bownas), Yushodo Co, 1961
Wilmer, Harry: Quest for Silence, Daimon Verlag, 2000
Yamakuse, Yoji: Heart and Soul of the Japanese (bilingual edition; transl. Michael A. Cooney), IBC Publishing, 2011

Yamazaki, Hiroshi: Space-Time of the Japanese Fine Arts and Architecture, Seizansha, 2011 (in Japanese)
Yasuda, Takeshi: Japan—Culture of Shapes, Asahi Shimbun Company, 1984 (in Japanese)
Yoshida, Yuko (ed.): Indigenous Japanese Language—A Collection of Modesty, Nagaoka Shoten, 2015 (in Japanese)

Chapter 4
Silence Takes Shape—The Birth of the Japanese Psychotherapies

To say nothing is a flower.
Japanese proverb

In the previous chapter we discussed briefly some aspects of the notion of silence—mainly its ontological and communication aspects within the Japanese cultural context. In this chapter we expound on the therapeutic power of silence and the way it is applied in the Japanese psychotherapies that are the subject of the present work.

Silence appears to have never been the hottest topic in the Western psychological science and psychotherapeutic approaches. This is especially valid for the verbal approaches where the phenomenon of silence is often discussed predominantly in negative terms, e.g., as a gap that has to be filled or a challenge that has to be overcome after being interpreted as a defense mechanism, an indicator of hostility, withdrawal, resistance, shyness, embarrassment, or all of these at once. In any case, for most of the verbal approaches silence during the therapeutic session is considered one of the "typical technical problems", together with prolonged interviews and canceled appointments (Edinburg et al. 1975: 41–60). Silence is further described as a phenomenon that "can frighten both therapists and clients" and make clients feel uncomfortable or even anxious; but, in other cases, "when used appropriately, silence can be soothing" or even be "the most therapeutic response available" and "a major tool used by psychoanalytic psychotherapists to facilitate free association" (Sommers-Flanagan and Sommers-Flanagan 2014: 71–72). However, even when considered positively, silence remains a "bordering notion" in psychology because it transcendes the "communicative capacity of language" (Lehmann-Oliveros 2016: 1). As such, it functions as a mere response or tool, not an end in itself.

Whatsoever the case is, such an understanding leaves no room for a full-fledged reflection upon the phenomenon of silence and its possibilities within a broader psychotherapeutic context. In order to reflect on silence, we first need to remember that it as a self-sufficient phenomenon such as birth, life, and death; hence its essence is liminal. "Certainly", the Colombian psychologist Olga Lehmann-Oliveros emphasizes, "different phenomena labeled as "silence", evoke the awareness of human boundaries" (Lehmann-Oliveros 2016: 2). For this reason, silence needs to be redeemed in the context of psychotherapy as far as any psychotherapeutic situation can be considered a liminal one—a situation which, despite the concreteness of the

V. Chervenkova, *Japanese Psychotherapies*,
DOI 10.1007/978-981-10-3126-7_4

problem or ailment, can always attain a more general existential and spiritual character. This is the basic rationale which we adopt when discussing the essence of the three Japanese psychotherapies and their relation to the phenomena of seclusion and silence.

4.1 When "Therapeutic" Has Less to Do with Health

We start this chapter with the awarenss that discussing the therapeutic power of silence may turn out to be a challenging task. This is so because, as previously mentioned, silence is often acknowledged one-sidedly as "a lack of…" and is thus not attached a therapeutic value, if it has anything in common with healing. To this end, first we need to define what "therapeutic" means.

The word "therapeutic" originates from the New Latin *therapeuticus*, which means "curing, healing." This word is derived from the Ancient Greek *therapeutikos*—"attentive, curative, helpful", hence "therapeutic" signifies "the art of healing" or "a curative agent" (Oxford English Dictionary 1978, Vol. XI: 280). "Healing", in turn, originates from the Gothic *hailjan* and Old High German *heilen*, which mean "whole; to become whole" (Oxford English Dictionary 1978, Vol. V: 153). All these meanings imply the presence of a disease or disability—physical or mental, or both. "Therapeutic" is therefore something that has positive effect on body or mind, something that has the power to restore the condition before the onset of the disease, or at least to alleviate the present ailment. On a deeper plane, "therapeutic" refers to a process required when one's wholeness has been dented or lost.

In this train of thought, we need to also discuss what a disease means as an existential situation that most of the humans share: first, diseases and disabilities take us out of the stream of daily life into a space where we suffer and experience discomfort—physical, mental, and social—all alone. It is a paradox, indeed, that even though there are people around us to care and console, the core of our own suffering and our response to it remain "ultimately a personal matter—something whose presence and extent can only be known to the sufferer" (Cassell 2004: 33). At the same time, diseases are situations which inevitably remind us of our own finitude, for which reason they might be likened to small-scale deaths, to general rehearsals before the hour strikes—at the bare stage with no audience we find ourselves robbed to the skin of the roles we have been acting. This is the moment when the totality of our being is put to the test.[1]

[1]It is worth mentioning here that the Japanese term "clinical"—*rinshō* (臨床)—uses the combination of the characters for "to face" or "gear oneself up", and "bed, couch". That is, in many cases being sick is a time when one "faces the bed", i.e., they lie down and adopt the same body posture as the dead. The same apllies, the Japanese psychiatrist and Jungian analyst Takao Oda suggests, to clinical psychology where mental problems put client closer to issues of death, thus calling them to a deeper, fuller experience of what it means to be alive (Oda 2005: 56–57).

All these turn the situation of disease and disability from a mere question of suffering and a quest for overcoming it to a liminal situation—a situation which, along with its frightening aspects, also has the potential of *transforming* the injury in a way that would grant the patient a far larger scope for spiritual growth. It is true that many of the therapeutic approaches we know today rarely address anything beyond the concrete injury to personhood—physical and/or mental. What the contemporary human sciences do is an attempt to fight off a particular manifestation of suffering, but they rarely address the individuality and totality of the individual concerned. In the era of idolizing knowledge, such an attitude is easy to explain: finite can approach only the finite, remaining helpless in the face of the infinite. That is, we have this and that medicine against this and that disease, or this and that psychotherapy is allegedly efficacious for this and that condition; and their common goal is removing the symptoms, i.e., the major cause of the suffering. However, we can never be completely sure if our intervention has brought forth the expected effect. It would be too naïve to believe that we can keep the process of healing under total control for "it is absolutely impossible to prove that a cure has ever cured a patient" (Sartre, as cited in Hora 1959: 239).

If we search for a profound response to the totality of human being put in a liminal situation—what we defined any disease as, i.e., a state which is betwixt-and-between the ordinary—than we should be aware that liminal situations can be addressed constructively and efficaciously by self-sufficient phenomena alone. It appears that the only phenomenon of this kind, which we can always approach and which does not surpass the capacity of our intelligibility, is silence.[2] Silence is not a mere negative condition that sets in when the positive is removed, but it is a phenomenon which, similarly to life and death, does not need anything else to manifest itself. But while we cannot create life *ex nihilo* or provoke a natural death, we can seek silence and voluntarily enter its world whenever and wherever we want. Therefore, we can assume that by exposing the disease as a liminal situation to the phenomenon of silence, we not only broaden the perspective for both therapist and patient, but we also give the numinous nature of healing its due. In this context, we use the word "exposing" because silence offers a modality of healing reverse to our common understanding, that is, we do not bring silence to symptoms and attempt to treat them with it, but quite the contrary: symptoms are brought to the world of silence, requiring us to take a step back, give up our fighting-off attitudes and then let the silence "speak".

As a phenomenon that is difficult to be exploited, silence appears to be completely useless. Paradoxically, however, it is through this very "uselessness" that silence can perform a healing function: silence becomes an interruption "which binds and joins" (Dauenhauer 1980: 134); "it interferes with the regular flow of the purposeful. It strengthens the untouchable; it lessens the damage inflicted by exploitation. It makes things whole again by taking them back from the world of

[2]Hereafter we use "silence" in the broad sense of the word, implying also stillness, seclusion, and lack of verbal communication.

dissipation into the world of wholeness" (Picard 2002: 19). Referring to the ontological qualities of silence as a self-sufficient, non-dualistic and non-pragmatic phenomenon which could be supposed to thus restore lost balance and wholeness, we outline also some of its possible therapeutic qualities:

- *possibility for constructive reconnection with one's symptoms*—diseases and disorders, psychiatric ones included, have rather strong material-like component and it is therefore common for us to sense them as entities foreign to who we are. We are difficult to admit that they belong to the total picture of our being and we usually hasten to part with them. We "think that symptoms appear out of nowhere" (Moore 1992: 158) and we rarely attempt to "listen" to the symbolic language they speak. However, once we enter silence and entrust ourselves to it, "our relationship to symptoms changes drastically. Symptoms become for us unrecognized possibilities rather than indications of something gone wrong" (Sardello 2008: 66). Our task therefore is to respond constructively to the symptom as a *significant coincidence*, as "body and life falling together" (Moore 1992: 161), rather than to attempt blindly to get rid of it.
- *possibility for recognizing the totality of one's own unique being*—the conflict between us and our symptoms belongs to the world of duality and so do we. Once the symptoms are being exposed to silence, they are allowed a voice that we cannot hear otherwise amidst the chaotic noise of both our Ego and the world. In silence we have the chance to stop attempting desperately to fight the symptoms off and to *see* the direction toward which they guide us—this is the unique path of our own life, which could be different had this "body-life coincidence" not happened. By overcoming the conflict between us and our symptoms, we may attain naturally a much deeper level of self-knowledge thanks to which we recognize ourselves as an inseparable body-mind unity; we experience our bodies from within as spiritualized entities.
- *possibility for constructive reconnection with the world*—in an age obsessed with countless means of communication, solitude and silence are often equated negatively with loneliness. This understanding is supported by notions in the human sciences that we are "social animals" and that our capacity to build interpersonal relationships on equal terms is a criterion for emotional maturity.[3] However, it is often the case that exactly "in deep solitude it can happen that the boundaries between self and nature dissolve" (Koch 1994: 124). Such an experience not only enhances the "appreciation of, and sympathy with, one's fellow men" (Storr 1988: 60), but it also evokes sensations of fusion with the world—an experience probably akin to the religious-like *oceanic feeling* discussed, although

[3]As previously mentioned, psychology rarely discusses issues of silence and solitude outside of their interpretations as defense mechanisms, or in the context of the *fear* or the *wish* to be alone. One of the exceptions, which comes from the psychoanalytic circles, is the British psychoanalyst Donald Winnicott who in his seminal paper "The Capacity to be Alone" (1958) discusses the *ability* to be alone as "one of the most important signs of maturity in emotional development", whereas a silent phase or a silent session may turn out "to be an achievement on the part of the patient" (1990: 29).

in a different context, between Sigmund Freud and Romain Rolland as a feeling of "an indissoluble bond, as of being connected with the external world in its integral form" (Freud 1961: 65). Such reconnection with the world occurs in a rather paradoxical way: the individual experiences the privacy of their own being, yet without loneliness. There is a unity between the world with its suchness and the individual in the consistent totality of their body-mind. While prompting the development of a more flexible and accepting attitude toward the paradoxes of life, such a unity appears to be also one of the most beneficial effects that silence can work upon one's soul—to restore it to wholeness, i.e., to *heal* it.

However, the therapeutic potential of silence does not necessarily open rose-tinted pathways to eternal wellness nor can it provide dictionary-type explanations and easy solutions to one's ailments. As we discuss in Part IV, experiences of silence are rather rich in emotional polyvalency, prompring subjects to talk about silence as being soothing and relaxing, but also as frightening or even unbearable.[4] Moreover, "making the claim for symptom alleviation would entice many people into working with Silence" (Sardello 2008: 68), thus exposing them to the risk of relapsing to Ego-driven quests for immediate recuperation. This would likely halt the opportunity for spiritual growth and shift the focus back to issues of injured personhood. If we use the Japanese metaphor of the Way, it would mean to miss the chance for "tuning" oneself with the greater picture of life. Working with silence without the necessary competence may involve risks, indeed, but, on the other hand, studying it may offer ways in which silence can be channeled in constructive direction—by maintaining the focus on more significant goals, i.e., integrating a broader concept of health into one's own life as an opportunity for self-transformation and for making one's disease biographically necessary.

In the next section we explain how this specific focus is attained and maintained in the context of the three Japanese psychotherapies—Morita, Naikan, and Dohsa-hou—and we also discuss them briefly within both the Western and the Japanese cultural and sociohistorical context of their respective times.

4.2 The Quiet Counterparts

In the previous chapter we explained that the Japanese are not very inclined to metaphysical reasoning, yet their life and culture are immersed in sophisticated spirituality that is difficult to find its equivalent elsewhere in the world. Although contemporary Japanese culture resembles in many ways that of the West, the immutable essence of this spirituality still resides in the notion of silence. "When my mind turns to Japan", the British painter John Lane writes, "I think of silence. At one time (and that was before the influence of the American culture), silence had

[4]Note that we do not discuss silence itself as having positive or negative aspects, but we discuss one's personal responses to it.

entered into every phase of the life of its people—their landscapes, their temples, their gardens and, in the rural areas, their homes. It was the spare clarity of Zen" (Lane 2006: 24).

In traditional Japanese culture silence holds a central place, indeed, and it is intimately related with the contemplative and intuitive nature of its people who tend to focus on direct experience rather than on analysis and intellectual learning. As the individual considers themselves part of the divine order of Nature, their lifelong task is to follow and internalize this order. "The point is not to be purposeful but to be natural," the renowned Japanese potter Shōji Hamada notes about his art (Hamada, as cited in McLuhan 1994: 189). This *naturalness* on all levels—body and mind, and intra- and interpersonal relationships—guarantees harmonious life, whereas straying from it inevitably results in a variety of problems: physical and/or mental disorders, and sense of meaningless in life considering that, as previously mentioned, the natural patterns attach meaning to life; they help one taste life.

This understanding seems to permeate the entire Japanese culture to become an essential part of the concepts of sickness, health, and healing as well: no matter how frightening or unwelcome a disease is, it requires a *constructive response* that may lead the person to further growth and self-integration. In this sense, what a Western woman—the mother of modern nursing care Florence Nightingale—suggests seems to perfectly summarize the centuries-old wisdom of Japanese culture regarding issues of disease: "all disease, at some period or other of its course, is more or less a reparative process" (Nightingale 1860/1969: 7), which "Nature has instituted" (Nightingale 1860/1969: 8). What we need is to become aware of this process and follow it. "Although it is often thought," Nightingale continues, "that medicine is the curative process, there is no such thing" because "nature alone cures. Surgery removes the bullet out of the limb, which is an obstruction to cure, but nature heals the wound" (Nightingale 1860/1969: 133). A fighting-off attitude, therefore, could be a beneficial answer for it brings solution to a concrete problem, especially in cases of emergency. On the other hand, it nevertheless remains a temporary solution because it does not take into account the patient and their life story in their entirety. In so doing, such an attitude threatens to rob the patient of the spiritual boons that the unique "pilgrimage" of their disease has been meant to bring forth.

Despite the strong Western influences the field of mental care in Japan has been experiencing since the early 1870s, when Western psychological thought was first introduced to the country,[5] indigenous forms of dealing with mental suffering have been practiced for many centuries. Before the modernization the Meiji Restoration initiated in 1868, there were no psychiatric hospitals in Japan in the modern sense of the word. Instead, there were asylums, most of which located within temple and shrine precincts, where patients with mental ailments were treated by monks through a wide variety of methods such as hydrotherapy, Chinese herbal medicines, fasting, and even rituals of incubation and reading of holy scriptures, to name only a

[5]This is the time when the term "psychology"—*shinrigaku* (心理学)—appeared among academic circles in Japan. For further details, see Ohyama and Uemura (1998: 80–82).

few (Omata 2003: 200–206; Kawai 2009: 18–19; Reynolds in Norbeck and Lock 1987: 110).[6]

In ancient Japan treatment seems to have never occurred outside of the body-mind interconnectedness notion and, regardless of the nature of the concrete disease—physical and/or mental—it was the body-mind unity that was always addressed. As Yuasa points out referring to a myth depicted in *Kojiki*, the oldest written chronicle of Japan, since ancient times the Japanese have recognized the body as a vessel in which the mystic wellspring of life is hidden (Yuasa 1994: 2). That is why the body is not rejected as "simply" a biological entity for the sake of mind, but is recognized as having the capacity to become spiritualized and transcendentalized. Hence the Japanese phrase *shinshin-ichinyo*(心身一如), which can be translated as *body-mind oneness* suggesting a possible solution to the logical difficulty of the body-mind dualism.[7]

In fact, such a dualism has never existed in Japan. As Carter points out, "in Japan, it is not that the typical man or woman on the street does not think of mind and body as separate and distinct, just as we in the West tend to do, but beneath this "commonsense" belief there is a long-standing tradition in which the goal of living, and of any discipline and practice, is to "reunite" what was already united at birth but was separated in the process of growing-up" (Carter 2008: 10–11). Although modernization has influenced all strata in Japan, in the orthodox forms of the Japanese psychotherapies we can still find intact the concept of the firm interconnectedness between body and mind, health and spirituality. Just as any of the *Dō*-practices, the Japanese psychotherapies, too, believe that healing as a process of inner transformation can be attained if the individual in their totality—body, mind, and spirit—involves themselves in diligent training.[8] Again, similarly to the *Dō*-practices, the Japanese psychotherapies are conveyed as living traditions and,

[6]For further details on the rituals of incubation—*incubatio*—referring to "prehistoric caves and megalithic monuments where one should remain for a certain period of time in order to receive, usually in a dream, some sort of revelation, inspiration, or healing", see the Italian philologist Francesco Benozzo's paper "Sounds of the Silent Cave. An Ethnophilological Perspective on Prehistoric "Incubatio" (Benozzo in Dimitriadis 2010). Even though the topic is discussed in ethnophilological terms with no particular relation to the East Asian cultural context, it further elucidates the importance of seclusion and silence when non-ordinary experiences, healing included, are sought after.

[7]In her work *The Japanese Self in Cultural Logic*, Takie Sugiyama Lebra explores Japanese idioms, which signify the affinity between body and spirituality as spiritual anatomy and/or embodied spirit (2004: 186–191). For further details on the *shinshin-ichinyo* concept, see the Japanese physician Hiroji Naka's paper "A Study on the Origin of "Shinshin-ichinyo" with Reference to the Source Texts of Dogen and Eisai" (2011). Naka concludes that *shinshin-ichinyo* has its origin in the term *shinjin-ichinyo* (身心一如)with emphasis on the first character—*mi* (身) —which generally means "body". This concept, Naka emphasizes, is essential for the Japanese psychosomatic medicine (Naka 2011:37).

[8]This is revealed unambiguously through the language used in the Japanese psychotherapies. For example, the places for intensive Naikan therapy are called *training centers*, while the therapist–client pair in Dohsa-hou is called *trainer–trainee*. For further details, see the respective chapters of Part III of the present book.

although indirectly, they imply the notion of a lifelong journey. Their clients can be likened to *Dō*-practitioners or pilgrims on their own unique way to wholeness, natural outcomes of which are physical and mental health as well.

However, as mentioned in Chap. 1, exactly this distinctive feature makes some scholars doubt if these approaches are psychotherapies in the Western sense of the word, and accuse them of lack of scientific basis and clear-cut theoretical frameworks.[9] As the British psychotherapist David Brazier aptly points out, "the idea that therapy can be a spiritual path is not the usual one. Generally, therapy is seen as a job or a quasi-medical activity" (Brazier 1995: 262–263). Indeed, when we think about healthcare, hospitals, white gowns and medical equipment are probably among the first images to surface in our minds. This generalized image often symbolically transmits to the field of psychology and psychotherapy an erroneous common understanding based on the prevailing healthcare model that the doctor is the one who "fixes" the ailment, whereas the patient is a passive recipient of the intervention; in Kawai's words, the patient is simply "being fixed" or "cured" (Kawai 2009: 15).

As we discuss in detail in the respective chapters, the Japanese psychotherapies seem not to fit this medical model; quite the contrary, they adopt what Kawai terms a *natural therapeutic model*, for which the proper verb should be "to get cured," "to recover" (Kawai 2009: 21). This model presupposes the mystic, yet active participation of a third party in the therapeutic process—the natural healing forces within the patient which only should be unlocked through a particular practice[10]; hence the proverbial humility of, for example, Naikan therapists.[11]

"Put the patient in the best condition for nature to act upon him" (Nightingale 1860/1969: 133). For the Japanese psychotherapies this "best condition" appears to be seclusion and silence. There, in the "incubator" of silence, the individual and their potential become the focal point, rather than their concrete suffering. Suffering is then considered a unique opportunity for spiritual growth. In a sense, seclusion and silence foster this potential and, in sharp contrast to the prevailing healthcare models which treat the finite with finite, the Japanese psychotherapies address the infinite with infinite. Indeed, if we aim to reach beyond the concrete ailment to issues of personal growth and the totality of one's being, which correlate naturally to healthier and better functioning in life, a manual-based diagnosis and a handful of pills could hardly do the job.

---

[9]Such accusations are most often leveled at Naikan therapy, which emerged from a religious practice (see Chap. 6; also, footnote 1 in Chap. 1).

[10]The American historian of medicine Erwin Ackerknecht notes that "the Japanese, who took over Chinese medicine together with Chinese culture in the ninth century A.D., did not show the same conservatism" (Ackerknecht 1968: 48) as India and China. "During the sixteenth century, probably under the stimulus of foreign contact, they developed a more direct clinical approach and a greater reliance on the healing forces of nature" (ibid).

[11]Naikan therapists usually bow in front of the client before and after every interview (see Sect. 6.2).

However, presenting the Japanese psychotherapies predominantly as methods for spiritual growth threatens to make light of their otherwise unquestionable therapeutic aspects, which have been proved over decades of practice and evident-based research in a wide clinical spectrum. These aspects allow us to line them side by side with the world's major psychotherapeutic approaches. Despite a number of culturally bound peculiarities they share, the Japanese psychotherapies are not some quasi-religious teachings, but well-structured approaches with roots extending deep into the Japanese history and spiritual culture. At the same time, they belong equally to the global current of the human sciences and offer adequate answers to the most burning questions of both their respective times and of the present days.

In Table 4.1 we present a brief outline of the context within which the three Japanese psychotherapies evolved:

Table 4.1 A comparative table presenting the Japanese psychotherapies within the context of the global tendencies in the psychological science, and within the local and the Western cultural and sociohistorical contexts

Japanese psychotherapeutic approaches	Western psychotherapeutic approaches	Japanese cultural and sociohistorical context	Western cultural and sociohistorical context
Morita Therapy (1910s–1920s)	Psychoanalysis and theory of neurosis in the works of Sigmund Freud and Alfred Adler become the cornerstones of the psychological science	After more than 260 years of national isolation enacted by the Tokugawa shogunate, the 1868 Meiji Restoration urges on the country's modernization and Westernization. The national identity confusion thus triggered results in the onset of various neurotic symptoms among the populace	World War I rages across Europe as one of the largest and deadliest conflicts in history; Modernism thrives, reflecting a wide-scale social and psychological transformation
Naikan Therapy (1950s–1960s)	Jungian psychology and the concept of archetypes and collective unconsciousness are in their heyday. Viktor Frankl's Logotherapy, too, gains popularity	Japan struggles to recover from its World War II capitulation and the Hiroshima and Nagasaki atomic bombings. These appear to be even more powerful as psychological weapons and the immediate need for self-reflection upon the Japanese national behavior becomes evident	Peak of structuralism (end-1950s) and its key concept of the interrelation between the elements of human culture; increasing interest toward Eastern philosophy and religion

(continued)

Table 4.1 (continued)

Japanese psychotherapeutic approaches	Western psychotherapeutic approaches	Japanese cultural and sociohistorical context	Western cultural and sociohistorical context
Dohsa-hou Therapy (1960s–1970s)	Owing mainly to Wilhelm Reich and Maurice Merleau-Ponty, the concept of body awareness is systematically brought into psychotherapy and different body-centered approaches are developed (for example, Postural Integration, and Dance and Movement Therapy)	Japan enters a period of rapid economic growth and gradually adopts the materialistic and comfort-oriented values of the Western societies (for example, the opening of the Tokaido Shinkansen bullet train line and Expo'70)	The counterculture advances with New Age and antiwar movements, and brings to the fore various social issues, many of which concern the physical body (for example, issues on human sexuality and experimentation with psychoactive drugs)

By placing the Japanese psychotherapies in such a broader context, we realize that they are not some isolated phenomena intended only for an island nation which values nonverbal communication and retreats in silence to soothe its ailments. Moreover, if we arrive at the understanding that silence, after all, "sharpens" our senses and enhances our *mindfulness*, we realize that silence could not lead to sterility, but to a deep insight about our common human condition. This, we suggest, is the cornerstone of the Japanese psychotherapies, which are worth due attention as the quiet, yet eloquent counterparts of the Western approaches.

In the next part we take a closer look at the intriguing world of the three Japanese psychotherapies—Morita, Naikan, and Dohsa-hou—a world where walking in silence helps us recognize our true nature of *Homo Viator* on the never-ending road of Life: unique and, at the same time, shared by all humans.

References

Ackerknecht, Erwin H.: A Short History of Medicine, Ronald Press Co, 1968

Brazier, David: Zen Therapy, Constable and Company Limited, 1995

Carter, Robert E.: The Japanese Arts and Self-Cultivation, State University of New York Press, 2008

Cassell, Eric J.: The Nature of Suffering and the Goals of Medicine (Second Edition), Oxford University Press, 2004

Dauenhauer, Bernard P.: Silence—The Phenomenon and Its Ontological Significance, Indiana University Press, 1980

Dimitriadis, George (ed.): Archaeologies and Soundscapes (BAR International Series), Archaeopress, 2010

Edinburg, Golda M., N.Zinberg, W. Kelman: Clinical Interviewing and Counseling: Principles and Techniques, Appleton-Century-Crofts, 1975

Freud, Sigmund: Civilization and Its Discontents (transl. and ed. James Strachey), Vol. XXI, Hogarth Press, 1961

Hora, Thomas: Tao, Zen and Existential Psychotherapy, Psychologia—An International Journal of Psychology of the Orient, Vol.II (2), Psychologia Society, 1959

Kawai, Hayao: Introduction to Psychotherapy: Psychotherapeutic Approaches—Collection IV, Iwanami Shoten, 2009 (in Japanese)

Koch, Philip: Solitude—A Philosophical Encounter, Open Court Publishing, 1994

Lane, John: The Spirit of Silence—Making Space for Creativity, Green Books, 2006

Lebra, Takie Sugiyama: The Japanese Self in Cultural Logic, University of Hawai'i Press, 2004

Lehmann-Oliveros, Olga V.: Something Blossoms in Between: Silence-Phenomena as Bordering Notions in Psychology, Integrative Psychological and Behavioral Science, Vol. 50 (1), Springer Verlag, 2016

McLuhan, Teri C.: The Way of the Earth—Encounters with Nature in Ancient and Contemporary Thought, Touchstone, 1994

Moore, Thomas: Care of the Soul—A Guide for Cultivating Depth and Sacredness in Everyday Life, HarperPerennial, 1992

Naka, Hiroji: A Study on the Origin of "Shinshin-ichinyo" with Reference to the Source Texts of Dogen and Eisai, Japanese Journal of Psychosomatic Medicine, Vol. 51(8), Japanese Society of Psychosomatic Medicine, 2011 (in Japanese)

Nightingale, Florence: Notes on Nursing—What It Is, and What It Is Not, Dover Publications, 1860/1969

Norbeck, Edward, M. Lock (ed.): Health, Illness, and Medical Care in Japan—Cultural and Social Dimensions, University of Hawaii Press, 1987

Oda, Takao: Psychotherapy and the Japanese Soul—Living the Myths, Baifukan, 2005 (in Japanese)

Ohyama, Tadasu, Y. Uemura: History of Psychology, Foundation for the Promotion of the Open University of Japan, 1998 (in Japanese)

Omata, Wa'ichiro: Origin and Typology of Psychiatric Hopsitals in Japan (before the Meiji Restoration), The 12th Congress of the World Psychiatric Association, Psychiatria et Neurologia Japonica, Vol. 105(2), Japanese Society of Psychiatry and Neurology, 2003 (in Japanese)

Oxford English Dictionary, Vol. V (H-K), Oxford University Press, 1978

Oxford English Dictionary, Vol. XI (T-U), Oxford University Press, 1978

Picard, Max: The World of Silence, Eighth Day Press, 2002

Sardello, Robert: Silence: The Mystery of Wholeness, Goldenstone Press, 2008

Sommers-Flanagan, John, R. Sommers-Flanagan: Clinical Interviewing (Fifth Edition), Wiley, 2014

Storr, Anthony: Solitude—A Return to the Self, Free Press, 1988

Winnicott, Donald: The Maturational Processes and The Facilitating Environment: Studies in the Theory of Emotional Development, Karnac Books, 1990

Yuasa, Yasuo: Cosmology of the Human Body—Eastern and Western, Iwanami Shoten, 1994 (in Japanese)

Part III
The Sun Rising at the Gate

In this part we introduce the theoretical frameworks of the three Japanese psychotherapies—Morita, Naikan, and Dohsa-hou—the interpretation of which is partly based on the author's personal experience with them. The phenomenon of silence and the image of the traveler/pilgrim that we brought up in Part II are now stripped off of their symbolic associations and are discussed in the concreteness of their therapeutic faculties: silence, which renders coldness to the therapeutic situation, corresponds to the empty-centered structure of *ma*—the space between the therapist and the client, which is needed so that the warm sunrays may shine through and heal the wounded (see footnote 5 in Sect. 3.1); and the image of the pilgrim who leaves their daily life and set off on a long and challenging journey—until they see the Sun rising at the gate.

Chapter 5
Morita Therapy—Chopping Wood, Carrying Water. Life Happens

Sweet is the lore which Nature brings;
Our meddling intellect
Misshapes the beauteous form of things:
We murder to dissect.

William Wordsworth

Chronologically, Morita therapy is the first among the three Japanese psychotherapies presented in this book. It emerged at the beginning of the 20th century almost at the same time when in Europe Sigmund Freud was introducing his psychoanalytic theory. The location of Morita therapy in respect to the Western psychology, psychiatry, and psychotherapy is subject of controversy: some recognize it as a natural continuity of the occidental psychotherapeutic tradition, whereas others consider it "clearly and deeply rooted in Japan's distinctive environment and traditional culture" (Fujita 1986: 5). While explaining the key philosophical and therapeutic principles of the approach, we elaborate on this issue too.

5.1 Origins and Development of Morita Therapy

Although it contrasts the "folk" therapy" (Lebra 1976: 215) of Naikan in the sense that it emerged within the academic circles, Morita therapy neither can be completely detached from its apparent cultural determinants. Its development took its founder Shōma Morita nearly 20 years—he "blended a large measure of Buddhistic thought with the personal accounts of his neurotic patients' problems, and borrowed some ideas from Western psychotherapies" (Reynolds 1980: 4). Similarly to the Naikan's founder Ishin Yoshimoto, Morita too referred to his firsthand experience, i.e., his own encounter with neurosis. This experience gives the therapy a taste of both authenticity and universality, posing questions of suffering and well-being that are common to all humans. Shōma Morita, David K. Reynolds summarizes, "was thinking on a basic human level, not only about the problems of Japanese people" (Reynolds 1980: 5).

V. Chervenkova, *Japanese Psychotherapies*,
DOI 10.1007/978-981-10-3126-7_5

5.1.1 Who Was Shōma Morita?[1]

Masatake (alias Shōma) Morita (森田正馬) was born on January 18, 1874 in the village of Fuke (now Noichi city), in Kōchi prefecture on the island of Shikoku. He was the first son of a sericulture farming family—Masafumi and Kamejo Morita—who called the small boy Mitsu (光), i.e., Shiny. Shōma had one elder and one younger sister, and one younger brother—Tokuya—that he was especially fond of.

In his early childhood, Morita was very even-tempered—he almost never cried and whenever left alone in the room, he played and fell asleep on his own. His paternal grandmother was worrying that the child was stupid, making this way his maternal grandmother feel indignant and snap back at her, "No fools can be born in our family!" (Iwata 2003: 218). Indeed, the young Shōma had a sharp mind and a sensitive character: he eagerly learned to read and write at the tender age of four. When he was nine years old, in the local temple—a one of the Shingon Buddhism—he saw a vivid painting of Hell with lakes of blood and needle-shaped mountains. This experience made Shōma constantly think of and fear death during daytime, and turn and toss in frightening nightmares at night; soon afterwards he began suffering from enuresis, which continued until he became 14 years old.

When Shōma was 10, his father started teaching him Chinese classics and forced him to stay all night to memorize the endless rows of characters. Besides doing sericulture business, Shōma's father was also a teacher at the local elementary school who was rather strict with the education and discipline of his children. By contrast, Shōma's mother was a warmhearted person who doted upon her son and with whom she often exchanged letters later in their life. Morita himself stated that all the neurotic symptoms such as enuresis that he suffered from during his youth resulted from a distorted parent–child relationship (Ohara and Ohara 1990: 17).

The father's stern attitude repelled Shōma from reading and writing—around the end of his elementary school education he played truant and run away from home. In September 1887 Shōma left for the prefectural capital of Kōchi where he entered junior high school. However, he was not motivated to study and his grades were rather poor. At that time he started suffering from headaches and also thought there was something wrong with his heart; his mother told him that he himself thought out his headaches (Iwata 2003: 219). His complaints made him visit regularly a local hospital where he was diagnosed with neurosis. As his grades, especially those in mathematics, continued to be poor, his father got angry and limited his tuition. Morita felt indignant with his father's decision and in 1892 he went with a friend to Tokyo to study at a cram school and gain his independence; but on the second month he got beriberi, which made him return home where he apologized to his father for rebelling against him, and returned to school. In the winter vacation of the

[1]All the biographical data in this section are summarized from Nomura (1974), Miura and Usa (in Lebra and Lebra 1974: 407–409), Usa and Kinoshita (1987: 191–197), Ohara and Ohara (1990:3–39), Kitanishi (1999: 179–183), Iwata (2003:15–31; 217–239), Hahakigi (2013), and Nakayama (2014).

next year, Morita began to keep a diary. He did diligently so until the end of his life, writing a total 36 notebooks, and even incorporated the Japanese tradition of diary keeping in his therapeutic approach.

In February 1894 Shōma got infected with typhoid fever which kept him bedridden for two months. Before fully recovering, he went for a bicycle ride and his quickened pulse made him think again there was something wrong with his heart. All these experiences made Shōma remember the frightening painting of Hell he saw back in his childhood and think of death again. With the time he became especially interested in mysticism and started studying magic, fortunetelling, and phrenology. He came across a book by the prolific Buddhist philosopher Enryō Inoue, which inspired his wish to solve scientifically mysteries such as superstition and evil spirit possession; but he was also eager to solve the mystery of life and death, and the body-mind duality. Later, this wish prompted him to begin studying medical psychiatry at the university.

In 1895 Morita graduated from the junior high school in Kōchi. Considering the poor health of his son, his father did not allow him to advance to high school and refused him tuition. However, Morita received a scholarship from Denryū Ōguro, an Osaka-based wealthy physician, on the premise that Ōguro would adopt him, and thus entered the Kumamoto Fifth High School. When the young man's father realized about this, he headed for Kumamoto immediately: he agreed to provide his son's tuition on the condition that Shōma would marry Hisai Tamura—daughter of Shōma's aunt; a Meiji Era father would not let his first son to be adopted that easily. That is how in July 1896 Morita married the 21-year-old Hisai. She worked as an embroidery and sewing teacher known among their relatives as a skilled and intelligent woman. Albeit raised in a family indifferent to education, Hisai used every moment free from household duties to read books and educate herself. Until the end of her life in 1935 she admired everything her husband was doing and consoled him wisely anytime he was dispirited. However, Morita did not find her beautiful and sophisticated enough, and felt as if something were missing in his marriage. Especially during their youth the couple often quarreled: "I did not intend to marry such a plain woman as you," Morita once said. In his "Memoirs about Hisai," which Morita started writing after Hisai's death, he reflects that he was selfish back then and made her feel bad by reproaching her for nonsenses. Once the couple began to live together in Tokyo, Morita started helping her study calligraphy, literature, and arts. "One day I will be a somebody and I want you to match me," Morita said to her (Ohara and Ohara 1990: 22–23).

After Morita secured his high scool tuition from his father, he devoted himself to studying. In 1898 Morita graduated from school and entered the Medical Department of Tokyo Imperial University (now University of Tokyo). Over the first two years in Tokyo, the young couple lived separately, but Shōma's mother visited him and took care of him. Nevertheless, his health remained rather poor: he was diagnosed again with neurosis, combined with beriberi due to which he could even hardly walk at times. Every day he took medicines and had injections, but to no avail. "This may be also one reason why he took an interest in psychotherapy" (Miura and Usa in Lebra and Lebra 1974: 408). On the top of it, his father, who had already abandoned his teaching profession and had entirely devoted himself to the family's sericulture business, was late with sending him money. At that time, Morita's annual examinations were already knocking at the door. Being brought to the edge of despair and also out of anger to his father, Morita decided to quit all his medicines and started preparing to die. While doing so, he studied fervently day and night. Before long, his efforts resulted in increased grades, and, miraculously, his neurotic and beriberi symptoms alleviated significantly. This experience was crucial for the development of Morita's therapeutic approach (Kitanishi 1999: 181)—"the unintentional effect on his mental and physical health through productive activity helped guide Morita in his subsequent understanding of anxiety disorders" (Ogawa 2013: 24).

Morita grew up as a timid young man with a fine sense of humor, strong perfectionist streak, and a never-give-up attitude. He was known as much of an eccentric (Kitanishi 1999: 180) who wore a self-sewn quilted *haori* with red lining and pulled a two-wheeled cart to bring his luggage to the dormitory. His character wonderfully combined his father's sharp and penetrating mind with warmheartedness as inherited from his mother. Was it not for Morita's personality, the therapy he developed would end up as too stern; but it was the "loving smack" that made the approach successful and this success likely resulted from the immeasurable influence of Morita's mother (Ohara and Ohara 1990: 18).

At the end of 1902 Morita graduated successfully from the university. Soon afterward he became an assistant at his home department and also began working at Sugamo Hospital in Tokyo. At that time he was already attending the lectures of Shūzō Kure (1865–1932), the founding father of psychiatry in Japan known as the "Japanese Philippe Pinel" because he "prohibited the use of fetters and other restraints on mental patients and finally ordered the destruction of such equipment" (Powell and Anesaki 1990: 41); he also ordered that inpatients should wear ordinary clothes instead of hospital gowns with the character for "insane"—(狂)—on the back (Iwata 2003: 155). On the cusp between the 19th and 20th century, Kure studied in Western Europe where he "immediately grasped the value of Kraepelin's research, which had just become systematized" (Fujinawa in Mezzich et al. 1994: 82). It was through Kure that Morita got influenced by the concepts of the prominent German psychiatrist. In August 1903, under the guidance of Kure, Morita headed for his native island of Shikoku to carry out a research among local people who were considered possessed by evil spirits, particularly by that of *inugami* (犬神)—the dog god—which made them speak and behave in a strange way, or get in a stupor or delirium. The symptoms of these people Morita classified as "invocation-induced psychosis" (祈祷性精神症) and, according to the Japanese psychiatrist Kazuhiko Nakayama, this research was an overture to the development of Morita therapy (Nakayama 2014: 53).

At that time the Japanese psychiatry was dominated by the German school, which instilled research on the possible physical causes of mental disroders (Kitanishi 1999: 182); however, there was no efficacious treatment for neurosis and this *status quo* prompted Morita to start treating his patients on a trial-and-error basis—from medical thearpy to hypnosis—but to no avail. He had especially hard times with patients suffering from erythrophobia: after many unsucessfull cases, he finally gave up to an extent that one day when such a patient visited the hospital to seek help from Morita, Morita ran away (Kitanishi 1999: 182). In parallel, he began applying actively occupational therapy (see footnote 3), and daily life-regulation method as inspired by the Swiss psychiatrist Otto Binswanger, in which labor and rest, reading, walking, etc., follow one after another in strict order. These attemps were a success, but only a temporary one especially to patients with acute psychiatric symptoms. To cope with the symptoms, Morita prescribed to patients total bed rest, which eventually proved efficacious but not satisfactory enough. Morita needed to continue his trial-and-error methodology.

In May 1904 Morita's dear younger brother Tokuya was called out to the Russo-Japanese war. Three months later he was killed on the filed; this brought a tremendous shock to Morita, but he continued to work hard and before long managed to send for the first time his own-earned money to his father. Two years later, Morita started working also at Negishi Hospital in Tokyo. There he showed such a fervent enthusiasm and innovative thinking that when the hospital's director carried out a personnel reform, he took into account Morita's suggestions. In his personal life Morita experienced sheer happiness: in September 1911, on the 15th year of his marriage, his first child—Shō'ichirō—was born. Right from the beginning, Morita started keeping a diary on his son's development, naming it *The Golden Boy Diary* (「金太郎日記」) (Iwata 2003: 226).

A brilliant theorist and prolific academic author and translator, in 1917 Morita was elected councilman of the Japanese Society of Psychiatry. Before long, in 1919, he began examining patients with neurotic and obsessive symptoms at his home and also hospitalized some of them there. It was the same year when Morita had his first successfully cured patient with erythrophobia. "Among some patients whom Dr. Morita was taking care of at his home there was a certain female, Miss Yatabe. She suffered from obsessive neurosis of mysophobia. She had been treated at the Sugamo Psychiatric Hospital for a long time, and had left the hospital without being cured. At his home Dr. Morita tried hypnosis, other usual methods of treatment, and his own method of persuasion, but had no success. He told me that sometimes he had lost his temper and struck her. To his surprise, however, the patient had been cured suddenly by herself when she abandoned herself in agony and despair. Dr. Morita studied this accidental case, and found the necessary conditions for this wonderful cure, which became the basis for his unique therapeutic method" (Shimoda, as cited in Miura and Usa in Lebra and Lebra 1974: 426). At that time, Morita's wife Hisai helped him with everything needed for the proper treatment: as Morita was rather busy also with his academic duties, it was Hisai who was more familiar with the patients and paid attention to the details of their daily life. Many of them, especially patients with mysophobia, got cured thanks to her straightforward instructions. Morita, on the other hand, influenced his patients and disciples with personal examples in his daily life, emphasizing that things and time should be used to their utmost: on the backs of advertisement handbills he wrote his manuscripts; the worn-out wooden clogs he burned to boil bathwater; when sick, he read books; at the entrance of his house he put up a list of presents that would trouble him—for example, melons and sweets, and presents that would make him happy such as money, soy sause and soybean paste. Even when in 1920 a recurrent colitis put him close to death, he though out to conduct a memorial service himself while still alive. In his later years when he was difficult to walk, he went outside in a stroller, all smiles. Morita continued writing his papers and examining patients even during the Great Kantō earthquake in September 1923, stating that one should do the things that have to be done regardless of the external circumstances. "I was probably the only one who kept on working when the earthquake occured," Morita wrote down in his diary (Iwata 2003: 231). It was seven months after Morita had lost his father.

Two years later, in 1925, Morita was appointed professor at the Jikei University School of Medicine in Tokyo. Around that time he started disputing the theory of psychoanalysis with Kiyoyasu Marui (1886–1953), Professor of Psychiatry at Tohoku Imperial University and the founding father of psychoanalysis in Japan. This made Morita especially popular among the academic circles; his popularity augmented further when in 1927 he, together with Sansei Hospital's founder Dr. Genyū Usa (see Sect. 10.1), cured the famous essayist and playwright Hyakuzō Kurata (1891–1943) from his obsessive disorder within only three months. This experience inspired Kurata to write *The Paradise of a Neurotic* (1932). In 1928 Morita's seminal work *The True Nature and Therapy of Anxiety-Based Disorders (Shinkeishitsu)* was published and in 1933 it was translated to German. A year earlier, in 1932, Morita opened "Morita Clinic"—a new building adjacent to his house where he examined and, when most necessary, hospitalized his patients.

In April 1934 Morita held a lecture entitled "The Origin of Obsessive Thoughts" at the congress of the Japanese Society of Psychiatry in Tokyo where he entered into heated arguments with Prof. Marui over psychoanalytic theory again. Prof. Marui reproached him that his concept was a vulgar belief, to which Morita replied that the psychoanalytic interpretations were nothing but superstitions (Iwata 2003: 203). However, the next day his clinic was visited by Tohoku University's professor Heisaku Kosawa (1897–1968), another key figure in the Japanese psychoanalytic circles known as the originator of the Ajase complex theory. After this visit, Morita said to some of his patients that should they want to undergo psychoanalytic treatment, he would introduce them to Prof. Kosawa; in return, he would like to know the effects of the treatment. In a sense, Morita relented toward psychoanalysis and acknowledged it; otherwise, he would not react so emotionally and would not compare his theory with that put forward by Sigmund Freud (Iwata 2003: 203–204).

At the beginning of 1935 Morita's health worsened significantly, for which reason he spent some time in Atami, a hot spring sea resort near Tokyo. In May of that year he returned to Tokyo, but his health remained poor, fixing him to bed over the summer months. In October of that year, his wife, Hisai, who had miscarriages and stillbirth in the past, passed away suddenly of cerebral hemorrhage; Morita started writing *Memoirs about Hisai*. Earlier, in 1930, Shōma and Hisai Morita lost their only son, the 19-year-old Shō'ichirō, because of tuberculosis. Morita's grief was enormous: he clung to his son's death body and lamented over him bitterly; when his concerned relatives attempted to move him away from the coffin, he returned immediately, crying. However, right after the funeral was over, Morita immersed himself in conversations with the others and looked as another person to whom nothing had happened. "I express my emotions the way they are, as a small child…If I cry when I am sad, the emotions "discharge" and my heart lightens," he explained (Iwata 2003: 180).

Morita continued doing his works and in April 1937 he was elected professor emeritus of Jikei University School of Medicine; but three months later he contracted dysentery, which required his hospitalization. His serious health problems were topped by the death of his mother in February 1938. Two months later, in April 1938, the 64-year-old Morita followed her to the other world. In his last hour he was surrounded by his relatives and disciples to each of whom he bid farewell. He donated his body to medicine.

Three days before passing away, Morita said to his disciple Akichika Nomura, "I will die holding the same spirit as that I was born with. Just watch. I always feel free to cry or to be angry. I wonder how false and painful the last hour of all heroes, geniuses, and high priests is. Ordinary people die naturally" (Iwata 2003: 239). Morita was an apostle of naturalness, who adviced his patients and disciples to be run-of-the-mill persons and considered himself being such one; a true *Homo Ludens*, he was as simple and free as a child who loved to entertain people. As such, Morita was a living example of the deeply humane philosophy behind the psychotherapeutic approach he developed: suffering is an experience that can enrich our inner world and bring out our creative power—if we taste pain thoroughly, we would never become its slaves; relying on our innate will to live, we must set a purpose in life and strive to accomplish it despite the external circumstances. This, as Morita demonstrated personally throughout his life, is what it means to be a human.

5.1.2 In-Hopsital Treatment Methods of Morita Therapy—Key Characteristics and Purposes

Shōma Morita was a child of the turbulent years spanning the Meiji (1868–1912) and Taishō (1912–1926) eras of the Japanese history. As shown in Table 4.1 (Sect. 4.2), it was a time when the Western culture was overwhelming Japan, triggering drastic changes in the worldview of its people, attitudes to healthcare among both professionals and clients included. The conflict that the Japanese intellectuals of that time experienced resulted in the simultaneous rediscovery of Eastern wisdom and the proactive adoption of Western concepts (Kitanishi 2000: 48). Shōma Morita, too, was not an exception: he studied Western medicine fervently, but not blindly—he reffered to the values of his native culture, and also to his own firsthand experience and clinical observations.

Considering this background—both sociohistorical and personal—Morita therapy was conceived to deal primarily with what Shōma Morita defined as *shinkeishitsu* (神経質—"nervous, high-strung") or "anxiety-based disorders involving a high degree of perfectionism" (Tanaka-Matsumi in Gielen et al. 2004: 285), which, in general, are indicative of the civilized individual's inflated sense of almightiness that they transfer from the external world to their soul (Ohtani 2002: 53). In this sense, Morita did not considered *shinkeishitsu* a disease, but a peculiar trick of mind (Iwata 2003: 33), and, as it will be explained in detail later, he established his approach not to combat the neurotic symptoms themselves, but to help his patients gain insight about their own obsession with the symptoms.

In his attempt to classify the *shinkeishitsu*-related disorders, Morita proceeded from their elemental characteristics, rather than from their particular manifestations, suggesting that they all share the same origin and that "autosuggestion is also one cause for the acceleration of adherence to those symptoms" (Miura and Usa in Lebra and Lebra 1974: 411). Morita felt sorry that some of his medical contemporaries did not understand this concept completely and distinguished the *shinkeishitsu*-related conditions only through their external manifestations, the symptoms. In so doing, they considered, for example, ordinary neurosis and obsessions to be completely different conditions (Morita 1960: 50). However, symptom-based classifications are nothing but a desk theory, which does not reveal the true essence of the disease, much less the methods it should be treated with (Morita 1960: 51). Morita proposed the following three types of *shinkeishitsu*, which "may grade or combine with one another" (Miura and Usa in Lebra and Lebra 1974: 411):

- Ordinary neurosis/neurasthenia(普通神経質)—manifests itself in complaints of psychosomatic nature such as headaches and stomachaches, insomnia, nausea, tremor, and fatigue with no physiological abnormalities observed. These complaints are underpinned by *an excessive anxiety* toward one's own health and physical condition.
- Paroxysmal neurosis/anxiety neurosis(発作性神経質)—this is a kind of fit—for example, palpitation, shivering, or even fainting—which evokes fear of the occurrence of a next fit. The *self-reinforcing fear* is essential to this condition, which in most of the cases becomes chronic and is often accompanied also by depressive symptoms.
- Obsessions/phobias(強迫観念症)—these conditions arise from a *mental conflict*, which manifests itself in the form of defensive behavior, for example mysophobia, nosophobia, erythrophobia, acrophobia, claustrophobia, etc. Obsessions and phobias Morita considered as being the most time-consuming and difficult to cure conditions (summarized from Morita 1960: 49–56; Miura and Usa in Lebra and Lebra 1974: 411–412; Iwata 2003: 33–34; and Kitanishi 2016: 42–45).

During the early years of the therapy's development, the approach was named in many different ways such as "neurosis therapy," "self-awareness therapy," "nature therapy," "home therapy," "occupational therapy," "experience therapy," "training therapy," and "discipline therapy." Although it is rare for a psychotherapeutic approach to be named after its founder—and Morita himself opposed it—his devoted disciples coined the name "Morita therapy" after Morita passed away (Ohara 1997: 30). Morita himself most often called his approach "reeducation" (再教育)

(Maruyama 1995: 1) or "specific treatment for *shinkeishitsu*" (神経質の特殊療法) (Ichikawa 2008: 84), stressing the importance of how the suffering individual should change their usual attitude toward their health condition and learn the meaning that "cure" has, i.e., "it does not mean removing the symptoms but living productively in spite of them" (Reynolds 1980: 7). For Morita the ultimate goal of education is not imposing a "should-do" attitude and bringing about lifestyle stability, but rather the development and improvement of one's personality toward the accomplishment of a certain goal (Morita, as cited in Maruyama 1995: 181–182).

The idea of reeducation permeates both the approach's therapeutic philosophy and clinical application. In order to serve this purpose, in-hospital Morita therapy is divided into four treatment phases, which are organically interwoven through strict rules and strong self-discipline. These phases are isolation and total bed rest, light occupation, heavy occupation, and resocialization, generally divided into bed rest therapy and occupational–communal interaction therapy:

****First phase—total bed rest and isolation (four to seven days)***—as the name suggests, this is the first phase during which the patient is isolated in a private room where they have to lie down in bed and not leave it, except for eating (meals are brought to the room) and bathing. Similarly to the intensive Naikan practice, patients are not allowed to entertain or comfort themselves with reading, writing, listening to radio, watching TV, or talking with other people, excluding their doctor, with whom each patient has interviews every evening. The client may think about whatever they want and sleep whenever they can no matter whether during the night or in the daytime, but *doing* something is strictly prohibited. Even if their symptoms aggravate and unbearable thoughts and images start flooding their mind, patients are advised not to try to fight off, analyze or think them away, but simply to observe them and let them pass—this, Morita therapy suggests, is the shortest way to getting rid of them.

The phase has two main aspects, namely a *diagnostic* and a *recuperating* one. First, during this phase doctors can observe the patient's behavior and eventually give a differential diagnosis (Morita 1960: 103). Isolation speaks volumes about the client's psychopathology since it creates a specific environment in which all inner conflicts emerge easily and the client is cornered to face them directly. As Usa emphasizes, by lying down for long hours the patient is forced to do what they do not like, and, at the same time, they are not allowed to do what they would like to. This is an "activity" through which the patient is being taught to part with the habit of explaining their emotions and sensations.[2] Therefore, letting the patient experience to the utmost their own suffering helps them live *with* it, not *against* it, and leave hold of their idealistic images of themselves, others, and the world. In this difficult process, the severity of the suffering becomes a kind of prognostic tool, i.e., the more severe the pain, the more likely the patient is to get cured (Kondo 1962: 16). Indeed, being all alone in silence "is a valuable resource when changes of

[2] In private communication with former Sansei Hospital's director Dr. Shin'ichi Usa (May 2013). Although the characteristics of this phase could be ascribed to the Zen Buddhist influences in Morita therapy, Shōma Morita took his cue from Montessori education, which was becoming popular at that time (Morita 1974: 104, 213).

mental attitude are required" (Storr 1988: 29) because "where silence is, man is observed by silence" and "silence puts man to the test" (Picard 2002: 17).

Second, being isolated from the external world and its stimuli, the client can recover from both physical and mental fatigue. After this period, however, usually around the third or fourth day, suffering is replaced by boredom and most of the patients are possessed by a strong desire to get up, move, and be active. This is an irrefutable evidence that there is a desire for life (Ohara 1997: 32), which already means the client is on their way to recovery (Kondo in Miki and Kuroki 1998: 28). Indeed, the client's recumbent body posture during this phase evokes parallels with a dead body, in sharp contrast to which the desire for getting up and being active becomes tantamount to being alive. Once this desire is present, that is, the client has sufficiently tasted the anguish of the extreme quietude and seclusion, they are considered ready to proceed to the second phase—that of light occupation.

**Second phase—light occupation (three days)*—this is the first time when the client comes into contact with the world again after having been totally isolated from it. Yet, to certain extent, they remain isolated, performing only light and monotonous work—for example, handpicking dead leaves in the yard—which is conducted *in silence*. This phase plays a key role in reaffirming the client's ability to experience directly their inner conflicts and unpleasant emotions the way they are. At the same time, this phase also tests the client's creativity and their ability to interact with the world, i.e., how their "starvation" for external stimuli can be transformed into creative voluntary actions. The key point therefore is that the client is supposed to find tasks themselves and perform them spontaneously, not because they are forced to do them.

This transition process is supported by the doctor who encourages the client to pay close attention to the minutest details of the world outside and describe in their diaries only what they *observed* and *did* during the day; by so doing, they learn to discern their thoughts and feelings from their real-time actions and become more aware of reality as it is, not as it should be as modeled in their mind. Observation of small objects such as flowers and insects is strongly recommended, but paying attention to and writing down about one's feelings and emotions, even about those evoked by the observation itself, is not encouraged (see Sect. 10.2). The aim is "to break the contradiction of thought by making the patient concentrate on unrelated activities, and help him get insight into the dynamics of the paradox" (Ikeda, as cited by Miura and Usa in Lebra and Lebra 1974: 418), while leaving them "in doubt about whether they will recover or not" (Miura and Usa in Lebra and Lebra 1974: 417). At the same time, the silent observation of the natural world around helps one reconnect with it and eventually internalize its order (see Sect. 5.2.4).

At the end of this phase, the client usually does not feel the need to think about or discuss their health condition and many people report they feel "lighter" and "healthier" both physically and mentally. According to Morita, this is just a sensation to which patients are not recommended to attach, because this is the reverse side of the same coin, the other being the symptom itself. Rather, clients are encouraged to transcend the pleasant–unpleasant dichotomy of their own sensations (Morita 1960: 114). Technically, the second phase serves as a bridge between the first phase of total inactivity, isolation and silence, and the third phase of more intense physical activity. In so doing, this phase guarantees the smooth transition from the horizontal to the vertical dimension; from inside to outside; from privacy to community; and also—figuratively and literally—from darkness to light.

***Third phase—heavy occupation (10 days or more)**[3] —this phase is one of more intense outdoor work assigned to clients in accordance with their individual physical condition. The phase is aimed at testing the client's capacity to face their anticipatory anxiety and follow rules without questioning them, rather than at testing the task performance itself—therapsists have to be mindful "not to let the patients be concerned with how they appear to others or with the dignity of their task" (Miura and Usa in Lebra and Lebra 1974: 417). The client's capacity for endurance, too, is tested and further cultivated. The purpose is the establishment of such physical and mental environment where clients can experience the joy of performing a certain activity and even to taste the sacredness of labor (Morita 1960: 115), regardless of their inner discomfort, struggle, or pain (Kondo in Miki and Kuroki 1998: 29). This process represents a transition from the world of self-conceived images to that of reality the way it is. Such a transition, as it will be discussed later in the text, underlies the entire therapeutic framework of Shōma Morita's approach. In other words, the client has to learn to take their inner sensations the way they are, allowing them not to interfere with the immediate daily tasks, because "too much dependence on ratonality and too little use of the therapeutic benefits of manual labor contribute to the persistence of mental illness" (Fujita 1986: 3). Through labor, patients "come to realize that happiness lies not far away, but in the immediate experience of daily life" (Miura and Usa in Lebra and Lebra 1974: 417); when they are "so fully occupied with their work that they are unconscious of the passage of time, they are ready for the next stage"(ibid.).

At the same time, the guidance on diary keeping continues, and the clients are now allowed to read, but only factual treatises such as ones on the natural sciences and history, not literature and philosophy. Additionally, clients are encouraged to spare time on creating art—calligraphy, painting, or wood carving—whatever reconnects them with their own creativity; also, this is the first time when patients are allowed visits from family members and friends, which, together with the intensification of the work assignments, helps patients prepare for the final stage of gradual returning to daily life.

***Fourth phase—resocialization (non-specified, but at least 10 days)**—this is the time when the doctor sends patients outside the hospital, allowing them to stay home overnight for one–two days, and commute to work or school. As this is not a

[3]The application of occupational therapy within a mental hospital setting in Japan began in 1901 when Shūzō Kure, Professor of Psychiatry at Tokyo Imperial University, opened two sewing rooms in the female ward of Sugamo Hospital, Tokyo. There patients were allowed to sew pillow cases and hospital gowns for use at the hospital. Three years later a workroom was built and occupational therapy became an official activity in the hospital (Honda et al. 2009: 1047). It is very likely that Shōma Morita was influenced by Kure's pioneering initiative and introduced it as part of his own approach.

mere returning to their former lifestyle, the clients have to apply what they have learned through their own experience over the first three phases and use it to cope with the challenges of reintegration of their "new self" into the non-treatment world. "The responses of the patients show much more variety and complexity that in the previous stages. The theory of neurosis in the Morita school has not taken up the problem of character structure which underlies the symptom and has no hypothesis concerning it. The goal of treatment here is rather to bring about conditions under which the patient can develop his capacities to the utmost, keeping his native character as it has been" (Ikeda, as cited by Miura and Usa in Lebra and Lebra 1974: 418). In order to foster a smoother transition to daily life, many patients refer to their hospital diaries and/or regularly consult their doctors to find out coping strategies that will help them advance further on their path to recovery and self-integration.

The four-stage structure of Morita therapy, with total isolation and gradual reintegration as its key characteristics, "is designed to engage the client in Nature, which in turn, reveals how "self" mimics nature" (Fujita, as cited in LeVine 2017). As the Australian clinical psychologist and Morita therapy specialist Peg LeVine points out, "this sequence of moving from isolation to ecological engagement to social reintegration is like a sandwich. Essentially, one's relationship to self is one piece of bread, and one's relationship to other people is the other slice of bread—but one's relationship to the eco system is the core filling" (LeVine in Bordes 2011: 252). Considering this, a "therapeutic alliance between client, therapist and Nature (ecosystem) can occur" (LeVine and Ogawa 2014).

Needless to specify, the establishment of such a therapeutic alliance requires plenty of time—the entire treatment process usually spans a period of approximately 40 days. This period may differ in duration depending on each individual case and on the specificities of the treatment facility as well—for example, 90 to 120 days as suggested by one of Morita's disciples, Tomonori (alias Chijun) Suzuki (1970: 40). In most of the cases, aftercare practice in the form of outpatient consultations with the doctor, regular meetings of doctors and ex-patients, and the publication of journals are available to all clients who have undergone the intensive course of Morita therapy.

5.2 Eastern Wisdom in Practice—The *Arugamama* Principle

As previously mentioned, Shōma Morita did not "concoct" Morita therapy in an instant, but needed a trial-and-error period of about 20 years to develop and refine his approach. Morita's ideas emerged as a natural consequence to the concepts of his predecessors in the field of Japanese medical psychiatry. These included Genyū Imaizumi and his concept of the transfer of mental energies, strongly influenced by the traditional Chinese medicine; Enryō Inoue known to have written Japan's first book on psychotherapy, *Psychotherapy* (「心理療法」) (see footnote 2 in Chap. 1); Shūzō Kure and his pioneering work in the field of occupational therapy (see footnote 3); as well as Morita's contemporaries such as Teikichi Ishikawa and his seminal work *Nervous Breakdown and Its Treatment* (「神経衰弱及其療法」) (1912) influenced by the French psychologist Pierre Janet; and Jō Nakamura and his theory on neurotic temperament—*shinkeishitsu* (神経質)—as presented in his book *Shinkeishitsu and its Treatment* (1912) (Okamoto 2013; 2015: 76–79).

At the same time, Morita's ideas unfolded within the religious and cultural setting and lifestyle in Japan, all of which are especially influenced by Zen Buddhism (Suzuki 1977: 219). Even though the approach did not emerge from a religious practice or experience, as Naikan therapy did, certain similarities between Morita therapy and Zen draw attention (Kondo in Miki and Kuroki 1998: 31). There is no evidence that Morita was a devoted Buddhist, but still from his youth he was interested in Zen Buddhism and especially liked paradoxical statements, *kōan* (see footnote 2 in Sect. 10.1). He calligraphed many Zen proverbs and often guided his patients using Zen allegories. When accused of being unscientific, Morita responded in spite of his teeth that his approach was not grounded on Zen Buddhism and the similarities between the two were simply a coincidence (Okamoto 2010: 51). At the same time, he considered Buddha and Shinran the "seniors" of *shinkeishitsu* in the sense that they addressed the profound anguish of human existence (Okamoto 2010: 63). Additionally, Morita was strongly influenced by the Zen Buddhist priest and Sansei Hospital's founder, Dr. Genyū Usa, who was his disciple and collaborator in the systematization of the therapy (see Sect. 10.1). Morita also experienced the influence of the renowned Zen Buddhist philosopher Daisetz Teitarō Suzuki (Maruyama 1995: 154–155). Some Morita therapy specialists such as Tomonori (alias Chijun) Suzuki even draw parallels between this approach and the religious doctrine of Dōgen, founder of the Sōtō school of Zen Buddhism. Although it seems Morita was not well versed in Dōgen's teachings, Suzuki finds striking similarities between (i) their concepts of inner transformation attained through immersing onself in life as it is and (ii) a Zen Buddhist temple—in the case of Dōgen, the Eihei-ji—and the original Morita therapy clinic in terms of austerity of their physical environment and stringent daily schedule (Suzuki 1977: 253). On the other hand, Morita was influenced by the works of prominent European psychiatrists such as Emil Kraepelin and Otto Binswanger, and only later, over the course of his research, he realized that his approach was somewhat akin to Zen Buddhism in terms of the enlightment-like experience that it fosters, rather than the religious doctrine itself (Suzuki 1977: 214). Indeed, certain Zen Buddhist flavor is manifested in Morita therapy in the way the approach helps its clients to "pay attention to the quality of ordinary daily actions; stressing the value of service to others; not being primarily centered on feelings; valuing tranquility; not accepting a victim mentality; and putting the client in situations where the opportunity for experiential learning (*taiken*) will be maximized" (Brazier 1995: 110).

Considering all of the above reasons, it will be well justified to use Kora and Sato's definition of Morita therapy as "psychotherapy in the way of Zen" or "psychotherapy in the Zen mode of thought" (Kora and Sato 1958). In the next sections we discuss how this culturally determined "mode of thought" is applicable to psychotherapeutic setting.[4]

5.2.1 Shōma Morita's View on Human Nature

Among Shōma Morita's concepts, there are two which can be considered the main pillars of Morita therapy and which are directly related to Morita's firsthand personal experience (Usa and Kinoshita 1987: 4): first, this is the theory of the *hypochondriac predisposition* (ヒポコンドリー性基調説) and, second, that of the mechanism of *psychic interaction* (精神交互作用説). The hypochondriac predisposition refers to a specific semi-congenital semi-environmentally induced attitude, which makes the individual fear or feel anxious about their own physical and/or mental health without an evidence that something might be wrong—for example, Morita's episode of paroxysmal palpitation during his youth (ibid.).[5] This predisposition is underlied by a strong fear of death and of becoming sick—*shi-no-kyōfu* (死の恐怖), which in some individuals with especially perfectionist and intellectual streak may turn into pathological symptoms that prevent one from performing almost anything. In other words, "the degree to which this fear is present determines the degree of abnormality" (Morita 1928/1998: 101). One of Morita's direct and most prominent disciples—Takehisa Kora—who became his successor at the Jikei University School of Medicine, named this tendency "inadaptability" (Miura and Usa in Lebra and Lebra 1974: 410) to the present conditions of reality and an inability to leave hold of one's own mental constructs. Such inadaptability turns one's mind into a battleground where reality as it is and the mental constructs of what it should be fight with each other to bring forth a contradiction of thought—*shisō-no-mujun* (思想の矛盾); but "thoughts are somewhat like images reflected in a mirror. In themselves, they have no objective substance, no concrete reality" (Fujita 1986: 67–68). The mental antagonism thus induced makes one suffer; it can even lead "to the development of an obsession" (Fujita 1986: 65). By the same token, the attempt to supress artificially the way one feels or to rationalize it—for

[4]According to Okamoto, whether there are or not Zen Buddhist influences on Morita therapy is a fruitless discussion. Morita's personal interest could not be detached from the process of establishment of his approach, for which reason Morita therapy can indeed be considered "Zen therapy" (in private communication with Prof. Shigeyoshi Okamoto, Director of Kyoto Institute of Morita Therapy, January 2016). Psychiatrist Susumu Oda corroborates this statement suggesting that Morita therapy's first phase—the total bed rest phase—shares certain common aspects, for example elimination of distracting thoughts, with the Zen Buddhist practice of sitting meditation, *zazen* (坐禅) (Oda 1990: 112); and so does the Morita therapy specialist Kenji Kitanishi for whom the Buddhist thought, especially the Zen Buddhist one, is the therapy's "weapon of treatment" (Kitanishi 2016: 24).

[5]Some scholars such as psychiatrist Mitsuzō Shimoda "emphasized the element of environment and considered that one factor for its creation is overdiscipline or overprotection in infancy" (Miura and Usa in Lebra and Lebra 1974: 410).

example, "Death is nothing to fear" (Miura and Usa in Lebra and Lebra 1974: 414) —is also a state of *shisō-no-mujun*.

However, referring to his firsthand experience—the time of despair during his student years when he studied hard despite his poverty and sickness—Morita emphasized that such an attitude not only does not help in solving the problem, but it further entangles the individual in their own torments, creating a vicious circle of stronger and stronger subjective pathological sensations (Ohara and Ohara 1990: 190). This is what Morita called *psychic interaction*, i.e., the more attention one pays to a certain sensation, the stronger the sensation would become to an extent that it culminates in a fixation. For example, if someone with a hypochondriac predisposition experiences paroxysmal palpitation due to lack of sleep or physical exhaustion, they would become anxious that there might be something wrong with their heart. Anxiety, in turn, would generate more tension and make the heart palpitations faster and stronger, which would draw the individual's attention more and more to their condition, thus trapping them into a sensation-attention vicious circle (Okamoto 2013). This circle can be compared to drug addiction: the more drugs the user takes, the stronger the addiction becomes because their craving for the initial pleasant sensations intensifies; this is the basic mechanism that underlies all neurotic and obsessive behaviors as well (Hahakigi 2013: 177).

To clearly describe this vicious circle, Morita used a Zen Buddhist allegory, known as *keroketsu* (繋驢桔), which tells about a donkey tied with rope to a pole: the more the donkey tries to free itself by moving around the pole, the more the rope tightens until it prevents the poor animal from moving altogether. This allegory depicts very well the mentality of individuals with neurotic symptoms: the more one tries to escape from one's own fears and anxiety, the more intensive they become, to an extent that they bring one to their knees and make them totally incapable of doing anything. Even though tided to the pole, if it did not make pointless attempts to free itself, the donkey would at least be able to walk around and graze grass. Similarly, even if tied by the rope of their fears or anxiety, individuals with *shinkeishitsu* can keep performing various activities if only they can manage to endure being tied for a while, i.e., *to accept* the natural flow of their own emotions (Kitanishi 2007: 36).

In cases of patients with neurosis who embrace high ideals, perfectionism, and a proclivity to abstract thinking, it is excactly the preoccupation with their condition that aggravates further their symptoms. In Morita therapy, such a preoccupation is named *toraware* (とらわれ)—"to be biased toward; to be preoccupied with." For example, if someone is afraid that they might be having a heart attack, this fear is the fact of the matter for them (subjective truth) although medical examinations clearly indicate there is nothing abnormal (objective truth). The incapability of distinguishing the objective from the subjective is what Morita defines as the essence of all neurotic disorders: when attention is biased, its natural flow is blocked to cause cognitive rigidity, i.e., *toraware*. The individual pays too much attention to certain subjective thoughts or sensations, but remains unaware of their own preoccupation with them and therefore suffer, much too often both physically and mentally (Morita 1960: 238–240) (Fig. 5.1).

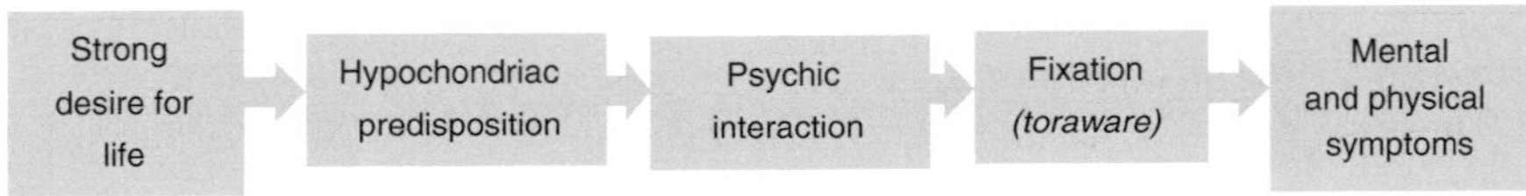

Fig. 5.1 *Toraware* and the development of neurotic symptoms (adapted from Morita 1960: 241)

As previously mentioned, this attitude is fuelled by fear of death and of becoming sick. However, such a fear is the one side of same coin, the other being the will to live and to preserve the self—*sei-no-yokubō* (生の欲望) (Watanabe 2003: 556). These two factors epitomize the very essence of human nature: the stronger the desire for life, the stronger the fear of death, and vice versa—those who do not want to live are not afraid of death. Consequently, "anxiety occurs when this desire to "preserve self" is exaggerated" (LeVine in Bordes 2011: 248), for which reason "the doctor should start by increasing the natural mental activity of the patient, enlarge the sphere of this activity and guide him to a free mental attitude" (Miura and Usa in Lebra and Lebra 1974: 415), i.e., not the patient's reasoning faculties are targeted, but their performance of concrete physical actions, which are supposed to result in a free mental attitude. As the renowned Japanese potter Kanjirō Kawai describes it, this is a state when one "thinks with hands and legs" (Hahakigi 2013: 142); when one rides on their will to live, which light up the destination of their life and help them stay alive (Hahakigi 2013: 135).

Through the *shinkeishitsu* concept thus developed, Shōma Morita in fact addressed fundamental issues of life and death in the broad sense of the word: life understood also as an endeavor to grow further, to learn and know more, and to self-actualize (Ohara and Ohara 1990: 56), and death understood as a blockage or negation of such an endeavor (Watanabe 2003: 556). Considering this, we can conclude that "Morita's theory has a positive, constructive content" (Fujita 1986: 179), represented by a fundamental trust in human nature: there is a drainless vital force that all humans share, "a strength to live as exhibited by children, who are engaged in activity all the time" (Fujita 1986: 19). The *sei-no-yokubō* concept is therefore representative for Shōma Morita's view on human nature: it spans to a vision of the individual as capable of attaining a higher plane of existence by immersing themselves into the flow of life and tasting it to the utmost even amidst illness and fear of approaching death—as Morita himself demonstrated through his personal experience.

5.2.2 *Toraware* and the Body–Mind Interconnectedness

"Although humans are prone to mental attachments, prolonged and intensified *toraware* is viewed as pathogenic" (Ishiyama 2003: 219). When it becomes such one, *toraware* rarely remains limited to the area of mental suffering alone, but it can also hamper certain physiological processes and the proper functioning of some organs.

Similarly to the majority of his contemporary medical doctors, Morita embraced the Eastern concept of body–mind unity: he never thought of mind and body as separate entities but likened them to an incense stick and fire—none of them alone can emanate the scent, but only their unity (Morita 1922: 369); the static aspect of this unity is the body, the dynamic one is the mind (Morita, as cited in Iwata 2012: 35). Over his clinical practice, Morita noticed that many of his patients with neurosis shared certain physical complaints, for example

- heaviness in the head as if there were lead inside; feeling of emptiness and sluggishness in the head
- face looks as if twisted; the individual often looks askance at other people
- stuffed nose; feelings of pressure on the nose bone
- when talking to other people, the individual stammers, blushes, or loses temper
- squeezing sensations in the chest; difficulty breathing
- paroxysmal palpitations; feeling low
- tachycardia and/or skipped heartbeats; feelings of imminent death
- stomachaches varying from dull to cramp-like pains; patients often keep their hand(s) on the abdominal area
- palpitations echo throughout the body, especially in the abdominal area, preventing the individual from laying down peacefully
- dull pains in the bladder; feeling the need to urinate becomes more frequent
- sensations of coldness and numbness in the limbs, etc. (Morita 1960: 242–243)

To these specific complaints, Morita added also more general ones such as insomnia, dizziness, and nausea (ibid.). When one or several of these symptoms are manifested, a patient with *shinkeshitsu* is very likely to seek professional help from somatic medicine specialists. During the course of the examination, however, the doctor may come across psychological symptoms like antropophobia or pathological fixation on one's body image, whereas physically the individual may be completely healthy; but addressing only the physical manifestation of an ailment would not be sufficient if the *neurotic fixation* behind it remains unidentified (Morita 1960: 51). Considering that any physiological disease has a psychological component, "psychological difficulties are often manifested in physical symptoms and complaints" (Ogawa 2007: 120). This is especially valid for individuals "with so-called personality disorders who adapt themselves poorly to circumstances and respond to the external world with extreme sensitivity or dullness" (Morita 1928/1998: 132).

The physiological complaints of the patients with *shinkeishitsu* could be compared to dream-like sensations or to illusions (Morita 1960: 243–244). These are activated under the force of *toraware*, but, as previously mentioned, the patient remains unaware that they themselves are the driving force behind this vicious circle. The process of development of unpleasant physical sensations Morita explained with the so-called internal projection—*naibu-tōsha* (内部投射): it is not the organ itself that suffers some physical dysfunction or abnormality, but the patient's anxiety is projected on it and creates certain (unpleasant) physical sensations in it (Morita 1960: 244–245). "According to Morita, assessment of a client's character requires a clinician's attention to the context of the client's concrete daily life and a careful history of the onset of symptoms; he advises therapisis to use both qualitative and quantative measures for evaluation" (LeVine in Morita 1928/1998: xxi). For this reason, even if specialized medical treatment is not applied, but only the individual's mental attitude and lifestyle is transformed, the symptoms are very likely to disappear naturally (Morita 1960: 51). Considering also Morita's view on body–mind unity, it is not a surprise that patients who have undergone Morita therapy got cured also from their insomnia, headaches, ringing in the ears, and even hemorrhoids (Iwata 2012: 34).

If an individual with *shinkeishitsu* visits a Morita therapy clinic, they would be surprised to realize that there is no immediate relief provided from the outside. Paradoxically, they would be left to experience their symptoms to the utmost and encounter their fears and anxiety the way they are. Through the total bed rest therapy, diary keeping, and garden work, the patient would be guided toward the understanding that, in fact, they fuel their own suffering and that the healing forces lie within them.

5.2.3 The Healing Forces Within

One of the distinctive features of Morita therapy is its general concept of healing, which spans beyond the fighting-off attitude that many Western therapeutic models adopt. As previously mentioned, for Morita the cure is paradoxically hidden in the very opposite attitude, i.e., not in rebelling against symptoms or attempting to get around them by devising all sorts of intellectual tricks, but in accepting them directly as they are. Morita emphasized the idea of healing as reeducation: neurotic symptoms are self-made constructs that results from narrow, inflexible, and inappropriate attitudes toward reality, or from too much conceptualization of reality. These attitudes can be transformed through training or learning of more *mindful* ways of living, i.e., ways that respond to reality as it is. Hence, Morita therapy clients are usually called *disciples*, whereas therapists are *teachers* who only provide key reference points on the way to such mindfulness. Morita therapists never put their clients into the passive position of mere recipients of healing from outside; rather, they teach their patients to assume a *passive attitude toward symptoms* and an *active attitude toward their own life and immediate duties*.

If we return to Morita's tough firsthand experience during his student years, we can see how important this experience was for the development of a whole therapeutic approach—so much so that some authors consider it the origin of Morita therapy (Iwata 2003: 29). A natural consequence of immersing himself in intensive study, Morita was not paying attention to the unpleasant feelings and sensations related to his diseases and also to his long-lived anger toward his father and his father's austere education. By so doing, i.e., studying hard while being anxious and afraid, he broke the vicious circle of psychic interaction between symptoms/feelings and attention, and "opened up" space for his *sei-no-yokubō* to manifest itself—a process which eventually resulted in getting cured and in heightening his grades.

Through this experience, Morita realized the paradox that remaining in the midst of our most intense emotions/symptoms and accepting them as they are give us the chance to broaden our self-knowledge: we realize that no matter how strong our fear or anxiety might be, there is always a vital force inside of us that helps us continue to create and make achievements in the world. This is a moment when, as Morita defined it, we "unlatch" ourselves and attain complete cure—*zenchi* (全治). The complete cure, however, is not related to some profound personality change or improved health condition, but to the awareness that one can do or achieve something one has not been able to perform before. It becomes possible not when the symptom disappears—for example, "If it were not for the disease, I would be able to do this or that"—but when our *toraware* toward it is gone (Morita 1960: 262). For this reason, *toraware* can be likened to a cork which hinders the manifestation of the vital force within us—once the cork is removed, i.e., not paid attention to, the vital force naturally starts gushing out.

It appears that Morita did not entertain much the concept of illness as "the necessary evil" nor did he try to analyze the role of the symptoms in the patient's life (Iwata 2003: 157–158): this is one of Morita therapy's key concepts and techniques called *fumon* (不問)—strategic inattention to the symptom used for preventing the psychic interaction in patients with *shinkeishitsu* to intensify further (Iwata 2012: 227) and for thus broadening out the patients' "visibility range", that is, from fixation on thier disease and their inner world to flexibility and *mindful* attention toward the external world. To this end, Morita therapy offers its clients a powerful tool that helps them in the tough process of attention shift, deconceptualization and, consequently, of releasing the healing forces within—this is the *observation* of the external world (from the second phase onward). The development of the patient's ability to observe occupies a special place in the Moritistic world where art, creation, and beauty are done their justice. As Usa and Kinoshita report, many of the cured Morita therapy clients use phrases such as "The world looks more beautiful now" or "It seems as if scales fell off from my eyes." These statements are not based on some visual experience that is then conceptualized and verbalized nor are they related to some aesthetical categorization. Rather, they refer to a breakthrough in consciousness prompted by the observation of phenomena in the purest mode of their existence; phenomena are observed without the mediation of one's judgment and intellectualization (Usa and Kinoshita 1995: 42–43), but through the observer's pure heart—*jun-na kokoro* (純な心).

This kind of observation in Morita therapy is indicative of a change in one's mental attitude, because "it is your mental attitude that determines whether you experience the projecting or the revealing power. The world is here in both modes. It is not that the world changes, it's your consciousness" (Campbell 1991: 252). Experiencing the world through the projecting power may involve judgement, conceptualization, and aestethic arrest, whereas the revealing power refers simply to "a marveling recognition of the radiant Form of forms that shines through all things" (Campbell 1991: 244). This specific process of observing with pure heart plays a key role in the Morita therapy practice and becomes the *sine qua non* of the successful treatment. Another aspect of this concept refers to one's ability to sympathize: a story tells that one day a dog entered the rabbit cage in the Morita clinic and ate the poor animal. The patient who looked after the rabbit said that the cage was not strong enough. "You don't need to say this," Morita reproached him. "Don't you have pity on the rabbit?," he asked. Morita used every situation to foster his patients' love and sympathy toward every living creature, i.e., to foster their *jun-na kokoro* (Okamoto 2010: 64). On the other hand, *jun-na kokoro* is neither a moral imperative to be imposed upon patients nor a criterion for positive mood that patients should pursue (Ichikawa 2008: 83). Rather, it is a state of mind in which the individual is true to their authentic nature (Morita, as cited in Ichikawa 2008: 82) or it is even a sense of belonging, of complete identification with the whole universe similar to that of a newborn infant to their mother as a fundamental human experience (Ushijima 2005: 56). Even though *jun-na kokoro* remains one of the most difficult to comprehend and least discussed among Shōma Morita's concepts (Iwata 2003: 167), it can be defined as the "tangible" aspect of Morita's therapeutic philosophy—the ability to accept one's own emotions the way they are (*aruga-mama*) and interact with the world from the perspective of one's own genuineness thus reconfirmed.

5.2.4 "The Willows are Green, the Flowers are Red" and the Art of Resilience

One of Morita's patients wrote the following: "The pure heart is a heart for which the willow is green, the flowers are red, the unpleasant things are unpleasant, and the pleasant things are pleasant. The pure heart can always find an on-the-spot solution, accepting any unfavourable circumstances the way they are. But if one pretends that the unpleasant is pleasant, one risks one's genuineness and soon entangles oneself in difficulties. The pure heart is the one that obeys reality" (as cited by Kitanishi in Kawahara et al. 2004: 84). Usually used as an expression for beautiful spring scenery, in Zen Buddhism the phrase "The willows are green, the flowers are red" (柳緑花紅) is a synonym for enlightenment, stressing the idea that the enlightened individual is the one who always approaches and experiences reality in a childlike way, without idealizations. The willows are green. The flowers are red. That is.[6]

The Japanese word that describes this attitude is *arugamama* (あるがまま). It consists of the words *aru* (ある)—the existential verb "to be", and *mama*(まま)—a derivative of *sono-mama* (そのまま), which means "as-is", "directly", "without any

[6]According to psychiatrist Tonao Sakurai, Shōma Morita often used this and other such phrases to describe the *arugamama* concept (Sakurai 1969:13).

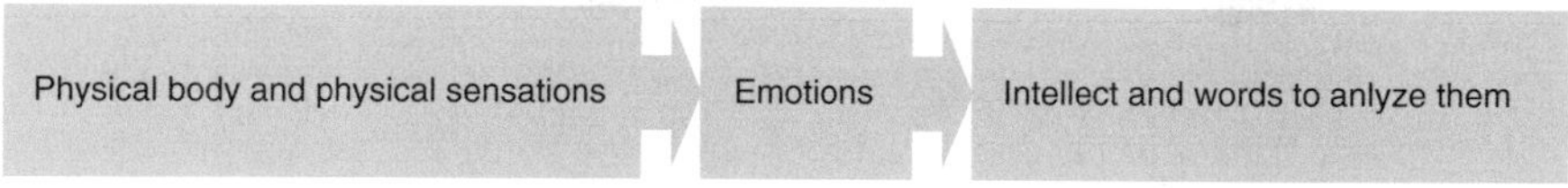
Physical body and physical sensations
Emotions
Intellect and words to anlyze them

Fig. 5.2 A common misconception often instilled by the Western psychotherapies is the application of the intellect for analyzing the phenomena of the inner world. This, however, may further exacerbate an already existing psychological problem (summarized from private communication with Sansei Hospital's director Dr. Shin'ichi Usa, May 2013)

change". That is, with *arugamama* we first say that, for example, there is a mountain, a tree, a house, etc., and then we confirm that it exists the way it is (Hahakigi 2013: 171). It is interesting to note, however, that among all living creatures, it is only humans who are difficult to exist "the way they are" because of their intellect, which they constantly direct to their bodies, their sensations, behavior, interpersonal relationships, etc. Moreover, humans often ruminate over, interpret, and judge what they have found out. That is how they themselves lay the foundations of the vicious circle that Morita called psychic interaction and turn themselves into the poor donkey of the Zen Buddhist allegory. However, as shown in Fig. 5.2, it is inappropriate to apply one's intellect to the world of self-consciousness in an attempt to put it in words and analyze it. Rather, the process should be halted at the "Emotions" phase, whereas the intellect should be directed to the external world and used only there. The inner world then should remain silent and free of theorization; it can only be observed and tasted—simply as when one looks at the starry sky in the night: probably with awe, but never with a desire to change the position of the stars and the planets.

How can one control and direct their intellect so as to attain the harmonious state of *arugamama*? As Kora points out, the *arugamama* concept has a paradoxical nature: it requires the client to give up their conceptualized images, and face directly their problem and the fear and anxiety it engenders. On the other hand, this is not a mere docile behavior or resignation, because while accepting their disease the way it is, the client has to release their innate vital force to perform a constructive behavior (Kora in Kawahara et al. 2004: 85). To this end, they have to adopt three key aspects of Morita therapy, which, according to Lebra, "are either derivatives or components of the *arugamama* principle" (Lebra 1976: 225).

The first aspect is *disregarding issues of one's past*, which puts Morita therapy in a sharp contrast to, for example, Freudian psychoanalysis and even, although in a different way, to Naikan therapy. In Morita therapy, ruminating over the past in search for the causes that have led the patient to their morbid condition is believed to further reinforce their conceptualized self-image and the vicious circle of psychic interaction. Needless to specify, one's past could not and should not be dissociated that easily from one's present and Morita therapy's aim is far from such superficial conceptualizations. What the approach stresses is the patients' respond to reality as it is here and now, and also the way they relates to their present emotions and sensations. The way the patients respond is indicative of attitudes and mental constructs the patients have entertained in their past, and their response to the present reality indicates which among these attitudes should be revised and eventually transformed (Kitanishi 2000: 49–50).

The second aspect of *arugamama* is related to the so-called *taitoku* principle (体得)—"to realize through bodily experience"; "to learn or master through one's own experience"; or "experiential embodied understanding" (Morita 1928/1998: 6). Again in contrast to the "talking" therapies of the West, Morita therapy does not rely on words, neither does it encourage the patient to ask questions or seek the therapist's interpretations—the only exchange of words remains limited to the brief evening examinations during the first phase and the diary entries as from the second phase onward. If the patient verbalizes their suffering, again they will fall prey to the vicious circle of their self-conceptualized images. Rather, the patient is encouraged to taste the immediate reality through their own experience, i.e., what it is like to be afraid or to have certain symptoms while performing a daily life activity. Such an attitude is likely to bring the patient much closer to life and, hence, to the healing forces within them more than any sort of theoretical interpretation of their condition.

Relying on one's personal experience is closely related to the *arugamama*'s third aspect known as *jijitsu* (事実)—"fact", "truth", "reality". This aspect "is supported by the conviction that facts, and facts alone, can be relied upon, and that whatever operates within the mind, whether intellectual or emotional, changes constantly, never stayes fixed even for a moment" (Kondo, as cited in Lebra 1976: 226). That is, thoughts are unreliable. Morita pointed out that thoughts usually run against real facts and likened them to "intellectual toys" (Morita, as cited in Iwata 2003: 68). He himself often wrote down in his diary minute details of his daily life, for example, how many sweets he ate on his way to work or how many times a month he had sexual intercourse with his wife. He did not feel the need to hide or be ashamed of the realities of his life (Iwata 2003: 66). This attitude speaks volumes not only about Morita's personality but, paradoxically, gives a specific metaphysical nuance to his therapeutic approach: neurosis could be considered a clear indicator that we do not "participate" completely in life; we are outside the "flow" of life. For life happens, as the Zen Buddhist saying goes, while we chop wood and carry water, that is, while we are consciously present in the reality of that very moment, here and now.

Thus the *arugamama* principle with its three aspects functions first as a countermeasure against cognitive rigidity and conceptualized self-image, which are considered the main cause of mental suffering. However, although *arugamama* is an important concept in Morita therapy, "therapists refrain from presenting such mental conditions to clients as goals to strive towards because of the danger of clients becoming preoccupied with such psychological states and losing sights of concrete tasks at hand" (Ishiyama 2003: 219), i.e., clients may walk again into the trap of *toraware*. Rather than a goal to strive toward, *arugamama* signifies a proactive attitude of "frank acceptance of facts as they are" (Fujita 1986: 331) and it differs this way "from submission and is clearly not resignation. It is an absolute acceptance" (ibid.).

For this reason, second, with the *arugamama* principle in practice Morita therapy turns its clients *from mere passive observers of the flow of life* (because of the symptoms) *to active and creative participants in it* (despite the symptoms). This is where we become aware of the metaphysical meaning of the observation process during the second phase of Morita therapy's in-hospital treatment—while observing the *arugamama* state of the natural world, it is likely that we return to where we have always belonged: to the natural universe, intrinsic part of which we all are; this state "endorses the union of the human self with the external, natural universe, in accordance with the Buddhist ideal.One should submit oneself to nature, be one with it, and face its reality" (Lebra 1976: 224). However, submitting oneself "does not mean a passive stance to give up one's efforts at problem solving, awaiting a miracle that would eliminate the emotional roadblock one is facing. Rather, one externalizes the psychological difficulty in a constructive manner" (Chen in Moodley and West 2005: 227). That is, simply by observing the organic growth and the natural state of being of plants and animals, the weather changes, and the succession of the seasons, etc., the client has the chance to experience their own self as part of the great circle of Life, where springing into existence and fading away harmoniously flow into each other; the client's symptoms and emotions, too, belong to this circle, they are part of the client's "internal Nature" (内的自然), which lies at the root of the will to live, *sei-no-yokubō* (Kitanishi 2016: 92-93).[7] Such an experience may consequently appease the client as they become aware that they *belong*—this is especially important for people with neurotic disorders whose mind often clings to the past or gets anxious about the unborn future, i.e., they *do not belong* to the here-and-now reality. However, we should emphasize that "seeking consolation in nature differs from seeing life reflected in nature" (Minami 1971: 62) and that Morita therapy strives toward the latter, thus making the concept of nature and naturalness one of its fundamentals together with that of *arugamama* (Ohtani 2002: 49).

The psychiatrist Hosei Hahakigi outlines three main benefits that observation of and contact with nature bestows on humans and which are extensively adoped in Morita therapy, namely (i) one shifts their attention to the world outside—in most of the cases it is the biased attention that brings forth a variety of symptoms; consequently, the working of nature fosters one's curiosity and imagination, (ii) one begins to notice the flow of time and the cycle of seasons: fresh green leaves turn

[7]An article by psychiatrist and writer Nariakira Moriyama (1991) suggests that in the establishment of his approach, Shōma Morita was influenced by the life of the renowned *haiku* poet Masaoka Shiki (1867–1902). Although Morita and Shiki have never met each other, essential Morita therapy concepts such as total bed rest, will to live, *arugamama*, and also the importance of keeping a diary are found in Shiki's lifestyle and in his literary theory. "An original view of nature was elaborated by Shiki, who did not cease to love the reality under his eyes even in a sick-bed. It is a frank and fresh look at nature. "Putting a sprig from a flowering plant at my bedside and sketching it naively, I feel myself gradually understanding the secret of nature ("A Six-foot Sickbed"). Eventually Shiki claimed the "theory of sketch-*haiku*", which considers *haiku* based on realism superior to imaginative haiku" (Moriyama 1991: 793). "It is eveident", Moriyama concludes, "that Shiki as well as Morita stand on the idea that only the fact is reality" (ibid.).

gold, then fall from the trees, then snow falls; yesterday's clear blue sky is now heavy with thick clouds and rain comes down in buckets—similarly to them, human emotions never stay the same, and (iii) one sees the grandeur and durability of Nature, compared to which their problems appear petty; consequently, a new vista opens up and the healing power of nature begins to work upon (Hahakigi 2013: 130–133).

Hence the explanation why many Morita therapy clients become interested and involved in creative activities such as painting, woodcarving, or photography, and find them soothing: it is a sign that the patient has already gained access to their innate vital force that has been hitherto blocked by *toraware* and this force fuels the true manifestation of their creativity. As the Japanese educational psychologist Takanori Akiyama aptly emphasizes, every human being possesses an innate creative force—no matter if it is expressed or is yet dormant, this force lies there as a possibility, turning every human behavior into an act of creativity (Akiyama 1962: 101). This act could be defined as a life-affirmative act *per se* since it urges the individual to shift their attention from themselves and their suffering to the world and help it change for the better; the individual can now tap their drainless creative energy and reconnect this way with the world in a more constructive way.

The deepened interest toward arts in the context of Morita therapy may also indicate that the client has mastered what we define here as the *art of resilience* that all natural phenomena "perform". For example, there is a time, albeit too short, for the cherry blossoms to bloom and then dramatically fade away. It is their "courage to be so exquisitely beautiful in the face of impermanence that fills the heart with sublime appreciation of the nature of reality" (Arai 2011: 194) and to which they owe their acclaimed beauty. But what if the cherry blossoms attempt to oppose the natural flow of the seasons and remain on the trees until mid-summer? Would there be anyone to appraise their tender beauty under the burning sunrays? It is hardly probable.

It therefore would not be exaggerated to state that the delicate sense for natural rhythms and seasonal changes typical for the Japanese *kokoro* has manifested itself in Morita therapy: "when one can see the beauty in impermanence, delusions dissolve, anger does not have a place to grip, and suffering loosens its tenacious talons" (Arai 2011: 197). While observing and experiencing firsthand the Nature's truth with the totality of their being, the client has the chance to experience their primordial affiliation with the world, seeing as if for the first time that, indeed, the "willows are green and the flowers are red." From the moment of that realization onward, the client will be a suffering stranger no more; they may still suffer, but they would never again allow their ailment to make them strangers to life and its beauty.

5.3 Morita Therapy and Metapsychiatry—A Brief Comparison

In the previous section we mentioned some contrasts between Morita therapy and psychoanalysis in terms of the way each of them considers the client's past. The contrast between the two approaches deepens further by the concept of consciousness against the unconscious: if psychoanalysis aims at bringing to light and rationalizing all unconscious content—hence the unconscious is given the negative connotation of an uncontrollable dark force—Morita therapy strives for quite the opposite. Harking back to the natural state of mind, which in Zen Buddhism is referred to as emptiness, *mu* (無), or primary consciousness, *honrai-no-ishiki* (本来の意識) (Morita 1960: 262), is equal to healing; hence the unconscious is given the positive connotation of a ubiquitous vital force.

Pointing out the contrasts between Morita therapy and psychoanalysis might be interesting enough, but considering the fact that the development of Morita therapy was influenced also by the Western psychology, we will search for similarities with Western approaches.[8] At first glance, such similarities can be found in the concept of the sensation-thought-emotion circle, on which the orthodox cognitive–behavioral therapy (CBT) is based. The so-called third wave CBT, which includes such approaches as mindfulness-based cognitive therapy, acceptance and commitment therapy, and dialectical behavior therapy, is focused on changing how people *relate* to thinking, not on changing thoughts themselves, and is this way quite similar to the Moritistic view (Okamoto 2012, 2015: 250).[9]

The German Neo-Freudian psychoanalyst Karen Horney's concept of basic anxiety, too, corresponds in a certain way to Morita's concept of the hypochondriac predisposition. However, "the anxiety called "basic" is not natural because the fear of death derives from the desire for existence" (Miura and Usa in Lebra and Lebra 1974: 410). Another similarity could also be found between Morita therapy and the Austrian psychiatrist Victor Frankl's Logotherapy: both of them advise the client not to flee their symptoms, but, on the contrary, to accept them and even to attempt to reinforce them—this is the so-called *paradoxical intention* in Logotherapy. Similarly to Morita therapy, Logotherapy is neither retrospective nor introspective. Rather, it focuses on the meaningful responses that the patient is able to give to reality—owing to them "the typical self-centeredness of the neurotic is broken up instead of being continually fostered and reinforced" (Frankl 2006: 98); the client is thus able to reach out beyond themselves for something other than themselves

[8]A brief comparison between psychoanalysis and Naikan therapy is presented in Sect. 6.3. For further details on the comparison between Morita therapy and psychoanalysis, see Takeo Doi's paper "Morita Therapy and Psychoanalysis" (1962) and "The Dialogue between Morita Therapy and Psychoanalysis" (2005) by Sadanobu Ushijima.

[9]An elaborated comparison between Morita therapy and contemporary Western modalities of treatment such as CBT is presented by the American Morita therapy specialist Brian Ogawa (2013: 49–65).

(Frankl 2000: 97). As Oda points out, Logotherapy is deeply rooted in the theistic existentialist philosophy and phenomenology (Oda 1992: 10), and as such it considers man an inseparable triunity of flesh, mind, and spirit. As a result, it puts any suffering in the context of the spiritual dimension, i.e., the purpose of transcendence. In Morita therapy, too, quite a similar mechanism is observed: the patient and all their suffering are entrusted to *arugamama* as a higher principle of existence where all life events find their ultimate meaning. It is therefore not a surprise that some authors call Logotherapy the Morita therapy's Western counterpart (ibid.).[10]

Considering all of these similarities, to draw parallels between Morita therapy and any of the above-mentioned approaches would then be well justified. However, we decided to turn attention to a relatively new but distinctive form of psychotherapy from the West, known as Metapsychiatry. The rationale behind this decision is that, as we elaborate below, the two approaches share striking similarities in their views on human nature and on the nature of disease. Although they differ in methodology and their therapeutic aspects cannot be readily transferred, a comparison between them would reconfirm that, indeed, Eastern and Western approaches to health and well-being are not developed entirely separately from each other.

Metapsychiatry was developed in the second half of the 1970s by the Hungarian-born American psychiatrist Thomas Hora. Similarly to Shōma Morita, Hora was influenced by both Western philosophical and existential psychological thought—that of Martin Heidegger and Ludwig Binswanger, to name a few—and Eastern traditions such as Zen Buddhism and Taoism. As a result, Metapsychiatry came to integrate principles from metaphysics, spirituality, and psychology, in an attempt, as its name suggests, to go beyond conventional psychiatry whose answers and solutions are oftentimes temporary.

Starting from this point, Morita therapy and Metapsychiatry share certain key points in their general understanding of human nature and the concept of healing:

- Both Morita therapy and Metapsychiatry tend to transcend past and future, i.e., *they operate beyond the temporal-spatial coordinate system of existence* into the dimension of timelessness or Truth—that is, *jijitsu* in Morita therapy and Reality or "omniactive Love-Intelligence" (Hora 1996: 60) in Metapsychiatry.[11] This tendency reveals their nature as ahistorical, acausal and non-teleological approaches for which therapy becomes possible and, hence, efficacious only to the extent it helps "the patient realize more and more what is real and what is not real" (Hora 1996: 82). The process of "cultivating" such a discerning inner eye is considered so important that it becomes tantamount to healing. In other words, mental health is defined as a state of consciousness characterized by the

[10]For further details on this comparison and also on the importance of the therapeutic setting, see Akio Kumano's paper "Morita Therapy and Frankl's Logotherapy—On the Meaning of Diversities in the Therapeutic Setting" (1969).

[11]For further details, see the author's concept of inner time in Morita therapy in Sect. 10.3 of the present book.

capacity "to see what is," i.e., "to cognize reality in its true essence" (Hora 1959: 242); to live in accordance with the *arugamama* principle, which is considered the ultimate remedy for neurosis in Morita therapy (Usa and Usa 1981: 6).

- We tend to ignore reality by allowing ourselves be distracted by our own *toraware* (in Morita therapy) or by the *five gates of hell* (in Metapsychiatry). Similarly to *toraware*, these "gates"—sensualism, emotionalism, intellectualism, materialism, and personalism—have specific pathogenicity responsible for a variety of disorders, from high blood pressure and skin problems to anxiety neurosis and interpersonal conflicts. It appears that Metapsychiatry confirms the Moritistic view that self-preoccupation and self-confirmatory fearfulness and/or ideations may often develop into a full-blown anxiety neurosis with all the broad array of mental, physical, and social pathology that accompanies it. For Metapsychiatry, too, the problem usually lies in the patient's misdirected interest, which Hora formulates as a *misdirected mode of being-in-the-world*. This mode often sprouts from certain values, "which may be socially and culturally acceptable but which are existentially invalid" (Hora 1996: 55).
- From this similarity another key concept common for Morita therapy and Metapsychiatry follows: *the concept of learning*. Let us remind that Shōma Morita himself called his approach reeducation. The patients of Metapsychiatry, too, "learn to perceive reality in a more valid fashion" (Hora 1996: 186). The ultimate goal of both therapeutic frameworks seems to be the attainment of such a state of mind that is not interested in what should be and what should not be, but one that adopts a well-developed faculty of discerning what *is*. Hence, both Morita therapy and Methapsychiatry's remedies are not operational, i.e., related to obeying some "should-ness", but *existential*, i.e., the rehabilitation process is essentially a *conversion process* launched through realization of the truth. It is not surprising that the Moritistic concept of complete cure—*zenchi*—is often likened to the Zen Buddhist enlightenment, *satori* (悟り). Indeed, there are many patients who describe their mental states after being cured through Morita therapy as if "Having just awakened from a dream," "The day has dawned," or "The world has changed" (Miura and Usa in Lebra and Lebra 1974: 421). It seems to be so because "the self-insight as devised in Morita therapy is not limited, in its deepest meaning, to an intellectual understanding" (ibid.), but it is a condition that can be called "intuitive vision" (ibid.), which dawns, gradually or in an instant, amidst the daily life.
- How is the above process of conversion achieved? In contrast to many psychotherapeutic approaches, especially the "talking" ones, Morita therapy and Metapsychiatry *are not analytical, but hermeneutic*, i.e., they require "a joint participation in a process of shedding light on the truth at hand" (Hora 1996: 140). This means that first, the therapist has to discern the patient's main mental preoccupation (*toraware* in Morita therapy), which "can reveal itself in the course of conversation, or just while being with someone for a while" (Hora 1996: 15). Second, the therapist needs to discover the set of invalid thoughts and ideas that underlie the clinical syndrome and reveal to the patient the erroneousness of their reasoning. When the patient is already aware of the

connection between their suffering and their erroneous mode of being-in-the-world, they naturally become interested in reorienting themselves in accord with mentality and principles of behavior that are more existentially valid, i.e., that match reality as it is. This therapeutic process, known as *hermeneutic elucidation* in Metapsychiatry—similar to certain extent to the rules of in-hospital treatment and diary guidance in Morita therapy—leads patients to the realization that whether they have a certain symptom or do not have it is not an essential issue. The essential issue is "to be a *beneficial presence in the world*" (Hora 1996: 16), which is the metapsychiatric definition of what a healthy person is. In other words, patient can be just as beneficial a person in the world with or without their symptoms and they always have the chance to respond to reality in a constructive way.

- Both approaches assume that the *therapeutic process is a phenomenon through which existence* reveals itself to the participants. Hence, the therapist's involvement in it becomes a way of life rather than a mere professional role. For Hora, "the existential psychotherapist does not "do" psychotherapy, *he lives it*. He meets his patient in the *openness* of an interhuman existential encounter" and "*openness (wakefulness) is the therapist's main qualification*" (Hora 1959: 239). In Morita therapy, Shōma Morita himself, as well as his disciples and adherents such as Genyū Usa, Shin'ichi Usa, Takehisa Kora, and Tomonori (alias Chijun) Suzuki, have dedicated almost all of their lives to their patients, creating an atmosphere of that *openness* and genuine humaneness which Metapsychiatry also talks about.[12] From this standpoint follows the next key characteristic that Morita therapy and Metapsychiatry share.
- *Pathology and sickness are referred to as one of the possible modes of being-in-the-world*, a way through which existence manifests itself. Since Metapsychiatry views all phenomena as modes of being-in-the-world, it assumes that if one is healthy, one has a certain mode of being-in-the-world. The same way, if one suffers from neurosis, psychosis, or schizophrenia, they express one of the possible modes of being-in-the-world. It is exactly this mode that needs to be addressed, not the personality. That is how Metapsychiatry leaves the framework of the conventional psychiatry, for it does not conform to the practice of labeling people with preconceived diagnostic categories and thus "obscuring the real issue" (Hora 1996: 217). Metapsychiatry seeks to "discern the specific and particular mode of being-in-the-world in every case" (ibid.). "In contrast to official diagnostic categories, which are based on symptomatology, the Metapsychiatric view is based on the meaning underlying the clinical picture. In other words, the mode-of-being-in-the-world is determined by an individual's belief systems, which may be conscious or unconscious" (Hora 1996: 218). Although Morita therapy makes use of conventional psychiatric categories, alike Methapsychiatry it does not rely on them for the ultimate treatment either.

---

[12]For further details about Dr. Shin'ichi Usa and the Sansei Hospital which he has been heading since 1957, see Sect. 10.1 and Appendix I.

- Since both approaches take the therapeutic process as a unique existential phenomenon, *they are "insured" against transference or countertransference reactions*, as well as against issues of resistance. This makes them offer a very clean work situation without interpersonal complications. "It is not the person of the therapist and not the person of the patient that is the issue, but Reality" (Hora 1996: 219). In such a situation, the patient's integrity is preserved. "He does not feel threatended. He is not in the position of being an object of tricky investigations and intrusions into his privacy" (Hora 1996: 186), but "participates as a total human being, not as Ego, Id, Superego" (Hora 1959: 240).
- Finally, "contrary to general belief, man cannot change himself. *Change happens to him*" (Hora 1959: 239). It is therefore naïve for us to claim or to aspire after curing a patient, because the act of curing is not a matter only of agency. For both Morita therapy and Metapsychiatry, "healing occurs through a meaningful shift in the world view of an individual brought about through genuine understanding of the structure of his existence, that is, through enlightenment" (ibid.). As Hora puts it poetically, "darkness cannot be removed from a room. It vanishes when light enters" (ibid.).

In conclusion, Morita therapy and Metapsychiatry share an atemporal, acausal, non-interpretative, hermeneutic, and holistic nature. Firmly anchored in the concept of Reality-as-it-is and attaching great significance to the patient's attitude toward it, they both agree that the designer of the client's problems is the client themelves. Hence neither of the two approaches "subscribe to the theology of suffering and affliction" (Hora 2013); rather, they proclaim redemption from the infinite sea of mental garbage—for which reason Morita therapy's total bed rest phase is of great importance—and development of sufficient understanding of reality and of oneself. Additionally, they both entertain the idea of healing as a mere "byproduct of the process of awakening and of giving up certain cherished ideas hitherto clung to" (Hora 1996: 149). They also admit that a symptom may signify the individual is not getting sicker, but healthier in the spiritual sense of the word as they are approaching Reality, the knowledge of which is healing itself; that a symptom is not something to be afraid of, but something to be completely accepted. For this reason, as Morita emphasizes, "a man of nervosity can not get well if treated as sick, but will soon get healthy when treated as if he were healthy" (Morita, as cited by Miura and Usa in Lebra and Lebra 1974: 419). In proclaiming disregard to the very object of healing—the symptom or disease—both approaches employ a paradox and thus take their clients beyond the health-sickness dichotomy to an opportunity for further personal growth.

5.4 Conclusion

Morita therapy is an "integrative therapy in that the psyche and soma are naturally rebalanced and the natural healing power is enhanced" (Nakamura, as cited in Ogawa 2007: 120). This clear-cut definition of Morita therapy reveals the approach's holistic attitude toward human nature and the concept of health and healing, all firmly grounded in the understanding that body and mind could not be intelligible outside of their unbreakable bond with Nature.[13] Therefore, unlike its counterparts approaches, Morita therapy "leaves" the closed-in therapeutic space of the consultation room and "goes" out to the open space of Nature, or, more properly, it considers Nature already a therapeutic space. "In this way", the Morita therapy specialist Akihisa Kondo points out, "Morita set a course that strays away from psychotherapies that ignore how Nature enhances our spontaneous and creative human nature" (Kondo, as cited in LeVine 2015). For this reason, it can be expected that "although Morita therapy has been one of the very few most recognizable non-Western therapeutic models in the realm of counseling and psychotherapy, its greater applicability and potential for therapeutic intervention remain to be explored" (Chen in Moodley and West 2005: 230).

Additionally, referring also to the Eastern concept of the cyclic nature of all phenomena—*enkan-ron* (円環論)—Morita therapy does not focuse on searching for the causes of suffering, but on the ways of restoring the lost balance between body and mind, on one hand, and between the individual and Nature on the other. To this end, and it makes the approach quite an astonishing one, Morita therapy manages with ease to combine contradictory elements such as total bed rest and isolation with strenuous work (occupational therapy) and communal engagement. Although "after the Second World War it was introduced into the United States by psychiatrists or clinical psychologists who has stayed in Japan as medical officers of the American army" (Miura and Usa in Lebra and Lebra 1974: 408) and it is today "incorporated into counseling and mental health activities" in North America and Australia (Nakamura in Hamanaka and Berrios 1999: 130), it was partly because of this eclecticism that Morita therapy has been running the gauntlet. Especially at the initial stage of its development, the approach was not taken seriously even in Japan "since at that time the influence of the German psychiatric line of thought was considerable and no great importance was attached to psychotherapy in general" (Miura and Usa in Lebra and Lebra 1974: 422), not to speak of "the psychogenic theory on nervous disease introduced by Morita, on which his psychotherapy was based and which was out of the main current of psychiatry for a long time" (Miura and Usa in Lebra and Lebra 1974: 408). The already mentioned psychiatrist Mitsuzō Shimoda (see footnote 5) was "one of the few who supported this therapy" (ibid.) at that time, stating that "it reached unfathomable heights in Oriental

[13]Kenji Kitanishi points out the Japanese concept of body-mind-nature monism (心身自然一元論), which lies at the root of the so-called realistic self (Kitanishi 2016: 96). For further details, see Kitanishi in Kawahara et al. (2004: 76) and Kitanishi (2008: 74; 2016: 95-96).

Medicine" (as cited in Kora 1995: 86). Criticism against Morita therapy, mainly from psychoanalytic viewpoint, included accusations "that it is not built up on a foundation scientific theory, and there is insufficient analysis of the complications occurring in the unconscious which may be the true cause for a neurosis" (Miura and Usa in Lebra and Lebra 1974: 423); that it does not "investigate the foundations and origins of neurotic behavior; sources of conflict material are not sought after and transference phenomena are not referred to". Finally, "suppression is the dominant theme in therapy; conformity the goal!" (ibid.).[14]

The structure of Morita therapy's in-hospital treatment may resemble, indeed, brainwashing with too much of obedience to authority and to stringent rules. Additionally, "if emphasis is put on the cultivation of "personality" (ibid.), the lack of analytical research may be a weak point of Morita therapy; but such arguments "show the difficulty in understanding the intrinsic value of Morita therapy" (ibid.), i.e., if there is no evident scientific validation to fit the existing intellectual schemes, then the method could not be therapeutically valid either. However, we should not forget that patients with neurosis and obsessive–compulsive disorders—the main target group of Morita therapy—more than anyone else need reference points to structure their lifestyle upon; more than anything else they need to be "grounded" in and "exposed" to reality, for which purpose stringent rules and obedience (to Nature) are used as tools through which patients have the chance to reflect on their limitations as human beings and thus reconsider their humility (Ohtani 2002: 53).

It can therefore be summarized that Morita therapy has contributed two very important concepts to the field of psychology, medical psychiatry, psychotherapy, and general healthcare practice. First, the uselessness of classifying the symptoms without a profound understanding of their origin—despite the multiplicity of symptoms manifested, diseases could be reduced to basic states of mind that all humans share, for example anxiety, fear, or anger. Second, the importance of transcending the health-disease dichotomy and using the very process of transcendence as a way to total healing. As Morita stated, true health comes at the moment when the indivudual transcends the pleasant–unpleasant sensation dichotomy (Morita 1960: 114); when the individual transforms the peculiar unnaturalness of their way of thinking and behavior as manifested in *toraware* to a natural one (Ohtani 2002: 49) and realize the intrinsic dynamism between the fear of death and the will to live to thus secure themselves flexible and more free way of life (Kitanishi 2012: 60). For this reason, causes and symptoms are not directly addressed in Morita therapy. In such a holistic context-based approach, "the goal is to improve functioning in real life, rather than self-centered mental health per se" (Matsuda, as cited in Ogawa 2007: 101), where functioning in real life means first of all a mindfull focus on the here-and-now reality. By so doing, regrets on past and fears of future diminish in a natural way (Kitanishi 1999: 106). Morita's "academic intentions were quite the opposite of the mainstream and represented the efforts of a

[14]As previously mentioned, Shōma Morita disputed heatedly with psychoanalyst Kiyoyasu Marui, Professor at Tohoku Imperial University.

pioneer spirit engaged in exploration of unknown territory" (Fujita 1986: 88). This unknown territory was not the mere elimination of symptoms—medical or behavioral therapy would sufficiently serve such a goal. Rather, Morita therapy aims to help its clients develop their human potential to the utmost regardless of their condition or external circumstances; to become like plum trees—one of the "three friends of winter" (see Chap. 2 and Appendix I)—that burst into blossoms of exquisite fragrance in the dead of winter. Paradoxically, the approach makes use of the same psychic energy that entangles its clients in neurotic symptoms, i.e., the excessive fear of death-will to live, suggesting that once this energy is redirected to constructive goals, elimination of symptoms would be a natural outcome (Okamoto 2015: 270). This perhaps explains as to why despite the anguish they experienced, many cured *shinkeishitsu* patients are grateful for having suffered—they had the chance to look at themselves more deeply and unbiasedly, and to gain insights about life as they never did before the onset of the symptoms (Ohtani 2012: 9-10).

Last, but not least, Morita therapy appears to be a deeply humane approach because it champions to the idea that being healthy or not should not have anything to do with our presence and "performance" as human beings in the world—it is only our mind that relates the two phenomena with each other. The onset of a symptom or disease is a mere *transient phenomenon*, which, like the seasons, will change and go away. It therefore should not prevent us from achieving our best and express *intransient aspects* of our existence such as creativity, freedom, and love. In so doing, Morita therapy teaches us that we are not sick individuals, but individuals with certain symptoms and these symptoms could not mar the core of our personality—unless we ourselves allow them to.

References

Akiyama, Takanori: Psychology of Creativity, Seishin Shobo, 1962 (in Japanese)
Arai, Paula: Bringing Zen Home: The Healing Heart of Japanese Women's Rituals, University of Hawaii Press, 2011
Bordes, Remi (ed.): Dire les Maux. Antropologie de la Parole dans les Médecines du Monde, L'Harmattan, 2011
Brazier, David: Zen Therapy, Constable and Company Limited, 1995
Campbell, Joseph: Reflections on the Art of Living—A Joseph Campbell Companion (ed. Diane K. Osbon), HarperPerennial, 1991
Doi, Takeo: Morita Therapy and Psychoanalysis, Psychologia—An International Journal of Psychology of the Orient, Vol.5 (3), Psychologia Society, 1962
Frankl, Viktor E.: Recollections—An Autobiography, Basic Books, 2000
Frankl, Viktor E.: Man's Search for Meaning, Beacon Press, 2006
Fujita, Chihiro: Morita Therapy—Psychotherapeutic System for Neurosis, Igaku-Shoin, 1986
Gielen, Uwe P., J. M. Fish, J. G. Draguns (ed.): Handbook of Culture, Therapy, and Healing, Routledge, 2004
Hahakigi, Hosei: The Will to Live—Fifteen Advices by Shōma Morita, Asahi Shimbun Publications, 2013 (in Japanese)

Hamanaka, Toshihiko, G.E. Berrios (ed.): Two Millenia of Psychiatry in East and West—Selected Papers from the International Symposium “History of Psychiatry on the Threshold to the 21st Century”, Gakuji Shoin, 1999

Honda, Yoshiharu, H. Suzuki, H. Honda, S. Irisawa: Pioneers in Occupational Therapy at Local Psychiatric Hospitals—Approaches at Shichiyama Hospital at the Beginning of the Taisho Era, Psychiatria et Neurologia Japonica, Vol. 111(9), Japanese Society of Psychiatry and Neurology, 2009 (in Japanese)

Hora, Thomas: Tao, Zen and Existential Psychotherapy, Psychologia—An International Journal of Psychology of the Orient, Vol.2 (2), Psychologia Society, 1959

Hora, Thomas: Beyond the Dream—Awakening to Reality, A Crossroad Book, 1996

Hora, Thomas: Who Designs Our Problems? (video), retrieved from www.pagl.org/main-landing/thomashoralanding/thomavideo/, PAGL Foundation, 2013

Ichikawa, Mitsuhiro: Outpatient Morita Therapy—An Intensive Short-Term Treatment of Neurosis, Hakuyosha Publishing, 2008 (in Japanese)

Ishiyama, Ishu: A Bending Willow Tree: A Japanese (Morita Therapy) Model of Human Nature and Client Change, Canadian Journal of Counselling, Vol. 37(3), Canadian Guidance and Counselling Association, 2003

Iwata, Mari: Morita Therapy as Described by Shōma Morita—Living with Pure Heart, Hakuyosha Publishing, 2003 (in Japanese)

Iwata, Mari: Flow and Movement in Morita Therapy—Morita Therapy’s New World, Hakuyosha Publishing, 2012 (in Japanese)

Kawahara, Ryuzo, S. Tatsumi, S. Yoshioka (ed.): Eastern Though and Psychotherapy—Encounters between Eastern and Western Spiritual Cultures, Nippon Hyoron Sha, 2004 (in Japanese)

Kitanishi, Kenji: Morita Therapy, Kodansha, 1999 (in Japanese)

Kitanishi, Kenji: Morita Therapy (in “Personal History and Psychotherapy”), Yasuda Life Welfare Foundation, 2000 (in Japanese)

Kitanishi, Kenji: A Book for Comprehending Morita Therapy Thoroughly, Kodansha, 2007 (in Japanese)

Kitanishi, Kenji: Past, Present and Future of Morita Therapy—Considering Its Origin, Jikei Medical Journal (Festschrift in Commemoration of the Morita Therapy Center’s Opening), 2008 (in Japanese)

Kitanishi, Kenji: Morita Therapy as an Outpatient Psychotherapy—Its Theory and Technique, Psychiatria et Neurologia Japonica, Vol.114 (1), Japanese Society of Psychiatry and Neurology, 2012 (in Japanese)

Kitanishi, Kenji: First-Time Morita Therapy, Kodansha, 2016 (in Japanese)

Kondo, Akihisa: On the Significance of Acceptance in Psychotherapy, Neurosis Research, Vol. 3 (1), Neurosis Research Meeting, 1962 (in Japanese)

Kora, Takehisa: How to Live Well: Secrets of Using Neurosis (transl. Gregory Peterson and David K. Reynolds), State University of New York Press, 1995

Kora, Takehisa, K. Sato: Morita Therapy—A Psychotherapy in the Way of Zen, Psychologia—An International Journal of Psychology in the Orient, Vol. 1(4), Psychologia Society, 1958

Kumano, Akio: Morita Therapy and Frankl’s Logotherapy—On the Meaning of Diversities in the Therapeutic Setting, Journal of Psychotherapy Vol.1(2), Japanese Psychotherapy Association, 1969 (in Japanese)

Lebra, Takie Sugiyama: Japanese Patterns of Behavior, University of Hawaii Press, 1976

Lebra, Takie Sugiyama, W.P. Lebra (ed.): Japanese Culture and Behavior: Selected Readings, University of Hawaii Press, 1974

LeVine, Peg: About the Classic Morita Therapy Institute, retrieved from http://www.aimoritatherapy.com/styled-4/index.html, Morita Therapy Foundation, 2015

LeVine, Peg: Brief Synopsis of Morita Therapy, retrieved from www.classicmoritatherapycentre.com, Classic Morita Therapy Centre, 2017

LeVine, Peg, B. Ogawa: Classic Morita Therapy Essentials with Special Consideration to Treating Anxiety and Trauma—Workshop for Professionals, retrieved from http://www.

aimoritatherapy.com/resources/Morita-Therapy-Workshop-Flyer-and-Outline-May-2014.pdf, Alachua County Department of Health Auditorium (Florida), 2014
Maruyama, Ouka: Shōma Morita's View on Human Nature, Naruto University of Education, 1995 (in Japanese)
Mezzich, Juan E., Y. Honda, M.C. Kastrup: Psychiatric Diagnosis: A World Perspective, Springer, 1994
Miki, Yoshihiko, K.Kuroki (co-ed.): Japanese Psychotherapies—Essence and Practice, Tokishobo, 1998 (in Japanese)
Minami, Hiroshi: Psychology of the Japanese People (transl. Albert R. Ikoma), University of Tokyo Press, 1971
Moodley, Roy, W. West (ed.): Integrating Traditional Healing Practices into Counseling and Psychotherapy—Multicultural Aspects of Counseling and Psychotherapy, Sage Publications, 2005
Morita, Shōma: Treatment of Neurosis and Neurasthenia, Japanese Society of Neurology, 1922 (in Japanese)
Morita, Shōma: Morita Therapy and the True Nature of Anxiety-Based Disorders (Shinkeishitsu) (transl. Akihisa Kondo and Peg LeVine), State University of New York Press, 1928/1998
Morita, Shōma: The True Nature and Therapy of Anxiety-Based Disorders (Shinkeishitsu), Hakuyosha Publishing, 1960 (in Japanese)
Morita, Shōma: Shōma Morita Collected Works (ed. Takehisa Kora), Vol. 1, Hakuyosha Publishing, 1974 (in Japanese)
Moriyama, Nariakira: Shōma Morita, Founder of Morita Therapy, and Haiku Poet Shiki: Origin of Morita Therapy, Psychiatry and Clinical Neurosciences, Vol. 45 (4), Japanese Society of Psychiatry and Neurology, 1991
Nakayama, Kazuhiko: Understanding Morita Therapy through Words—A Brand New Form of Morita Therapy, Hakuyosha Publishing, 2014 (in Japanese)
Nomura, Akichika: Critical Biography of Shōma Morita, Hakuyosha Publishing, 1974 (in Japanese)
Oda, Susumu: Writings on Eastern View on Madness, Shisakusha, 1990 (in Japanese)
Oda, Susumu: Religion and Psychotherapy—Parallels between Eastern and Western Cultures, Proceedings of the 15th Annual Congress of the Japan Naikan Association, Japan Naikan Association, 1992 (in Japanese)
Ogawa, Brian: A River to Live By—The 12 Life Principles of Morita Therapy, Xlibris/Random House, 2007
Ogawa, Brian: Desire for Life: The Practitioner's Introduction to Morita Therapy for the Treatment of Anxiety Disorders, Xlibris, 2013
Ohara, Kenshiro: Living in One's Skin—Soul Prescriptions by Morita Therapy, Kodansha, 1997 (in Japanese)
Ohara, Kenshiro, K. Ohara (ed.): Morita Therapy, Sekai Hoken Tsushinsha, 1990 (in Japanese)
Ohtani, Takayuki: The Concept of Nature in Morita Therapy, Annals of Humanities and Social Sciences, Vol. 2, Toyama University of International Studies, 2002 (in Japanese)
Ohtani, Takayuki: Cognitive Actions in Morita Therapy Considered from the Perspective of Language Use, Annals of Contemporary Sociology, Vol. 4, Toyama University of International Studies, 2012 (in Japanese)
Okamoto, Shigeyoshi: A Study on the "Zen-Morita Therapy"—History and Development of Sansei Hospital, Interdisciplinary Journal of Social Sciences, Vol. 3 (2), The Society for Interdisciplinary Studies of Social Sciences, 2010 (in Japanese)
Okamoto, Shigeyoshi: Wave after Wave—Buddhism, Morita Therapy, Cognitive-Behavioral Therapy and Meditation, retrieved from kyoto-morita.org, Kyoto Institute of Morita Therapy, 2012 (in Japanese)
Okamoto, Shigeyoshi: The Lost Thing of Morita Therapy—The Wisdom of the Hidden Sages of the Past, retrieved from kyoto-morita.org, Kyoto Institute of Morita Therapy, 2013 (in Japanese)

Okamoto, Shigeyoshi: The Forgotten Morita Therapy—Remembering Its History and Essence, Sogensha, 2015 (in Japanese)
Picard, Max: The World of Silence, Eighth Day Press, 2002
Powell, Margaret, M. Anesaki: Health Care in Japan, Routledge, 1990
Reynolds, David K.: The Quiet Therapies—Japanese Pathways to Personal Growth, University of Hawaii Press, 1980
Sakurai, Tonao: Random Thoughts on Morita Neurosis, Journal of Psychotherapy, Vol.1 (2), Japanese Psychotherapy Association, 1969 (in Japanese)
Storr, Anthony: Solitude—A Return to the Self, Free Press, 1988
Suzuki, Tomonori: Life Couching for Neurosis—The Reality of Morita-Type Personality, Seishin Shobo, 1970 (in Japanese)
Suzuki, Tomonori: Discussing Morita Therapy, Seishin Shobo, 1977 (in Japanese)
Usa, Genyū, S. Usa: Living in Truth, Sansei Hospital/Sansei-kai, 1981 (in Japanese)
Usa, Shin'ichi, Y. Kinoshita: The World as It Is—Buddhism and Morita Therapy, Toho Shuppan, 1987 (in Japanese)
Usa, Shin'ichi, Y. Kinoshita: The World as It Is(sequel)—Similarities between Religion and Morita Therapy, Toho Shuppan, 1995 (in Japanese)
Ushijima, Sadanobu: The Dialogue between Morita Therapy and Psychoanalysis—In Search of New Psychotherapeutic Horizons, Tokyo Jikei-kai Medical Journal, Vol. 120 (2), Jikei University School of Medicine, 2005 (in Japanese)
Watanabe, Naoki: The Cultural Background of Morita Therapy, Psychiatria et Neurologia Japonica, Vol. 105 (5), Japanese Society of Psychiatry and Neurology, 2003 (in Japanese)

Chapter 6
Naikan Therapy—*Memento Mori*

It is not the end of the physical body that should worry us.
Rather, our concern should be to live while we are alive.
Elisabeth Kübler-Ross

After Morita therapy, Naikan is the next representative Japanese psychotherapeutic approach from a chronological point of view. As it was already shown in Table 4.1 (Sect. 4.2), Naikan evolved amidst the turbulent postwar years of the 1950s and early 1960s and, in contrast to Morita therapy and Dohsa-hou, its foundation was laid not by an academic scholar but by a Buddhist priest, Rev. Ishin Yoshimoto (1916–1988). As such, it is not related to "any professional psychotherapeutic form, Eastern or Western" (Murase in Lebra and Lebra 1974: 388).

In the next sections, we trace back the roots of Naikan and shed more light upon its relation to religion. We do this in order to prepare the ground for an in-depth reflection on the method's therapeutic potential and its applicability to a wide spectrum of both mental and physical conditions.

6.1 Tracing Back the Roots of Naikan Therapy

Considering Yoshimoto's statement that Naikan is devoid of religious elements (Yoshimoto 1965/1989: 189; Miyazaki 1992: 6), it is not difficult to turn a blind eye to the fact that the method originated from its founder's firsthand religious experience. This experience, according to the founder's own words at the time, defied description (Yoshimoto 1965/2007: 99). On the other hand, such an experience was not peculiar to Yoshimoto's life story alone, but has been common for numerous spiritual seekers from different cultures since the dawn of human history. Moreover, Yoshimoto himself used to say that "It is not me who founded the Naikan method. Shinran and Buddha founded it. What I do is just advertising it." (Yoshimoto 1977: 1; 1983: 44).

V. Chervenkova, *Japanese Psychotherapies*,
DOI 10.1007/978-981-10-3126-7_6

6.1.1 *Jōdo Shinshū* and the Kamakura Zeitgeist

The term *naikan* (内観) was probably first used by the influential Japanese Zen Buddhist monk Hakuin Ekaku (1686–1768) in his work *Yasen-Kanna* (夜船閑話) —*Quiet Conversations on an Evening Boat* (1757)—referring to a method for self-discovery, which involve diaphragmatic breathing (Okumura et al. 1972: introduction; Kawahara 1996: 101). However, the Naikan method "advertised" by Ishin Yoshimoto is of a different origin.[1] We suggest its roots could be traced back far beyond the Edo period when Hakuin Ekaku lived to the time of the Kamakura shogunate (1185–1333)—a time when "with the sudden collapse of the Kyoto court and the onset of the feudal era, among the swift and bewildering changes that ensued was a sweeping redirection of the religious life in Japan" (Bary 1964: 185). This redirection marked the climax of a long period of penetration of the Buddha's dictum that life is suffering to all strata of Japanese society. It mirrored Japan's gradual shift "from the archaic to the historic type of religion, that is, from an affirmative world view to a world rejecting religious view" (Andrews 1977: 253).

After the country's Golden Age of Heian (794–1185) when literature, the fine arts, and high court life flourished, the Kamakura shogunate faced two attempts for Mongolian invasions—in 1274 and 1281—and bloody civil wars. These historical events likely helped the Buddhist conviction that this world is one of sorrow and delusion to capture the imagination of the entire populace. Over the dark medieval times of disunity and violence, the deepening pessimism among people gave an impetus to the search for "a radical salvation, thus propelling Japan into one of the most interesting periods in her religious history" (ibid.) and marking "a revolution in the development of Buddhism" (Dobbins 2002: 1) itself. "New forms of religiosity—specifically, Pure Land, Zen, and Nichiren Buddhism—rose to prominence and eventually spread throughout the nation. The simplified devotions and practices that they advocated offered an appealing alternative to the strenuous and complex systems of discipline that dominated Japanese Buddhism up to that time. So profound was the impact of those teachings and so dramatic was their departure from the past that Japanese scholars have come to describe them as New Buddhism, *shin-bukkyō* (新仏教), in contrast to the earlier eight schools of Old Buddhism, *kyū-bukkyō* (旧仏教)" (ibid.). The schools of Kamakura Buddhism thus established "ultimately became the largest and strongest religious organizations in Japan" (ibid.). The most evident and significant feature of this New Buddhism was that "it wast not preserved as a mere heirloom of the *ancien régime*, but elbowed its way out among the people and made itself at home in the households of humble folk" (Bary 1964: 185).

The Buddhist religion of the new age was not one of mystic ceremonies but a religion of simple piety and spiritual exercise. "Dogma gave way to personal

[1]For further references on Hakuin's Naikan practice, and the Naikan method introduced by Ishin Yoshimoto and Zen Buddhism, see Sato (1972: 169; Sato in Takemoto 1984: 168–172), Muramatsu (1991: 23–31), Igarashi (1991: 192–193), and Kurita (2001: 112–130).

experience, ritual and sacerdotalism—to piety and intuition, and this new type of religion exerted its influence beyond class limits" (Anesaki 1963: 168). Moreover, in contrast to the priests of Old Buddhism "who conducted the salvation of the emperor and nobility, and prayed for the protection of the nation, the priests of Kamakura New Buddhism put their efforts on the salvation of the general population" (Matsuo 2007: 53). That is how Buddhism "went down" among the masses and the balance of political power shifted away from the court toward the warrior class. With such a thorough transformation, new spiritual and aesthetic values also bloomed to play a key role in the formation of the entire Kamakura zeitgeist. These, we suggest, relate to the philosophical background of Naikan therapy and therefore they need a brief introduction in the context of the present book.

According to Addiss et al., the most enduring among the Kamakura values are the following hard-to-translate Japanese words (Addiss et al. 2006: 83–96):

- *Mujōkan* (無常観·無常感)[2]—sense of impermanence and mortality—considered one of the most important and influential values of the Japanese spiritual history (Kamei 1969: 6) and also the main culturally formative worldview of the Kamakura period (Nishio, as cited in Kusanagi 1973: 25), *mujōkan* refers to the insight that impermanence is the essence of life, and birth and death are therefore equally intrinsic to it (ibid.). Such an insight may function as an evaluative criterion that helps one discern between finite and infinite, relative and absolute (Kusanagi 1973: 27), and thus be more mindful of the limited time one is given on earth because, as the Buddhist doctrine suggests, it is very difficult to be born as human (人身受け難し—lit. "to adopt a human body") (Kamei 1969: 15). *Mujōkan* is further related to the Buddhist concept of sin, which considers sin being the result of one's earthly desires (Kamei 1969: 26); but earthly desires, too, are impermanent. In its aesthetic aspects, *mujōkan* relates to the next ideal of the Kamakura period—that of *aware*.
- *Aware* (哀れ)—the transient nature of all things; the poignancy of things. "Among Japanese aesthetic terms, *aware,*" also *mono-no-aware* (物の哀れ), "is a special case" (Richie 2007: 51). Having its origins in the preceding peaceful era of Heian when it "was akin to an interjection like "ah" or "oh" (Richie 2007: 52), in the medieval times *aware* came to represent mainly a sudden consciousness of the sad, even tragic nature of one's life and of the world itself, corresponding to the ancient Roman poet Virgil's *lacrimae rerum*, "the pity of things" (Morris, as cited in Richie 2007: 55). Especially "in the conflicting realities of the middle ages, it evolved to meet the needs of those looking for

[2]The second combination of characters appeared later to describe "the beauty of impermanence," *mujō-bikan*(無常美感) (Kamei 1969: 6). As Addiss et al. suggest, the awareness of life's impermanence, and of one's own finitude as both aesthetic and spiritual values produce "in a sensitive person the possibility of a sense for beauty" (Addiss et al. 2006: 85). The aesthetics of impermanence is depicted in masterpieces of the medieval Japanese literature such as *An Account of My Hut* by Kamo no Chōmei and *Essays in Idleness* by Yoshida Kenkō. Both authors renounced the world and became representatives of the so-called recluse literature (Hiekata 2009: 19).

salvation in the next world" (Yamakuse 2011: 185). *Aware* could be further defined as "emotional shorthand, instantly leading from the perception of beauty to a melancholy consciousness of the transience of human life" (Stanley-Baker 1984: 83); hence its relation to *mujōkan*.

- *Inton/Tonsei* (隠遁•遁世)—retreat, seclusion, withdrawal. "The ideal of retreat formed an essential component of the social and spiritual attitudes of the time" (Adiss et al. 2006: 90) of Kamakura period. Although, strictly speaking, no unified term was used in the Japanese language at that time to capture these convictions and beliefs, it remained a key concept, incorporating a preference of the past over the present. Undoubtedly, in the long aftermath of natural disasters, political conflicts, and devastating civil wars, "the present was often sensed as dreary, if not dangerous; only the past held one particular kind of beauty, that of nostalgia for something that could never come again" (Addiss et al. 2006: 92) (see footnote 2). One more perspective, whose historical background we will not discuss here, suggests that this ideal was also related to monks who distanced themselves from the official monasticism—*kansō* (官僧)—and engaged assiduously in Buddhist practices in isolated places. In spite of the fact that becoming a monk was originally identical to renouncement, the tendency for leaving the *kansō* ranks indicated that the latter had became yet another secular world. *Inton/tonsei* therefore has the meaning also of "re-renouncing the world as a kind of second retreat" (Matsuo 2007: 62).
- *Yūgen* (幽玄)—etherealness and subtleness, "a sublime, mysterious, veiled and profound beauty that points beyond itself" (Pilgrim 1981: 32)—probably the highest ideal for elegance, refinement, and sophistication in many Japanese arts and "a primary term in early Buddhist-influenced aesthetics" (ibid.), *yūgen* is said to have its origin in the aesthetic consciousness of the Heian aristocrats, especially in the concept of *aware*, but it delves even deeper (Fujiwara, as cited in Tanaka 2013: 49). As the combination of the characters for "dim" and "dark, profound" suggests, it comes to mean "something too deep either to comprehend or even to see" (Richie 2007: 54). *Yūgen* might also be understood as "unknowability," "mystery," and "beyond intellectual capacity," but not "utter darkness" (Suzuki 1988: 56). Another interpretation suggested by the American Japanologist William LaFleur links *yūgen* to the ineffable mystery of life "concerning the interdependency of all things" (Richie 2007: 54), the awareness of which may evoke awe to an extent akin to religious experience. *Yūgen* further connotes the aesthetics of tranquility born out of Japan's mild climate and beautiful nature for all four seasons (Hiekata 2009: 26); the aesthetics of silence, which in the Japanese arts is conveyed by Nature to the human heart (Hiekata 2009: 37–38); and even the aesthetics of death because *yūgen* lures the individual to heavenly worlds and evoke readiness to part with this life (Morigami 2015: 75–76).

These core values determined the Kamakura people's mentality and the ethical and aesthetical codes shared in that turbulent times. Needless to say, these values did not sprout in an instant—they emerged among the nobility of the late Heian period—but it was during the Kamakura period that they were "accommodated" within the spirituality of the new epoch. At the same time, the wind of change brought to the Kamakura's religious stage something essentially new: "Kamakura Buddhism had no starting point other than the direct, unflinching confrontation of life's negative dimension. The founders of the new faith grasped life in its gravely negative aspects" (Ienaga, as cited in Machida 1999: 134). What is more, against this background the founders of the new faith erected the figure of humanity in its ineradicable sinfulness. That sinfulness "called for an entirely new solution—one that can only come from *outside* oneself, i.e., from Other Power—*tariki* (他力), the Transcendent" (Keel 1995: 36), in an opposition to the self-power—*jiriki* (自力).

Among the avant-garde of the New Buddhism schools such as the Pure Land, Zen and Nichiren, it was the Pure Land school that exclusively dealt with the idea of transcendence and afterlife, and gave prominence to pietistic faith. That is how it gained popularity also as the Other-power (*tariki*) school. As such, it stood in sharp contrast with the other Buddhist doctrines of that time, especially Zen, which advocated rigorous spiritual training focused on self-discipline through *jiriki*.

Used even now in daily conversations, *tariki* and *jiriki* are among the key concepts of the Japanese religious thought, but their interpretation spans far beyond the subject of the present work. We only briefly discuss the concept of *tariki* as "the mother of *jiriki*" (Itsuki 2014: 19) considering that *tariki* is interconnected with the rest of the Kamakura's spiritual values and also that it likely provides clue to the philosophical basis on which seven centuries later Naikan therapy would develop.

6.1.2 The Three Pillars of *Jōdo Shinshū*: *Tariki*, *Muga*, and *Zange*

One of the main branches of Buddhism and also one of the strongest religious schools that have been tremendously popular for centuries throughout Asia is the Mahāyāna Buddhism (sanskr. महायान—"Great Vehicle"). Having its origins in India in the 1st century BC, the spirit of the Mahāyāna devotion spread to many Asian countries and captured the hearts of their peoples with its tenet for universal salvation through the worship of Buddha Amida (sanskr. अमिताभ Amitābha—Buddha of Infinite Light; jp. 阿弥陀如来—Amida Nyorai): sincere faith and faith alone can foster the Buddha nature that lies dormant in every sentient being so that everyone can become Buddha. In Japan, among other Buddhist schools this devotion "is most vitally and thoroughly embodied in Pure Land Buddhism" (Kaneko 1965: 54). The spread of the Pure Land doctrine in medieval Japan "represented a striking change in outlook for the Japanese people, and in the process of establishing itself, the doctrine too underwent profound changes" (Bary 1964: 186).

This change was probably related to one important feature of the Kamakura period: "the appearance of strong personalities both among the warriors and the religious leaders" (Anesaki 1963: 168) who "tried to reevaluate Buddhism through their own painful life experiences" (Matsunami 2004: 10). Among them there was a person considered one of the key philosophical and innovative minds of Japan. That was Shinran (1173–1263)—a former Tendai school monk and once a staunch disciple of Hōnen, the founder of the Pure Land school—*Jōdo Shū* (浄土宗). Shinran founded the *Jōdo Shinshū* (浄土真宗), a branch of the Pure Land Buddhism also known as Shin Buddhism or True Pure Land Buddhism.

Often called "the Japanese Martin Luther," Shinran shared the German theologian's concept that our salvation does not depend on our good works, religious practice, charity, or any of the acts we perform in our lives, but "is bestowed upon us when we have unwavering faith in God" (Itsuki 2001: 206). Similarly to Luther's religious revolution—the Protestant Reformation—which was to shake Europe in the 16th century, Shinran encouraged people by proclaiming that being reborn in the Pure Land—*jōdo* (浄土)—the ultimate goal for any believer, was attainable not through elaborate rituals or complicated philosophy, but through a simple practice that anyone could do anywhere: the invocation of Buddha, *nembutsu* (念仏).[3] What mattered to Shinran was no longer Amida Buddha as the object of worship, but simply the chanting "Namu Amida Butsu." "Amida Buddha as expedient device can be objectified, but not "Namu Amida Butsu", for it is the actual interrelationship between subject and object; it is not a static "thing," but a dynamic "event" (Matsunami 2004: 12). Only through reciting *nembutsu*, Shinran preached, we are able to cross the current of suffering at any moment because the foundation of salvation has already been laid millions of eons ago by Buddha Amida in his Primal Vow—*hongan* (本願)—to take everyone to his Realm of Bliss.[4] Furthermore, life of *nembutsu* is designed as a way that leads straight to that realm where enlightened beings live without knowing the sufferings of earthly existence. "There is no good that surpasses the *nembutsu*," Shinran said (as cited in Kaneko 1965: 62–63).

As previously mentioned, the tenets for universal salvation thrived on the Asiatic continent long before landing to Japan, where they assumed the form of *Jōdo Shū* and *Jōdo Shinshū*. These religious formations, together with Zen Buddhism, can be considered the true manifestation of the Japanese spirituality (Suzuki 1972: 20). That they emerged within a Buddhist context was a matter of historical chance, which only gave impetus to the development of true religious consciousness among the Japanese

---

[3]In the context of *Jōdo Shinshū*, *nembutsu* means repeating the phrase *Namu Amida Butsu* (南無阿弥陀仏—"Homage to Infinite Light" or "Adoration to the Buddha of Infinite Life and Light"). According to the Japanese religious scholar Masaharu Anesaki, "this formula had been in use before the time of Hōnen, especially among votaries of Buddha Amida, but it was Hōnen who exhorted an exclusive use of the formula as an expression of devotion and gratitude" (Anesaki 1963: 173).

[4]According to Daisetz Teitarō Suzuki, "it was not until the thirteenth century in Japan, during the Kamakura period, that the Primal Vow appeared on the center stage of history. The ripening of karmic circumstances, including sociopolitical disintegration, civil strifes and natural calamities, awareness of human finitude, and growing religiosity, prepared the way for the Primal Vow to become fully manifest and to play a crucial and lasting role in the life of the people" (Suzuki 1998: 14).

society (Suzuki 1972: 21) or even, as the Japanese Buddhist philosopher Kodo Matsunami suggests, helped the Japanese "religious consciousness to attain its highest peak" (Matsunami 2004: 14).

What is then innovative and essentially Japanese about the Pure Land thought, especially about the one introduced by Shinran through *Jōdo Shinshū*? According to the interpretation of the Japanese historian Saburo Ienaga, the innovative element in the Pure Land Buddhism was Shinran's concept of *akunin-shōki* (悪人正機), "which teaches that the evil person is the true object (the "right spiritual capacity") for whom Amida's compassionate Vow is meant" (Keel 1995: 5). This keynote Shinran expressed in *Tanni-shō* (歎異抄—*Notes Lamenting Differences*)—a collection of dialogues with Shinran compiled posthumously by his disciple Yuien: "Even a good person can be born in the Pure Land, how much more likely it for an evil person!" (*Tanni-shō* 1962: 22). By so preaching, Shinran turned upside down one of the fundamental teachings of his master Hōnen, "Even a bad man will be received in Buddha's Land, how much more a good man" (as cited in Anesaki 1963: 182). Although some followers of Shinran would interpret this provocative statement as a "negation of morality" (Anesaki 1963: 183), the *akunin-shōki* concept "does not mean that it is all right to do evil" (Itsuki 2001: 95). What Shinran actually did was to carry the idea of the faith in Buddha's grace (*tariki*) to extreme conclusions, thus marking "a very significant step in the history of Buddhism" (Anesaki 1963: 182)[5].

Through this step Shinran clearly pointed ways for deepening our relationship with the Other-power—the divine grace that invisibly, yet constantly supports our lives. However, *tariki* is not something that would easily reveal itself to us. In order to become aware of its ever-present blessing power, we need to clean up our hearts so as to open space for it inside of us—a conscious act that requires profound self-reflection and eventually repentance. This process, which, as we will elaborate later in the text, underlies the entire Naikanistic philosophy, relates in a way to the common Buddhist concept of selflessness, *muga* (無我).[6] Although *Jōdo Shinshū* rarely uses this concept in its doctrine, through the idea of total reliance upon *tariki*

[5]It is worth mentioning that in its teaching about faith, *Jōdo Shinshū* is astonishingly akin to Christianity. The *Jōdo* teaching "is believed by some scholars to have been influenced by Nestorian Christianity in China before it crossed over to Japan, and its modern priests readily borrow Christian ideas and terminology" (Shepherd 1937: 77). In this sense, Shinran's striking teaching can be interpreted as similar to the Biblical parable of the prodigal son in the Gospel of Luke (Luke 15: 11–32), or to the simile of the one of a hundred sheep gone astray (Anesaki 1963: 183). One more parallel could be drawn again with the Gospel of Luke, according to which Lord Jesus Christ says to the criminal crucified next to Him, "Truly I tell you, today you will be with me in Paradise" (Luke 23: 43).

[6]By no-self we should not understand a lack of self or of self-conscious faculties, but rather the direction of these faculties as we discussed in the chapter on Morita therapy. Psychiatrist Takao Oda suggests that *muga* means giving up one's Ego-driven intentions (Oda 2005: 47), whereas the American philosopher David Edward Shaner interprets it from "the more axiomatic consideration that nothing in this cosmos has been empirically verified as existing" (Shaner in Callicott and Ames 1989: 170). As "all things in this world are impermanent," the Buddhist tradition suggests, the self too "is subject to constant change" (ibid.). *Muga* can also be defined as a state of utmost peacefulness that a human being can attain (Kanamitsu 1985: 224).

"it nevertheless advocates the abandonment of all self-effort (*jiriki*) in reliance of the power of the Buddha (*tariki*)" (Dobbins 2002: 158). In other words, faith includes "by definition the abnegation of self" (ibid.). "Other schools of Buddhism," the American philosopher James C. Dobbins further suggests, "often link no-self to clerical life. The strenuous practices and discipline required of monks and nuns are intended to liberate them from any sense of an independent, controlling, and enduring self. Release from that view is part and parcel of Buddhism's ultimate realization. Shin, needless to say, stands in contrast to those traditions, for it rejects the clerical ideal. Instead, it advances a pragmatic selflessness largely in the form of gratitude. The person of faith looks on Amida, the world, and other people with a self-abandoning sense of indebtedness and thankfulness" (ibid.).

Faith as total trust requires a shift of our mental attitude that relies on self-power to an attitude of reliance on the Other-power, and this is a process of conversion, not a mere cognitive act. "Change of heart," says Shinran, "means to overturn and discard the mind of self-power" (as cited in Keel 1995: 91). The sincere faith in Buddha's grace is therefore the *summum bonum* for the *Jōdo Shinshū* believers, but, as previously mentioned, becoming aware of it is not an easy task. While walking the difficult path of faith, which is a path of self-abnegation, it is easy for one to say, "I cannot perceive the grace of Buddha. Is it not invisible?" To this Shinran would reply, "It is our grave sins that prevent us from noticing it. Although we are not aware, we are already embraced by the grace of Amitabha" (Nakamura 2002: 81). Even though "Shinran did not particularly support much the myth of the original sin, expressed by Christian thinkers" (Nakamura 2002: 85), he speculated upon sinfulness. In his interpretation, "sin hath no substance in itself, and is but the shadow of our illusion; and soul (lit. the essence of mind) is pure in itself" (ibid.), i.e., sin is devoid of own reality and the individual can therefore be liberated. That is why, when Shinran used the terms *zaiaku* (罪悪) or *zaishō* (罪障)—the Japanese equivalent for "sin"; the innate impulse "to justify ourselves and to blame others" (Kaneko 1965: 62), and *zange* (懺悔)—"confession," "penitence," he referred primarily to a "keener self-reflection of the innate sin of man" (Nakamura 2002: 80).

That is how *tariki* (the divine grace that is bestowed upon us), *muga* (selflessness) and *zange* (penitence) became the indispensable elements thanks to which the follower could "see their delusions by virtue of compassionate light; they have been touched by reality" (Suzuki 1998: 13). This insight-like process might be fostered by an act of profound self-reflection, but it appears that in some cases even such an act is not sufficient. As the Korean Buddhist philosopher Hee-Sung Keel suggests, "the realization of the true state of one's being is by no means a "natural" knowledge based upon self-reflection or self-consciousness. For a person thoroughly corrupt and false, such self-reflection can only be a mere camouflage and cannot reveal truth at all. Thus, for Shinran, the true realization of one's sinfulness paradoxically suggests that one is already under the light of grace and truth. To know the truth about oneself is already to be grasped by truth" (Keel 1995: 90).

Considering all of the above, in the next section we trace how the three pillars of *Jōdo Shinshū* as manifested together with the acme of self-exploration—an austere practice known as *mishirabe*—have likely influenced the development of Naikan therapy.

6.1.3 *Mishirabe*—The Courage to Face Death

Many articles and books about Naikan therapy, English-language ones included, open with statements that can be summarized as "Naikan was developed from an austere self-exploration practice known as *mishirabe,* which was typical for one of the branches of *Jōdo Shinshū*." However, it is difficult to find even a Japanese-language source that specifies which branch exactly was it, thus leaving *mishirabe*'s origin and evolvement veiled in mystery. Some authors claim that *mishirabe* was handed down to the generations after Shinran's death as a spiritual training in the *Kibe* school (木辺派)[7] of *Jōdo Shinshū* (Sato 1993: 234), while others state that it was applied over the centuries "for training newly admitted monks of the *Jōdo Shinshū* sect" (Shinfuku and Kitanishi in Verhagen et al. 2010: 185) or define it as a "very demanding Shin Buddhist self-cultivation practice" that was "aimed at achieving enlightenment" (Ozawa de-Silva 2006: 7). Nonetheless, the uncertainty about *mishirabe*'s origin remains.

Why do we need to explore the origin of Naikan therapy? We suggest that tracing back the roots of any psychotherapy and discussing it in the context of the socioreligious background it has evolved from is very important for two main reasons: first, it provides a deeper knowledge about the method and its therapeutic structure and functions; second, it gives us the opportunity to broaden our understanding of mental health in history and eventually to apply this understanding to modern realities. Moreover, in the context of Naikan such an exploration becomes a major task because, as previously mentioned, in contrast to Morita therapy and Dohsa-hou, Naikan was founded by a Buddhist priest. This makes the approach first of all a cultural phenomenon and then psychotherapy, i.e., a culturally embedded psychotherapy. For this reason, we consider it essential to elucidate as fas as possible the origin of *mishirabe*.

Mishirabe (身調べ—"to explore oneself"; "self-examination")[8] was a practice for reflecting on one's past in an attempt to realize which deeds prevailed—the good ones, referred in Japanese to as "seeds of virtue" (善の種子), or the bad ones,

[7]*Kibe* is one of the subsects of the orthodox *Jōdo Shinshū.* Its doctrine is the closest one to that of the *Hongan-ji-ha*(本願寺派) dominant sect.

[8]The first character of this word—*mi*(身)—is used nowadays to signify "body" or, in certain cases, "self," but in the past it referred to the entire human being as an indestructible triunity of body, mind, and spirit (Miki and Kuroki 1998: 284; Maeshiro 2010); also, a state of complete oneness. *Shirabe*, in turn, derives from the verb *shiraberu*(調べる), which means "to explore," "to examine," hence the whole word comes to mean "to explore oneself thoroughly." For further details on the concept of *mi*, see Hiroshi Ichikawa's work *The Structure of Mi* (1993) and Noboru Yasuda's work *The Body of the Japanese* (2014).

also called "seeds of evil" (悪の種子) (Iwaoka 2002: 25–26). The practice was based on the premise that we usually tend to justify and overrate ourselves and blame others, and considered self-justification being the epitome of sin and ignorance. The purpose of *mishirabe* is then to help one become aware of all the care and support one has received since birth till the present day from all people, all living creatures and even Nature, and, while trying to compare one's past deeds to this support, to realize one's self-centeredness and sinfulness. In *Jōdo Shinshū* terms, this process could be interpreted as the obedient acceptance of Buddha Amida's Primal Vow. Then, realizing that even such a sinful person could be saved by Amida's grace, one's heart starts to overflow with gratitude and joy. In other words, the deeper the *zange* is, the deeper the joy (ibid.).

What we know today about *mishirabe*, its history, and its dissemination is organically related to the life story of the founder of the Naikan method, Rev. Ishin Yoshimoto. However, this knowledge seems to remain somewhat confined to his direct disciples and Naikan professionals only. We suggest that exploring Ishin Yoshimoto's life story is essential for tracing back the roots of Naikan therapy, for which reason in the next section we outline it, referring to his autobiography *Naikan Method—Forty Years of History* (1965/1989), his book about Naikan *An Invitation to Naikan* (1983), the commemorative books *Devoted to Naikan—The Life of Ishin Yoshimoto* (1989) and *Shinobigusa—A Life Dedicated to Naikan* (1989), as well as to other reliable sources by authors who knew him in person, be they Naikan professionals or not.

6.1.3.1 Ishin Yoshimoto—A Life of Spiritual Seeking

Inobu (alias Ishin) Yoshimoto (吉本伊信) was born on May 25, 1916 in Yamato-kōriyama, a small town in northern Nara prefecture. He was the third boy out of five children of Ihachi Yoshimoto, a trader of fertilizers, and Yukie Yoshimoto. Both his parents were *Jōdo Shinshū* followers.

Ishin grew up as a "gentle and compassionate boy. One day when he was a first grader, he cried all the night upon hearing his teacher had to leave school because of a sickness" (Maeshiro 2009: 34). Additionally to his mild character, he was also known for being "a top student and was always appointed as a head of class" (ibid.); he was often applauded for performing *rakugo*—the traditional Japanese comic storytelling.

Several days before Ishin's eighth birthday, on May 12, 1924, his four-year-old sister Chieko passed away after a short illness. His mother's grief over her only daughter defied description. She remembered how every time Chieko heard the bell of the nearby temple chiming, she used to beg her mother to take her to the temple. However, being preoccupied with household duties, Yukie never managed to fulfill her little girl's simple wish. Crying desolately while holding Chieko's picture and reproaching herself for having been a bad mother, Yukie swore that from now on she would start visiting the temple duly. This tragic loss prompted Ishin's mother to become an even more fervent *Jōdo Shinshū* follower.

Over the years after Chieko's death, Ishin used to accompany his mother to the temple and spend his evenings trying to read with her the scriptures, for example Shinran's *Kyōgyō Shinshō* (教行信証)—*True Teaching, Practice, and Realization of the Pure Land Way*. To the surprise of everyone, he even memorized and recited parts of the text. These childhood experiences played a key role in his life, fostering his religious devotion and the further development of his personality. When Ishin graduated from school at the age of 17, he followed his mother's advice to study Buddhist scriptures seriously at the nearby temple. He also continued polishing his calligraphy skills and aspired to become a calligrapher after his works were awarded exhibition prizes several times; he got his wish fulfilled in 1935 when he opened a calligraphy schoolroom and started teaching.

In the summer of 1936 his elder brother's father-in-law—Zenkichi Morikawa—went to the town of Fuse in Osaka prefecture, where he practiced *mishirabe* at a religious group called *Taikan-an* (諦観庵).[9] Soon after that he visited the Yoshimotos and explained his experience in detail to the young man's father. At that time, Ishin was writing calligraphy in the adjacent room and heard everything the relative said, not knowing that his eavesdropping would establish his relationship with *Taikan-an* and eventually change the course of his life.

Having tasted the fruit of the knowledge, Ishin started eagerly seeking ways to learn more about *mishirabe* and eventually to try it himself. Before going directly to *Taikan-an*, he decided to pay a visit to Gijō Fukumoto—a distant relative in Nara prefecture whom he knew to be familiar with *mishirabe*—and asked him what *Taikan-an* and the practice were like. To this Fukumoto replied with several questions such as "Have you ever experienced the state of *muga*?" (Iwaoka 2002: 27). Yoshimoto did not manage to answer and they both realized that no matter how many scriptures Yoshimoto knew, he lacked authentic religious experience. This realization spurred even further Yoshimoto's motivation to go to the *Taikan-an* group and try *mishirabe*. However, Fukumoto did no consider Yoshimoto ready yet and decided to introduce him to his *mishirabe* senior Yasuyuki Inoue. After several days spent in religious discussions that were aimed at testing the novice's faith and determination, it was decided that Yoshimoto would undergo *mishirabe* at the Morikawas. Before starting, his wallet was taken as a symbolic act of breaking up all mundane bonds. The same was done with his belt and kimono sash so that to prevent him from committing suicide. It was October 1936.

At that time, the first one or two days before the practice started, the candidate had to undergo *chi-gatame* (地固め)—"to level the ground," "to pave the way to"—a preparation, which included familiarizing the candidate with *mishirabe*'s austerity—namely, no eating, drinking and sleeping allowed during the entire time of the practice—and listening to sermons and participating in religious discussions. During the practice the person would be seated in the corner of the room enclosed by a folding screen and deprived of sustenance and sleep. On every 2 hours the

---

[9]*Taikan* (諦観) is a Buddhist term, which means "to see the truth clearly"; *an* (庵) means "hermitage; humble cottage".

practitioner had to answer the interviewer's questions such as "Is your mind concentrated (on Buddha Amida)?" (一心一向—*isshin-ikkō*, Nagayama and Shimizu 2006: 11–12), "If you die right now, where your spirit will go?,"[10] and "Which of the deeds you have done until now prevail—those that would send you to Heaven or those that would send you to Hell?" (Yoshimoto 1983: 21). The practitioner also had to follow instructions such as "Forget yourself, your possessions and even your life, and reflect sincerely on your past" (ibid.). Apparently, a *mishirabe* practitioner was the one who was not afraid of death and had the courage to readily part with their life in the name of spiritual transformation (Usami 1988: 97).

The followers of the *Taikan-an* religious group used special words to refer to the practice's three stages: a yet inexperienced person was called *jōsan* (定散)—a one who has learned Buddhism, but lacked authentic religious experience and their mind was yet attached to mundane matters. The one who was undergoing *mishirabe* was called *byōnin* (病人), which literally means "sick person, patient." According to Yoshimoto's wife Kinuko Yoshimoto, *byōnin* was the one who worried about what was going to happen with them in the afterworld (Takemoto 1989: 32). That was evidently so because the practitioner had to answer the above-mentioned question many times during the practice, that is, to "weigh" their good deeds and their bad deeds in order to understand if they would go to Heaven or to Hell. The third term was *shinjitsu* (真実), which means "truth, reality." This was an individual who has attained enlightenment through *mishirabe* and was therefore allowed to interview *byōnin*-s. In the *Jōdo Shinshū* terminology, *shinjitsu* is also used to describe faith as a "consequence of Amida's transferring his "true and real" (眞実—*shinjitsu*)mind to our minds, which are full of falsity and selfish desires" (Keel 1995: 83). The *mishirabe* interviewers, in turn, were called *kaigo-nin*(悔悟人), which means "those who listen to one's repentance over past mistakes" (Nagayama and Shimizu 2006: 11).

At last, Yoshimoto started his first *mishirabe* experience completely aware of the harsh conditions. His first interviewer was Teishin Komatani, the *Teikan-an*'s head, who later became his master. When Komatani asked him what he came for, Yoshimoto replied bloated with pride, "To attain the state of *muga*" (Iwaoka 2002: 30). However, while trying to concentrate, he could not help but listen to the conversations in the adjacent room: "He is far off from exploring himself thoroughly," master Komatani said to the others (ibid.). Yoshimoto also knew that somewhere in the house there was Kinuko Morikawa, Zenkichi Morikawa's granddaughter and Yoshimoto's first love. Under these circumstances, the young man gave up the practice rather soon.

Although Yoshimoto felt ashamed of his half-hearted efforts, he soon regained his strong determination and asked for *mishirabe* once again—this time at the *Taikan-an* group in the town of Fuse. At the beginning the practice went well, but around the fourth day he felt very weak and realized that he could not bear to go on without food and sleep anymore. At that time, Riu Morikawa—an experienced *mishirabe*

---

[10]The word "spirit"—*tamashii*(魂)—is emphasized by Yoshimoto himself (1983: 21) and later by the Naikan specialists Masami Kusunoki (in Kawahara 1998: 5) and Masahiro Nagashima (2004: 44).

practitioner who later became his mother-in-law and his paragon of thorough self-reflection—was sitting nearby and encouraged him to continue; but Yoshimoto devised a plan and on the sixth day he started pretending he was insane. His mentors at *Taikan-an* took pity on him, gave him food and allowed him to sleep. That is how Yoshimoto's second attempt also ended in failure.

On top of that, his *mishirabe* senior Yasuyuki Inoue withered him by saying that he would never be saved by Amida's grace; but should he nevertheless wish to try *mishirabe* again, Inoue adviced him, he would better go deep in the forest and spend there five days in complete silence (Iwaoka 2002: 40). Yoshimoto did not wait a second: in the cold January of 1937 he headed for Yatayama, a low mountain near Yamato-kōriyama, where he knew a narrow cave. There—all alone amidst the cave bats—he started his third attempt for *mishirabe*, which appeared to be even more difficult without the help of an interviewer. On the morning of the fourth day, Yoshimoto realized how life threatening his endeavors were and he left. Outside the cave he came across his relatives who were looking desperately for him in the forest; some of them already considered him gone insane. The third time, too, was a fiasco. Then the next month Yoshimoto concocted a lie to his father and started planning his fourth attempt. His father, a Pure Land Buddhist who harbored doubts about *mishirabe*, soon became aware of his son's intentions and confined him to his home. Nevertheless, Ishin's zeal for practicing *mishirabe* was growing even stronger; also, falling in love with Kinuko Morikawa, who had already attained enlightenment through *mishirabe*, the young man "repeatedly asked himself the same question, "What should I do to be respected by her?" (Maeshiro 2009: 35). He loved her very much and wanted to marry her, so he was eager to follow the same path that she did. Later on, when they got married, he often heard her reciting in her sleep "Namu Amida…Namu Amida" (Iwaoka 2002: 49) (see footnote 3).

In May 1937 Yoshimoto married his beloved Kinuko, who was only 17 years old at that time, and in September of the same year, after gaining permission from Yoshimoto's father, the young couple went to work in Osaka. A few weeks later, at the house of a *mishirabe*-experienced relative of Kinuko in Nara prefecture, Yoshimoto started his fourth *mishirabe* with the strong determination that this time he would not leave the place even if it would cost him his life. "Kinuko is pregnant, so please take care of her if I die," he asked his parents-in-law prior to his departure to Nara (Iwaoka 2002: 53). Among the ineterviewers, there were Gijō Fukumoto and Teishin Komatani again. "Consider this a place for thorough *zange* through *mishirabe*, the same as that under the Boddhi Tree where Buddha attained enlightenment 2,600 years ago. Be careful not to profane it!," Fukumoto warned him. To this Yoshimoto replied, "Even if I am going to die, I will not move from here!" (Yoshimoto 1965/2007: 96). As the hours and the days passed, Yoshimoto explored his sins more and more diligently, but he admitted to the interviewers that he did not feel them deep in his heart. "If you die right now, where will you go?," they asked. "I will go to Hell," Yoshimoto replied. "This is not the same as to go out to enjoy the cherry blossoms," the interviewers despaired of his superficial self-exploration—so much so that on the fourth day of the practice they were about to give up. "That's it!," master Komatani said curtly, ready to walk off the folding screen; but Yoshimoto threw himself upon Komatani's knees, agonizing in fear of death and in the pain of his own sins. Then he fainted. "And then suddenly I awoke and felt extremely happy —so happy that I began to roll on the floor, cry out of joy and laugh from the bottom of my heart, impossible to cease. I felt as if I was saved after having run around the crater of an active volcano. Just a few minutes ago I was hardly able to walk on my own, but in the moment of enlightenment I felt as if I was walking above the clouds. In that moment I swore I would turn myself inside out to spread this sheer happiness throughout the world" (as summarized from Yoshimoto 1965/2007: 98–100; 1983: 37). It was 8 o'clock in the evening, November 12, 1937, the same day of the month and the same hour his little sister Chieko had passed away before 13 years.

This crucial personal experience sparked the development of one of Japan's representative psychotherapeutic approaches. However, we could never have Naikan therapy as we know it today if it had not been for two of Yoshimoto's predecessors: Taikan Nishimoto, the founder of the *Taikan-an* religious group, and Yoshimoto's mentor Teishin Komatani. Let us see who they were.

6.1.3.2 The *Taikan-an* Religious Group

The *Taikan-an* religious group was founded by Taikan Nishimoto (西本諦観),who was born in 1849 in Ehime prefecture on the island of Shikoku. During his teenage years he became a monk at Nishi-Hongan-ji, the main *Jōdo Shinshū* temple in Kyoto, where he eventually climbed up the ladder to become a priest famous for his eloquent preaching (Iwaoka 2002: 182). One day, while preaching in a temple in Tokyo's Asakusa, he heard an old man saying, "In the past, monks used to sacrifice their life and possessions to seek the truth; nowadays they sell the truth to provide for themselves." Nishimoto was struck. He immediately left the temple and set off on a journey in search of a spiritual mentor (Yoshimoto 1985: 103).

The road led Nishimoto to Nose in Ishikawa prefecture, where he met master Chiekō (智慧光). A person of great wisdom and erudition, Chiekō, too, had been a monk in Nishi-Hongan-ji (Kusunoki in Kawahara 1998: 2), but later in his life he had been tried in court over disseminating heterodoxy (Yoshimoto 1965/2007: 58). It was under his guidance that Nishimoto practiced *mishirabe* and attained *temmei-kaigo* (転迷開悟—"turn the illusions down and attain enlightenment")—the enlightenment he had pursued for so long. [11]

---

[11]According to Kusunoki, it was Taikan Nishimoto's enlightenment under the guidance of master Chiekō that made *mishirabe* popular for the first time, but the practice's very origin nevertheless remains unknown (see footnote 13). However, it is probably related with the history of *Jōdo Shinshū* (Kusunoki in Kawahara 1998: 1–2), especially judging by the fact that master Chiekō lived in Nose, which is located in the region of Hokuriku often called the "Pure Land sect kingdom" (Itsuki 2001: 117). Additionally, founder Yoshimoto defined *mishirabe* as a spiritual practice maintained by a special branch of *Jōdo Shinshū* and this practice served as a basis for the development of Naikan (Yoshimoto 1983: 21). However, Yoshimoto had in mind not *Kibe* or any other of the official *Jōdo Shinshū* branches, but exactly the *Taikan-an* religious group (in private communication with Mieko Hariki, head of Osaka Naikan Training Center and direct disciple of Ishin Yoshimoto from 1973 until Yoshimoto's death in 1988, October 2012). It is very

Then Nishimoto decided to go back to Nishi-Hongan-ji in Kyoto. There he served for some time the 21st chief priest of the temple—the Reverend Myōnyo (明如上人)—but he eventually left because of doctrinal differences. He moved to Osaka where he started the life of layman, but he continued preaching among people, guided them in practicing *mishirabe*, and eventually founded the *Taikan-an* as a group devoted to this religious practice. After Nishimoto passed away in 1912, his wife became the group's leader, while Nishimoto's favorite disciple—Teishin Komatani (駒谷諦信)—became her right hand (Iwaoka 2002: 184–185). After Nishimoto's wife passed away, the group was headed by Komatani. Under Komatani's guidance Ishin Yoshimoto started his spiritual journey that was to lead him to the establishment of the Naikan method.

As for Komatani, his disciple Yoshimoto did not tell much about his life story. He was probably born in Kobe and had a wife and children. However, it remains unclear where and when he met master Nishimoto and at what age he started practicing *mishirabe*. In contrast to Nishimoto, Komatani devoted less time to traveling and preaching, and concentrated on his own self-exploration. It is said that the years after attaining enlightenment he spent in weeping away his deep sinfulness. Komatani passed away from machine-gun fire at the age of 65 or 66 during the July 1945 air-raids over Osaka (Iwaoka 2002: 186–187).

It could be summarized that together with Yoshimoto's mother and wife, Komatani played a significant role in Yosimoto's life, hence in the development of Naikan. Yoshimoto himself even stated that master Komatani was the originator of the Naikan method (Yoshimoto 1983: 55).

6.1.4 From *Mishirabe* to Naikan Therapy

After the enlightening experience through *mishirabe*, Yoshimoto became the right hand of his master Komatani, who sent him to various places to interview people practicing the method. In the meantime, Yoshimoto's father found out about his son's activities and called him back home to help in running the family business. In February 1938 the young couple—Ishin and Kinuko—went to Yoshimoto's native town of Yamato-kōriyama; a month later their first child, a daughter, was born. In 1941 Kinuko gave birth to a son and in 1942—to another one, but both children passed away shortly after their first year of age. In the meantime, Ishin headed Morikawa Sangyō, a leather

(Footnote 11 continued)

likely that Yoshimoto preferred not to name this religious group since officially he was a *Kibe* monk and when in 1955 he registered his temple in Yamato-kōriyama—*Naikan-ji*(内観寺)—he listed it as a branch temple of this sect (Maeshiro in Miki and Maeshiro 2006: 201). Yoshimoto was aware that mishirabe "was seen as a "pagan activity" by many other Shin Buddhists" (Ozawa-de Silva 2006: 7) for whom the sincere *nembutsu* was the only path to salvation. Probably because of this, no particular relationship between *Taikan-an* group and the *Kibe* branch can be found out (Maeshiro in Miki and Maeshiro 2006: 201).

wholesaler in Yamato-kōriyama established by his parents-in-law—the Morikawas—in order to provide for his family and also to fund the dissemination of Naikan.[12]

At that time, some of Yoshimoto's relatives, including his mother and brother, underwent *mishirabe*. It made the number of *shinjitsu* people within the *Taikan-an* increase and this tendency reinforced the already existing cleavage between hard-liners and soft-liners, with each of the group obeying its own rules. Yoshimoto and his mentor Komatani belonged to the hard-liners for whom the *mishirabe* interviewer was considered a truth-seeker too. They claimed that what the practitioner reported could serve as a hint for the interviewer's own self-exploration. Moreover, even after having attained enlightenment, one had to continue their keen self-reflection; otherwise they would relapse to the initial state of *jōsan*. These statements opposed the rules of the *Taikan-an* soft-liners. However, with the time the number of people willing to undergo *mishirabe* declined gradually and the hard-liners decided to amend their rules. Still, the first rule stated that one should not hasten to attain enlightenment but focus on their keen self-reflection, placing special emphasis upon the sense of impermanence—*mujōkan*—and on that of guilt (Kusunoki in Kawahara 1998: 6–7).

At that time Yoshimoto was already aware of the wind of change: around 1941 he started pondering upon the transformation of *mishirabe* under the guidance of master Komatani. Yoshimoto thought that there should be a practice not as austere as *mishirabe* was—a practice available to everyone regardless of their age, sex, and religion thanks to which they could explore themselves thoroughly and thus attain personal growth. He started this initiative with changing the name of the practice—he coined the word *naikan* from the phrase *naishin-no-kansatsu* (内心の観察), which literally means "observation of one's inner world" (Miki et al. 2007: 109).[13] Yoshimoto got inspired also from *The Method of Naikan* (「内観の法」)—the title of a book by the prolific Japanese physician Yū Fujikawa (1865–1940) published in 1936 (Takeda in Sato 1972: 168).[14] That is how the young man began fulfilling the oath he had made to himself at the time he attained enlightenment.

---

[12]Hence in the English-language literature on Naikan Yoshimoto is often considered a businessman.

[13]Considering the Buddhist roots of *mishirabe*, the Naikan specialist Ryōji Takeda suggests that although no clear evidences can be provided, *naikan* may also be related to the Buddhist term *naibu-kanshō*(内部観照), which means "to contemplate inward" (Takeda in Sato 1972: 167); whereas the physical education researcher Hidemasa Yatabe referes *naikan* to an ascetic training handed down in the ancient Taoist tradition. This training required the practitioner to carefully explore the flow of energy throughout their bodies and the condition of their internal organs. Later on, the training was incorporated in *mishirabe*—a religious practice of the *Jōdo Shū* Buddhism (Yatabe 2011: 180).

[14]It should be noticed that Fujikawa used the term *naikan* only in the sense of "deep introspection" without referring to any particular method (Kawahara 1996: 103; Kawahara 1998: 8). On the other hand, Fujikawa, who was also a successful researcher of *Jōdo Shinshū*, suggested that the *naikan* practice was related to *myōkō-nin*(妙好人—"wondrous, excellent person")—an ordinary, but extremely pious *Jōdo Shinshū* devotee who lives a life of total dedication to Buddha Amida. Fujikawa described *myōkō-nin* as "the one who practices *naikan*" and it is probable that when

6.1.4.1 The Birth of Naikan

Some *mishirabe* questions and instructions such as "If you die right now where will you/your spirit go?, "Try to face death," etc., were rather obscure and limited to a certain religious doctrine. Therefore, Yoshimoto decided to transform them into "Explore yourself in relation to your close ones, starting with your mother." Over a week, the practitioner would be sitting in a narrow space surrounded by a folding screen; on every 2 hours an interviewer would come to whom the practitioner would briefly answer what they have remembered. Unlike *mishirabe*, Naikan embraced a caring attitude toward the practitioner, providing them with food and a place to sleep so that everyone could try it.

This was one of the major changes Yoshimoto introduced to *mishirabe* under the guidance of his master Komatani; the others included:

- Even if the person is not ready to face their own death, it is enough if they have the heart of spiritual seeker.
- The term *shinjitsu*—an individual who has already attained enlightenment—is replaced by "adviser" or "healer" (助言者•治療者), whereas the *mishirabe* practitioner (*byōnin*) is renamed "Naikan practitioner" or "patient" (内観者•患者). Also, the time for practicing is extended to seven or, in some cases, even to 15 days.
- From "Observe yourself" or "Reflect on your past," the instructions are specified to examining oneself over a concrete age span of the past regarding a concrete person, starting from one's mother.
- The number of practitioners is increased to more than one in the same room (Yoshimoto 1970: 2–3; Yoshimoto, as cited in Okumura et al. 1972: 15–19).

The gradual transformation of *mishirabe* into Naikan was already taking place, but up until 1942 the religious elements in the practice were rather noticeable, for which reason Yoshimoto was criticized that the method was in fact a religious one. He therefore started eliminating these such elements gradually and in order to defend the new method, he stated that

- Naikan does not deal with anything related to Buddha's mercy and salvation.
- Naikan is not based on any religious doctrine.
- Naikan does not deal with the supernatural nor does it rely on the oracle of a particular spiritualistic medium.
- Naikan is only a method for self-reflection; as such, it does not stipulate that the practitioner should join the ranks of a certain religion once they accomplish the practice (Yoshimoto 1965/2007: 189).

(Footnote 14 continued)

naming the approach Yoshimoto took his cue exactly from this definition. Therefore, as Takeda suggests, the goal of Yoshimoto's Naikan method is the becoming of *myōkō-nin* (Takeda in Sato 1972: 168). However important this topic might be, it requires yet another detour which is difficult to afford in this book.

However, it did not mean that Yoshimoto was no longer religious or that the practice did not involve any religious sentiments at all. In fact, Yoshimoto admitted to calling himself *jūshoku* (住職), i.e., "chief priest of a temple" (Lebra 1976: 202), but "he carefully distinguished his two roles, secular and religious" (ibid.).

6.1.4.2 The Dissemination of the Naikan Method

In July 1945 Yoshimoto published a booklet—*Self-Reflection (Naikan)* (「反省(内観)」)—and embarked on the vigorous dissemination of the method. While running his company, he carried out a one-week Naikan training among the company's staff: even if the participants have only repented themselves of some past mistakes, a great transformation in their spiritual life was observed. On a daily basis, the transformation resulted in smoother interpersonal relationships with both family members and co-workers, and also in increased production efficiency at work. This experiment, considered the first study of intensive Naikan, suggested that the method could be successfully implemented also in Japan's postwar reformatory schools and prisons.

As Yoshimoto needed to earn both money and social credibility, he worked at his company in Osaka knowing no rest; in the evenings he traveled to his native Yamato-kōriyama to guide there people in Naikan. Probably because of his hectic lifestyle, in 1949 Yoshimoto got tuberculosis; but even while in sickbed, he continued to run his company through the telephone. Four years later, in 1953, he quit his business activities once and for all and devoted himself entirely to Naikan—the dissemination of the method was his long-cherished dream and his mission. In the same year he, together with wife Kinuko, opened in Yamato-kōriyama the Naikan Dōjō (内観道場)[15]—a place where everyone was welcome to practice the Naikan method for free under the guidance of the couple. At the very beginning, only a few practitioners dared to try it, but Ishin and Kinuko Yoshimoto did not give up and kept running the *dōjō*. With the time, the number of people who managed to solve their problems and improve significantly their life after experiencing Naikan started to increase gradually (Miki et al. 2007: 109).

In 1954 Yoshimoto introduced Naikan to the Nara Juvenile Prison and the attempt was a success: the ex-inmate recidivism rate decreased significantly. Before long Yoshimoto was appointed chaplain of the prison and a special room for practicing Naikan was opened there. Although more than a decade ago Yoshimoto stated that Naikan was not based on any religious doctrine, he sometimes wore a Buddhist vestment and called the inmates who practiced Naikan "truth seekers." The method was still religiously tinted.

---

[15]Although *dōjō* (道場) can be translated as "training hall" or "training center," in this case we prefer to stick to using the Japanese word because it implies the original idea about *Dō*(道)—the Way—as a symbol of spiritual transformation, which is eventually Naikan's ultimate goal (the concept of *Dō* we discussed in Sect. 3.2). Hence one more possible translation of *dōjō* could be that suggested by Keel, i.e., "a place for cultivating enlightenment" (Keel 1995: 54). For further details on the topic, see Sect. 6.1.7.

After 1957 the introduction of Naikan in prisons and reformatory schools was launched throughout the country. In the same year Yoshimoto renamed the Naikan Dōjō to Naikan Educational Training Center (内観教育研修所) (Maeshiro in Miki and Maeshiro 2006: 185). In the 1960s Naikan already attracted the attention of the mass media, while more than 30 people a week were willing to try the practice (Miki et al. 2007: 109); among them there was even a *yakuza* godfather who repented his life hitherto and went straight after one week at the training center.[16] The method spread also to the education and business. However, the instruction "Explore yourself in relation to your mother (father, etc.)" remained obscure and the practitioners tended to lose focus easily. Using his experience as a successful entrepreneur, Yoshimoto took his cue from the balance sheets in the trading business and in 1967–1968 he formulated the three Naikan questions as we know them today, namely

- What have I received from X?
- What have I given/done for him (her) in return?
- What troubles and difficulties have I caused him/her?

6.1.4.3 Naikan Therapy

The positive outcomes that the newly developed method yielded soon drew the attention also of the academic world. The first scholars who applied Naikan to inpatients with psychiatric disorders were Kō Takeuchi, Professor of Clinical Psychology at Shinshu University, and Nikichi Okumura, Professor in the Department of Psychiatric Neurology at Okayama University (Hatano 1999: 2). Another key figure of that time—the Freudian psychiatrist Rokurō Ishida—applied intensive Naikan to a 42-year-old female patient diagnosed with dissociative disorder and reported remarkable positive changes (Kawahara 1998: 79).[17] In the psychology circles, the Naikan method was introduced by Kōji Sato, Professor at Kyoto University.

As a result, the interest toward Naikan grew and between 1968 and 1978 Yoshimoto was invited to give lectures at the medical departments of several universities across Japan such as Okayama, Kyushu, Tottori, and Osaka University. In the meantime, in 1971 Yoshimoto renamed the center once again—this time to Naikan Training Center (内観研修所)—to respond to the broadening scope within which the method was applied. Yoshimoto's unflagging activities brought him in 1975 Medal of Honor with Blue Ribbon—a decoration by the Japanese Government conferred upon individuals who have made significant achievements in the field of public welfare.

---

[16]In 1965 "Yoshimoto started charging a small fee for Naikan, taking others' advice that free Naikan might actually dissuade people from doing it, since Naikan might then be mistaken for an obscure new religion" (Ozawa-de Silva 2006: 8).

[17]These scholars are considered pioneers of the Naikan implementation outside of the Naikan *dōjō* into a hospital setting.

Then in 1978 with the joint efforts of Takahiro Takemoto, head of Ibusuki Takemoto Hospital in Kagoshima prefecture, and Yoshihiko Miki, Honorary Professor of Psychology at Osaka University, the Japan Naikan Association was established. The new entity held its first conference immediately after, in Kyoto. At the beginning of the 1980s, other Naikan training centers started opening doors throughout Japan. This boom was followed by the 1983 publication of Yoshimoto's book *An Invitation to Naikan*.

Now it seemed that Yoshimoto had fulfilled his long-cherished dream to help as many people as possible to taste the fruits of thorough self-exploration and transform their lives for the better. He passed away on August 1, 1988 because of pneumonia, doing Naikan interviews almost until his last breath. "Preparing a funeral is unnecessary; it would trouble so many people. Let's hold only a wake!," he said shortly before passing away (Japan Naikan Association 1989: 10). Yoshimoto donated his body to the Nara Medical University. An energetic person with a penetrating mind and warm heart, he was known for his proverbial humility and speech always seasoned with wit and humor, but also for his strictness both toward others and himself when it came for Naikan (Miki et al. 2007: 110). Rev. Ishin Yoshimoto—the Buddhist priest and tireless spiritual seeker—was posthumously conferred the Japanese Imperial decoration Fifth Class Order of the Sacred Treasure.

Three years after Yoshimoto's death, in September 1991, under the guidance of Akira Ishii, Professor at Aoyama Gakuin University in Tokyo, the first International Naikan Conference was held in the Japanese capital. The second one opened four years later, in September 1995, in Vienna. In April of the same year, the first issue of *Journal of the Japan Naikan Association*—a Japanese-language scientific journal of the Japan Naikan Association—was already available to all interested in the achievements of the Naikan therapy. In this way, the dissemination of Naikan overseas—to countries including the United States, Austria, Germany, and China—was reinforced after it was first introduced in Europe in the 1970s by two Germans, a prison pastor and a psychologist, in cooperation with the Japanese psychologist Isao Takino, now Professor at Kyoto Tachibana University (Kawahara 1998: 13).[18]

6.1.5 Naikan, Naikan Method, and Naikan Therapy

Although the method was applied successfully in different areas, Yoshimoto feared most that Naikan might be misinterpreted as a therapeutic approach. He even prohibited those who reported improved physical condition or cured disease after practicing Naikan to share it with others (Nagashima 1991: 72) out of fear that Naikan could be mistaken for some newly risen cult (Nagashima 2004: 44).

[18]We do not discuss in detail the spread of Naikan outside of Japan. For further references on this topic, see Ritter (2002: 3–18), Miki et al. (2007: 47–62), and Ozawa-de Silva (2006: 156–159, 165–167).

However, the transformation of the once religious practice into a therapy was on its way. With the rapid spread of Naikan and the beginning of its application also as a therapeutic method, a number of issues related to its scientific verification and terminology arose. One of them pertained to the term *naikan*. Some people tended to mix it with the meditative practice of the Zen Buddhist monk Hakuin Ekaku (see Sect. 6.1.1. and footnote 1), whereas others labeled it "Yoshimoto Naikan" because of the three questions that Yoshimoto had introduced; but as Yoshimoto did not consider himself a founder (Yoshimoto 1983: 44), he was extremely opposed to the usage of his name in this way and he himself never called the practice "Yoshimoto Naikan" (Muramatsu 1991: 24). Although "this therapy is generally called Yoshimoto Naikan to avoid confusion" (Shimazono in Harding et al. 2015: 154), most of the contemporary Naikan specialists, especially Yoshimoto's disciples, term the approach either Naikan therapy or Naikan method. As Yoshimoto's son Masanobu Yoshimoto points out, *naikan* refers to the method for inner observation itself and to the specific setting where it takes place. Then it is important to specify the purpose for which the method is applied. For example, if it is used in the field of correctional education, it should be termed "Naikan-based education" (内観教育); if it is applied for the treatment of psychosomatic diseases, it should be called "Naikan therapy" (内観療法); and when used as a means for personal growth, it should be called simply "Naikan method" (内観法) (Yoshimoto in Yoshimoto and

Table 6.1 Main differences between Naikan therapy and Naikan method

Naikan therapy	Naikan method
Applied at medical institutions and psychological consultative centers by medical and psychological professionals	Applied at reformatory schools, religious centers and Naikan centers; no specific requirements to interviewers
Depends on the specifications of the case	Anyone can practice
Understanding one's own mistakes and feeling sorry for them	Deep sense for one's innate sinfulness
Sense for oneness with one's family and close ones	Sense for oneness with the entire humankind
Improvement of one's interpersonal relationships	Reconciliation with the whole world
Focused on one's efforts during the intensive Naikan practice	Focused on receiving God's grace
Increased self-capacity and competence (from bottom to top)	Becoming open for and receive God's grace (from top to bottom)
Body and Soul	Spirit
Healing	Salvation, absolution
Inner transformation	Breakthrough into the transcendental dimension of human existence
Healthy life	Eternal life

Motoyama 2011). In the comparative Table 6.1 we clarify the main differences between the Naikan therapy and Naikan method.[19]

As previously mentioned, Yoshimoto stated that Naikan was devoid of religious elements and even listed several proofs to this statement. He did it in order to keep the practice's good image and prevent it from being condemned as one of the latest sectarian formations.[20] On the other hand, as Ihara points out, many Naikan practitioners report that their Naikan experience evokes religious or spiritual feelings (Ihara 2012) because in many cases the profound inner transformation itself helps the individual to transcend their "small, pathetic subjectivity and to see all pernicious, vexing contraries harmonized within the whole" (Cook in Callicott and Ames 1989: 222). Guiding his Naikan practitioners toward such a religious-like experience was probably Yoshimoto's ultimate goal (Ihara 2012) and it explains Yoshimoto's strong refusal to use either the name "Yoshimoto Naikan" or "Naikan therapy." Moreover, as he himself pointed out, Naikan's goal is nothing but one's ability to always be grateful, no matter what adversities they encounter; and if a disease is cured after a Naikan practice, this should be considered an accompanying effect but never an end in itself (Nagashima 2004: 44).

We can then define Naikan as a psychotherapeutic approach based on the Naikanistic philosophy, remembering that therapeutic ends have nothing to do with the practice's very origin. In the next section we explore further the term *naikan* and its connotations, which are likely related to the essence of the method's otherwise undeniable psychotherapeutic potential.

6.1.6 On the Term *Naikan:* To Look and *To Look*

As previously mentioned, founder Yoshimoto coined the word *naikan* from the phrase *naishin-no-kansatsu*. In most of the English-language sources on Naikan, *naikan* is usually translated by dividing the two characters it consists of—*nai* (内) and *kan* (観)—which respectively mean "inside, within" and "observation". Hence the whole term comes to mean "inside looking" or simply "introspection", which can be rendered by more poetic expressions such as "a trip toward the within" and "seeing oneself with the mind's eye".

On the other hand, the second character—*kan*—"carries a specific meaning in the context of the Japanese Buddhism. It implies observing or visually imagining an object during meditation with intensively integrated states of mind" (Murase in

[19]The comparisons in this table are partly based on "Naikan as Psychotherapy"—a paper presented by Dr. Shō'ichi Ihara, psychiatrist and Catholic bishop, at the 24th Naikan Workshop held in October 2012 in Kyoto, as well as on Teruaki Maeshiro and Mieko Hariki's paper "Ishin Yoshimoto—A Brief Life Story" (1995).

[20]In postwar Japan "a plethora of new religious sects began to emerge" (Befu 1971: 117) mostly because of "the turmoil and confusion which swept the country in the wake of a complete military defeat and unconditional surrender" (ibid.).

Lebra and Lebra 1974: 396). This specific meaning of *kan* appears in one of the three principle scriptures of the Pure Land Buddhism, which is also the most favored text among the Japanese believers (Morikawa 1984: 25)—the Amitāyurdhyāna Sūtra (Amitāyus Mindfulness Sūtra)—*Kan-Muryō-Jukyō* (観無量寿経). In this text *kan* refers to the proper development of *mindfulness* (Kanamitsu 1985: 219) so that seeing the invisible, i.e., the Pure Land paradise, becomes possible. Such a faculty is fostered by 16 visualization exercises, unified under the term *kampō* (観法), that need to be done in the order prescribed by Buddha should practitioners wish to draw closer to the Pure Land and eventually attain rebirth there. The exercises include the contemplation of real objects of the phenomenal world, for example, the setting sun, in a way that its projected image begins to "shine" in the disciple's mind even when the phenomenon is over, but also the visualization of invisible objects such as the lotus throne of Buddha (Morkiawa 1984: 26).

Additionally, in the past, the word *kansatsu* (from which *naikan* derived) has been used to express the process of "contemplating the appearance of the Buddha and of the Pure Land" (Oe, as cited in Machida 1999: 69). Therefore, the Japanese aesthetician Keisho Morikawa suggests, the concept of *kan* played a key role in the formation of the Japanese aesthetic sense over the centuries and contrasts, for example, the Western naturalistic realism, which focuses on the accurate expression of the visible phenomena. For the Japanese, the contemplation of the ordinary visible phenomena opens up a door to seeing—*kan*—the greater and more substantial world of the invisible (Morikawa 1984: 26–27). A classification of world cultures made by Richard Wagner into the *Augenmensch* and *Ohrenmensch* illustrates this further: "the Japanese are *Augenmensch*" (Anesaki 1974: 19), i.e., people who attach value to the visual faculties and to what is seen rather than to what is, for example, heard or touched.

Such a religious and cultural background provides an additional clue about the development of Naikan as a unique Japanese psychotherapeutic approach. In the context of its specific setting, on which we will elaborate later, the faculty of seeing the invisible (*kan*) and its effect upon the visible may refer to two major consequences for the practitioner. These can be respectively related to two planes, namely the personal and interpersonal, and the transpersonal one:

- *Personal and interpersonal plane*—in an attempt to answer the three Naikan questions, the practitioner tries to explore concrete facts of their past in relation to their close ones. In so doing, practitioner has the chance to perceive the invisible ties through which the very fabric of their existence, including personal relationships, health condition, etc., has been woven of. As a result, the practitioner may gain further clarity about their own personality and about their past and present, too, thus laying the foundations of a more constructive behavior and lifestyle in the future.
- *Transpersonal plane*—through the exploration of seemingly all-too-common facts, the Naikan practitioner also has the chance to gain insight into the interconnectedness of all phenomena in the world and recognize themselves as those who belong to this world on equal terms with all other beings. Such an experience paves the way to significant spiritual transformation that may eventually evoke deep gratitude and awe. These, as previously mentioned, founder Yoshimoto pointed out as the Naikan's ultimate goals.

In Sect. 6.2 we interpret Naikan's therapeutic potential considering these two planes. Before doing that, we will draw a brief parallel between Ishin Yoshimoto and *Jōdo Shinshū*'s founder Shinran, discussing the striking similarities between their teachings and the zeitgeist of their respective times.

6.1.7 Ishin Yoshimoto as the Twentieth Century's Shinran

As mentioned earlier in the text, in July 1945—immediately before the Hiroshima and Nagasaki atomic bombings and Japan's unconditional surrender in World War II—Yoshimoto published *Self-Reflection (Naikan)*, a booklet considered the first printed record where the term *naikan* is used to signify the approach in question. It was hardly a coincidence that in the booklet's preface Yoshimoto wrote that it was time for a deep, nationwide self-reflection, but he wondered about how many people were actually doing it (Yoshimoto 1945:2). "World War II was like a huge tidal wave that washed away the pre-existing culture of Japan. It surely washed away not only the physical heritages and life-styles, but also many of the traditional philosophies and value systems" (Uyeda 1991: 201). Even eight years later, in 1953, when Yoshimoto opened the Naikan Dōjō in his native Yamato-kōriyama—a place where everyone was welcome to practice Naikan—the wounds of the country's military holocaust were still fresh in people's hearts. A time when all illusions were uprooted and new hopes were yet to bloom—such is the broader sociohistorical context within which we should interpret the significance of Yoshimoto's mission. Despite a whole seven centuries that separate the two epochs, this context allows us to draw certain parallels with the Kamakura period, characterized by "a concatenation of disasters" that "sowed the seeds of lack, of blights, famines, and epidemics" (Machida 1999: 23). The pessimism thus deepened made the people of Kamakura period question the very foundation of their existence and to seek, consciously or not, for a spiritual beacon to guide them through.

Similarly to the Kamakura Buddhism, which was dedicated to the salvation of the masses as "opposed to the state-linked Buddhism of earlier times" (Itsuki 2001: 117), the birth and dissemination of the Naikan practice, too, targeted the populace. With its philosophy of reconciliation of the individual with the world, Naikan provided a refuge for the traumas, poor health, and suicidal inclinations that were rife in postwar Japan. It might not be an exaggeration to state that exactly this was the function of Yoshimoto's Naikan Dōjō: similarly to the adepts of the new faith (*Jōdo Shinshū*), the Naikan practitioners, too, met in a place called *dōjō* to "cultivate enlightenment" (see footnote 15). As Keel explains, "*dōjō* was not the traditional Buddhist monastery exclusively intended for the monks who had renounced the world. No such institution was now necessary for the new movement of faith, in which there was no distinction between monks and lay, men and women, high and low, young and old, and where the only requirement was sincere faith to give up one's self-power and rely on Amida's Other Power" (Keel 1995: 55–56). Such an open atmosphere, however, did not mean that the *Jōdo Shinshū* believers had not to follow certain rules while in the *dōjō*. The oldest set of congregational rules, dated 1285, which were formulated to act as guidelines for the behavior of the group members, included the following examples:

- "Do not be slack in your respect for rulers and parents.
- Do not enter the dojo laughing or whispering or with an air of haughtiness.
- Do not do such things as envy those who are superior or belittle those who are inferior. If people violate these, then even if they are called fellow believers or religious companions, you should expel them from the congregation and you should not sit with them or join them" (Dobbins 2002: 66–67).

A similar type of organization can be observed in most of the Naikan training centers in Japan today, where practitioners have to obey a set of rules regarding both their Naikan practice and daily schedule. These rules provide for a termination of the practice in case of misconduct.[21]On the other hand, the introduction of rules do not presuppose authoritarian attitude by a leader: Shinran did not consider himself founder of a religious school nor did he adopt the role of a master with disciples—he "denied having even a single disciple, placing himself on equal terms with his followers and describing them as companions and fellow believers" (Dobbins 2002: 64). "I am already neither a priest nor a layman," Shinran said. "Therefore, my surname should be bald-headed fool"—*gutoku* (愚禿)—"outwardly shaven, inwardly secular and polluted" (as cited in Nakamura 2002: 79). Shinran admitted that he was "a lost soul, unsure of himself and of all else in this life except the abiding grace of Amida. His only aim was to bring this faith in Amida to those like himself who needed it most, to those ignorant and illiterate souls who could not distinguish good from bad, to "bad people" rather than "good people" (Bary 1964: 203–204).

Ishin Yoshimoto, too, thought of himself in a similar manner. As previously mentioned, he rejected the name "Yoshimoto Naikan" and did not consider himself being the founder of Naikan but simply the one who "advertised" it. Such a humble attitude Yoshimoto expressed by joining his palms as if in prayer and bowing every time before and after he held a Naikan interview. Additionally, he stated that he was a deeply sinful person, who was grateful that practitioners shared with him their inmost secrets. "The voice of the Naikan practitioner," Yoshimoto said, "is a voice from Heaven" (Shimizu 1999: 80).[22]

If we remember Shinran's revolutionary statement "Even a good person can be born in the Pure Land, how much more likely it is for an evil person!" (*Tanni-shō*

[21]For example, the rules of the Nara Naikan Training Center include "Keep silence"; "Do not disturb the other practitioners"; "Do not enter other practitioners' rooms under any pretext"; "Do not scrawl on the walls or furniture"; "Handle the center's property carefully," etc.

[22]Although he himself did not state it clearly, Yoshimoto introduced the practice of joining palms and bowing in order to express reverence toward the Buddhahood that lies dormant in every Naikan practitioner (Ikemi, as cited in Nagashima 2004: 46). Indeed, considering that the practitioner sits in a narrow space all surrounded by a folding screen, this act resembles the ritual opening of a home altar where a statue of Buddha is kept (Nagashima 1991: 74).

1962: 22), it is not a surprise then that the first people among whom Yoshimoto applied the Naikan method were juvenile delinquents and prison inmates. That is how Shinran's doctrine of *akunin-shōki*, which takes the evil person as the proper object of Buddha's compassion, thrived once again in the 20th century's postwar Japan. This fact allows us to conclude that what Shinran did in the context of Buddhism by bringing it "down to the earth" for the salvation of the masses, Yoshimoto did seven centuries later by developing the Naikan method. Considering this, we cannot but agree with the Naikan specialist Mari Sengoku that the philosophical roots of Naikan therapy lie deeply in *Jōdo Shinshū* (Sengoku 2005: 89).

In the end, recognizing all the similarities between the epochs in which *Jōdo Shinshū* and Naikan emerged, as well as between the teachings of founders Shinran and Ishin Yoshimoto, Naikan could be defined as a sociohistorical and cultural phenomenon, out of which, in the later stage of its development, a successful psychotherapeutic approach evolved.[23] In the next section we explore the therapeutic structure and functions of this approach and the way they are applied within the contemporary clinical setting.

6.2 Naikan's Therapeutic Structure and Functions

"As I do not have academic education," Yoshimoto said, "I entrust the Naikan theorization to the scholars. My life-long task is to guide those who practice Naikan" (Takemoto 1984: 8; Miki et al. 2007: 110). Although Yoshimoto held lectures and wrote books and articles on Naikan, he remained fully devoted to Naikan and preserved the humility he expressed in this statement until his last breath. For this reason, the theorization of the method came relatively late (Miki et al. 2007: 110), providing a variety of opportunities for its evidence-based therapeutic achievements to be interpreted. Some of the most popular definitions of Naikan among the Naikan community in Japan include "technique for solving life problems" (Kusunoki 1980), "method for self-insight" (Yoshimoto 1983), "door to self-discovery" (Muramatsu 1995), "psychotherapy of love" (Yanagita 1997), "method for healing the anxiety and becoming happy" (Miki and Miki 1998), "science of self-insight" (Hatano 1999), "a way for encountering one's true self" (Nagashima and Nagashima 2001), and "a way to re-experience love" (Miyake 2006).

Some scholars as Takao Murase, who was posthumously named "the Naikan nurturing parent" (Takemoto, as cited in Nagashima 2004: 44), interprets Naikan in the light of traditional Japanese values such as *sunao* (素直—"authentic", "true to oneself") and *on* (恩—"obligation") (Murase 1970; 1995; 1996), whereas Yoshihiko Miki interprets it through *amae* (甘え—"emotional dependence")—a

[23]In this case we can borrow the Japanese-born American anthropologists Emiko Ohnuki-Tierney and Takie Sugiyama Lebra's terminology and define Naikan as "indigenous treatment" (Ohnuki-Tierney 1984: 82) and "ethnotherapy" (Lebra 2004: 31). Lebra's earlier definition of Naikan as "culturally based moral rehabilitation" (1976: 201) reads a little obsolete, but it nevertheless reflects the fact that Naikan "best elucidates the core values of Japanese culture" (ibid.).

key concept for understanding the Japanese personality structure as suggested by psychoanalyst Takeo Doi (Miki 1976: 282–287). Others view Naikan as a mourning ritual (Takino 1980) or interpret it from the standpoint of the Freudian psychoanalysis (Ishida, as cited in Okumura et al. 1972: 87–91, 82–198), dream analysis (Maeshiro 2001: 80–83; 2005: 79–80), cognitive-behavioral therapy (Sakano in Kawahara et al. 1999: 47–59), family and brief therapy (Kojima in Kawahara et al. 1999: 60–76), Jungian psychology (Tanaka 2004), and Morita therapy (Horii, as cited in Takemoto 1984: 173–177).

Regardless of the various definitions and interpretations, there is one key fact that, as the Naikan specialist Yō'ichi Motoyama suggests, should not be ignored under any pretext—this is the fact that Naikan therapy originated from founder Yoshimoto's firsthand religious experience (Motoyama 2002: 60). After having attained enlightenment, Yoshimoto spoke of two main things he felt at that very moment, namely guilt and gratitude. In fact, these are "the two basic pillars of Pure Land Buddhism, first formulated by Shandao (613–681) in seventh-century China" (Unno 2006: 161): "first, the limitless compassion that is bestowed upon us by life (*tariki*); and second, the inherent self-centeredness that permeates our actions and thoughts" (Krech 2002: 13). For this reason, Yoshimoto likened the Naikan practitioner to a *nembutsu* practitioner whose life is permeated by deep gratitude and deep *zange* (Yoshimoto 1983: 45). Later during the years, Yoshimoto used to say that Naikan's two main pillars were the sense of guilt and the sense of impermanence (*mujōkan*) (Maeshiro 2005: 31).

In the next section we attempt to find out how these pillars function as therapeutic tools, referring exclusively to the original form of intensive Naikan practice as established by Rev. Ishin Yoshimoto.

6.2.1 Naikan's External and Internal Therapeutic Structure—Key Factors

Together with voicing his simultaneous feelings of guilt and gratitude, Yoshimoto also reported that his physical condition altered from extreme weakness and dizziness during the practice to a sense of warmth, lightness, and total well-being, which were visible in his healthy appearance and vigorous movements. How could this sudden, almost magical change be explained? In search for an answer, we summarize three key factors of the Naikan practice, namely (i) characteristics of a Naikan training center's setting and overall physical environment; (ii) time frame and general rules of the practice; and (iii) Naikan interview rules. These we analyze in terms of their form and content, which respectively form the method's external and internal therapeutic structure.[24]

---

[24]What we suggest here is a possible interpretation of the Naikan's therapeutic structure. According to the psychiatrist Ryūzō Kawahara, for example, Naikan's therapeutic structure is based on four pillars: the three questions, maternal-like care and empathy, paternalistic rules, and strong concentration on the part of the client (Kawahara in Kawahara et al. 1999: 4–8).

6.2.1.1 External Therapeutic Structure

Characteristics of Naikan training center's setting and physical environment—most of the Naikan training centers that operate in Japan today follow the model of Yoshimoto's *dōjō* in Yamato-kōriyama. They are located in areas remote from the hustle and bustle of big cities, in quiet neighborhoods and relatively close to nature; such are, for example, the centers in Nara, Mie, Tottori, and Tochigi prefectures. The centers are accommodated in typical Japanese houses with plain façades and room floors of *tatami* straw mats. Some centers such as the two in Nara prefecture follow the Yoshimoto's model, i.e., the interviewers are a couple who lives on the center's first floor, prepares the meals for the practitioners, and keeps an eye on their conduct.[25]

The usual Naikan training room is bare and can hold several practitioners at a time. During the practice, every one sits in a comfortable posture on the floor on a Japanese-style cushion—*zabuton*—or on a blanket, all surrounded by a folding screen. In some cases, the use of a low chair is also allowed. The clients sleep at the same place where they simply spread a Japanese-style *futon* bedding on the floor.

Time frame and general rules—stringent schedule and rules during the one-week practice are among the key factors of the intensive Naikan. A typical daily schedule is presented in the Table 6.2 below[26]:

Table 6.2 Daily schedule for intensive Naikan (by courtesy of Nara Naikan Training Center)

First day	*
13:30–14 h	Reception—the interviewer shows the client the place where they will practice Naikan. In most cases, the client is asked to fill in a psychological questionnaire and, in some cases, to do projective tests such as Baum Test and Landscape Montage Technique
14–15 h	Orientation for all clients
15–18 h	Naikan practice and interviewing starts
18 h	Dinner[a]
18:30–21 h	One or two more interviews
21–21:30 h	Writing the Naikan diary
21:30 h	Going to bed

[a]At breakfast, lunch, and dinner time, audio-tape recordings of insights of Naikan practitioners, as well as lectures by founder Ishin Yoshimoto are broadcast over an intercom system. These are believed to serve as models for proper introspection and eventually provide hints for the clients' own Naikan practice.

[25]After a full renovation carried out in 2003, Yoshimoto's center in Yamato-kōriyama, Yamato Naikan Training Center, is now functioning under the guidance of Teruaki Maeshiro—Professor of Clinical Psychology at Bukkyo University and the center's third-generation director—and his wife, the Naikan specialist Naoko Maeshiro. The other center, the Nara Naikan Training Center, opened in 1983 with the direct support of Ishin Yoshimoto. It has been operating for more than 30 years now by Yoshihiko Miki, Honorary Professor at Osaka University, and his wife and the center's director, the clinical psychologist Junko Miki (see Appendix II).

[26]This is the schedule applied at the Nara Naikan Training Center. The schedules at other centers may vary slightly, but in general they all follow a common pattern.

Second to fifth (sixth) day	
6 h	Waking up by the sound of music
6–6:30 h	Washing one's face and cleaning up around, including one's own place in the room, as well as some common-use places such as the restroom, the corridor or the staircase
6:30–7:30 h	One Naikan interview
7:30 h	Breakfast
8–12 h	Two to three interviews
12 h	Lunch
13–18 h	Three to four interviews; taking shower for exactly 20 min
18 h	Dinner
18:30–21 h	One to two interviews
21–21:30 h	Writing the Naikan diary
21:30 h	Going to bed
Final day	
6–6:30 h	Waking up and cleaning
6:30–7 h	Round-table discussion with all the clients and interviewers
7–7:30 h	Breakfast
7:30–8 h	Preparation for going home
8 h	Leaving the center

While practicing Naikan, the client is not allowed to leave their place behind the folding screen except the time for going to the restroom and bathroom; meals they take in the room. Their mobile phone is collected at the reception and the client is allowed to use it only in cases of emergency; neither should the client read, listen to radio, watch TV, etc.

****Naikan interview rules*** (as summarized from Nagashima 2004: 47–48):

- A Naikan interview is usually held on every 1–2 hours, which means that eight to ten interviews are held daily. Yoshimoto suggested an interview should be done even on every 30–40 min so that practitioners do not lose concentration.
- One interview should be finished within 3–5 minutes, because the client should not waste their practice time on talking. Yoshimoto taught that the Naikan practice could not deepen through talking.
- The client is required to share one to two concrete facts for each of the three questions. This, however, does not mean that after having found one such, they should stop and wait for the interviewer to come. The Naikan specialist Masahiro Nagashima compares this process with calligraphy training—during the training the calligrapher fills many sheets, but in the end they show to their teacher one or two only (Nagashima 2004: 48).

- As a basic rule applied by Yoshimoto, the client should start the Naikan practice by answering the three questions in regard first to their mother and from the time they entered elementary school. According to Yoshimoto, doing Naikan about preschool age could be misleading since in most of the cases these memories are based on what one was told by their families and relatives later in life.
- After finishing with Naikan in regard to their mother, the client should progress to other significant persons such as father, siblings, grandparents, partner, children, teachers, colleagues, friends, etc. Depending on the purpose for which the client has come to practice Naikan, they might be required to do Naikan also on themes such as "lies" and "stealing," as well as to calculate the amount of money their parents have spent to bring them up and educate them.
- Naikan should be done for periods of three to five years of the practitioner's life. However, how these periods are divided depends on the client's age, experience, particular problem, and other personal and situational factors.
- The time spent on reflecting on each of the three questions should respectively be 20:20:60%, with special emphasis on the third question "What troubles/difficulties have I caused to…?" (Yoshimoto 1977: 12).
- As a basic rule, taking notes during the practice is not allowed. This, too, Yoshimoto considered a waste of valuable practice time.
- Every time before the interview starts, the interviewer should sit on the floor in front of the folding screen, join their palms as if in prayer in front of their chest, bow from their waist, open the screen's door and make eye contact with the practitioner, again join palms and bow, and then start the interview. The same procedure is repeated after the end of the interview; the interviewer should bow once again also after closing the screen's door.
- The interviewer only listens, but they should never analyze, interpret, or intervene on what the client reports. The role of the interviewer is that of a fellow-traveler (Kitami in Baba et al. 1990: 235), who simply observes if the practitioner follows the rules for practicing Naikan.

6.2.1.2 Internal Therapeutic Structure

All these key factors sharply distinguish Naikan from its Western counterparts. In an attempt to gain more profound understanding of the method and its therapeutic potential, we attempt to analyze these factors also from the standpoint of their content, with each of them being lined with a brief symbolic interpretation[27]:

[27]Terms such as "symbolic" and "archetypal", typical of the Jungian psychology, are used here to refer to factors or types of experiences that we all share as human beings. However interesting the comparisons between Naikan and Jungian psychology might be, lack of space prevents us from discussing them here. For further references on the topic, see Tanaka (2004) and Chervenkova (2013).

***Naikan training center's setting and physical environment:**

- A Naikan training center is usually located in a quiet and relatively secluded place—this is the very first step that helps the practitioner detach themselves from their daily routine, adapt gradually to *seclusion and silence*, and direct their attention to their inner world.
- The center is accommodated in an ordinary house where the interviewers cook and provide for the practitioner's physical comfort—leaving the comfort zone of one's daily routine could be frightening, but such a home-like atmosphere helps the practitioner cope with their initial fears and resistance. On a deeper plane, experiencing the warmth and coziness of home life provides the practitioner with the sense that they are being taken care of, especially if the interviewers are a couple, which perhaps reflect the protective aspects of the *mother–father* archetype.
- The room for practicing Naikan is usually a Japanese-style one—the simple atmosphere of a Naikan room corresponds on a symbolic level to the idea of encountering oneself the way it is, without "decoration." It is a place where attaining the state of selflessness—*muga*—eventually becomes possible.
- The practitioner sits on the ground in a comfortable position, but preferably in Japanese-style *seiza* posture with folded legs neatly tucked under the upright torso —the style of sitting on the floor in Japanese culture is the primary standard for coordinating bodily movements between sitting and standing. In sharp contrast to the Western chair culture, where standing is a sign of respect, in Japan it is the *seiza* posture that conveys respectfulness and humility. Furthermore, "*seiza* is considered not only a social gesture but also a starting point of spiritual training" (Lebra 2004: 198–199). On the other hand, as Takemoto points out, it is not the type of sitting posture that is important, but using it as a means for concentrating one's mind on the practice (Takemoto 1984: 15).
- The practitioner is surrounded by a folding screen in a way that neither they can see beyond it nor they can be seen from the outside—instead of providing a sense of protection, for some clients spending almost 15 hours a day in such a confined space might be frightening and could evoke feelings of oppression or even claustrophobia. As Maeshiro suggests, the client's capacity to stay secluded behind a folding screen becomes a litmus test for their pathology, emphasizing the contrast between "being/feeling lonely" and "being alone": the former is difficult to bear because of a sense as of detachment from the world, whereas the latter speaks of psychological maturity as manifested through one's ability to reconnect in a healthy way with others and the world (Maeshiro 2005: 45). As we will discuss later, this process of reconnection underlies the therapeutic structure of Naikan and perhaps explains the method's positive outcomes in a surprisingly broad range of application. Moreover, considering the meaning of the Japanese word for folding screen—*byōbu*—we suggest that the screen also contours the space to mark a protected, sacred-like area where a non-ordinary

event takes place.[28] Although inside the screen it is rather dim, shafts of indirect light appear from above, making the space inside neither too dark nor too bright, i.e., appropriate for the practitioner to concentrate exclusively on their inner world (Nagayama and Shimizu 2006: 53). This key factor corresponds directly with the next one.

- The practitioner's rigid posture—the look of the Naikan practitioner's rigid posture surrounded by a folding screen evokes associations with a baby in the womb or a dead body in its tomb, hence with the *birth–death* dichotomy. In the context of Naikan therapy, this dichotomy synthesizes "to form a new symbol—that of rebirth" (Ozawa-de Silva 2006: 28). Not surprisingly, many practitioners report a feeling as of being reborn or compare the tranquil space behind the screen with a mother's womb (Maeshiro 2005: 42–43). Also obvious are the parallels with traditions of seclusion observed in some indigenous ethnic groups, formally enunciated as *rites of passage*. These rites include the stages of separation, transition, and reincorporation (Van Gennep 1961). In our understanding, the therapeutic process in Naikan passes through stages similar to them, especially if we consider the strong ritualistic aspects of the Naikan interview, to be discussed in detail later in the text.[29]
- More than one client can practice in the same room—this may appear totally unacceptable or even wrong from the perspective of Western psychotherapy, especially because of issues of confidence. However, hearing what the other clients report is believed to serve as a hint for the practitioner, stimulating further their own process of self-reflection (Takemoto 1984: 15); similar is the function of the lectures broadcast at breakfast, lunch, and dinner time (see table footer a, Table 6.2). Additionally, the process of facing one's own sinfulness appears not so frightening in the presence of others as compared to the seclusion and silence of individual practices—the collective practice requires a common space to be shared with others, thus suggesting to practitioner that they are not alone on their challenging way to self-discovery.

Time frame and general rules:

- Time frame—once set, the time frame during the Naikan practice could not be subject of significant changes and should be strictly followed. What is very important about Naikan therapy is that its time frame follows the natural circadian rhythm, i.e., practitioners get up at sunrise, go to bed shortly after sunset, and take their meals three times a day at fixed hours. Although natural to

---

[28]*Byōbu*(屏風)literally means "a wall that protects from wind", while the closed space thus created by the screen is called *hōza*(法座)—"a place where the teachings of Buddha are preached and listened to," i.e., "a sacred space."

[29]Takie Sugiyama Lebra suggests that the phases of the intensive Naikan process can be summarized as "initial confusion or resistance; "awakening"; self-repulsion and depression; and hopefulness and tranquility" (Lebra 1976: 212).

humans, circadian rhythm is almost completely forgotten by contemporary people who have somehow adjusted to a hectic lifestyle, in which the lack of natural order reflects and further aggravates the disordered state of their inner world. The Naikanistic time frame addresses not only one's physical well-being, but it also serves as the first step toward inner order, i.e., it functions as an external model which the psyche can, through the mediation of the body, gradually internalize (Chervenkova 2013: 39). On a symbolic plane, this time frame brings to the fore dichotomies of night–day and darkness–light, to help further the client resonate with the natural circadian rhythm.

- General rules—the stringent rules could be considered the psychological equivalent of the confined space behind the folding screen. Using the above-mentioned interpretation of the folding screen as a litmus test for the client's pathology (Maeshiro 2005: 45), following or refusing to follow certain rules, too, may speak volumes of the client's general attitude toward others and of their capacity to establish healthy interpersonal relationships. Furthermore, the rule that stipulates house cleaning not only helps the practitioner to concentrate on a certain activity, but it also assists them in "cleaning up" their mind.

Naikan interview rules:

- The practitioner is asked to remember and report only concrete facts regarding the three Naikan questions—this rule brings to the fore the idea that there are no trivialities; however trivial a fact may seem, it has already been stored in the warehouse of our past, reflecting the uniqueness of our personal hitherto experience. The function of this Naikan factor, which we later formulate as *existential grounding* (see Fig. 6.2 in Sect. 6.2.2.1), provides the practitioner with the chance to face reality as it is and, as the Japanese medical ethics researcher Sawako Hattori puts it, to re-experience their past here and now in a new way (Hattori 2011: 55). In other words, the Naikan clients explore their past through the prism of tangible facts only, not through their own emotions about these facts (Ishii 2000: 67–68). On a deeper plane, the process of entering the warehouse of our past and discovering seemingly trivial facts there is what verifies our existence in the universal flow of *interdependence* as a basic law of life, i.e., we become aware that we are not victims of random circumstances; that we live a meaningful life in a meaningful world. In the end, this process confirms that we *are*, we are *connected* and we *belong*, and this is a joyous participation in the world, not a compulsive relationship.
- The practitioner should spare 20% of their time on the first question ("What have I received from…?"), 20% on the second question ("What have I done for/given to…?"), and the remaining 60% on the third question ("What troubles and difficulties have I caused to…?"). As previously mentioned, when formulating the three Naikan questions, Yoshimoto took his cue from the balance sheets used in trading business. He decided to place special emphasis on the question "What troubles/difficulties have I caused to…?", presuming that it could help the practitioner realize their own sinfulness, which is one of the key points about

Naikan. However, if the practitioner starts with this question, it is very likely that their psychological defenses will block the entire process. That is why, Yoshimoto decided to introduce the question "What have I received from…?" considering that when the practitioner realizes the troubles they have caused despite all the benevolences they have received, their sense of guilt would grow even more. In the end, Yoshimoto introduced the question "What have I done for/given to…?" to balance the other two questions. Finally, he arranged the three questions in the present order, leaving the toughest one, i.e., "What troubles/problems have I caused to…?" for last and assigning it more than half of the total time (Takemoto 1989: 33). As it could be expected, a fourth question such as "What troubles/difficulties have I been caused?" is totally disregarded in Naikan.

We suggest that the three questions and the special emphasis on the third one clearly reflect Yoshimoto's personal experience in *mishirabe*—realizing what we have been given will make us realize the infinite love and compassion we constantly receive so as to be alive (*tariki*); whereas realizing the troubles we have caused will help us face our own selfishness. The latter could be considered one of the key points of Naikan's inner therapeutic structure, for which reason a special emphasis is placed on it.[30] As many Naikan practitioners, the author included, report, it is difficult to find out what they have given to or done for others, but it is easy to recall what they have been given and especially the troubles they have caused.[31] Through the reflection upon seemingly trivial matters, the practitioner has the chance to experience the unconditional maternal love or even the universal cosmic love (Takemoto 1989: 33) that silently, yet powerfully nourishes their spirit (Murase 1996: 222).

- The practitioner should start doing Naikan first about their mother or, if that is the case, about their caregiver. The role of the mother figure, the psychological aspects of the mother image, or that of the Great mother archetype are too broad to discuss here.[32] In the context of Naikan, there are several possible

[30]It is worth mentioning that during the interview the interviewer uses the verb "explore," i.e., "Which relationship did you explore over the past 2 hours?" instead of "think about" or "remember" (on the meaning of *mishirabe*, see footnote 8). As the Naikan specialist Kakusei Yanagita suggests, the third Naikan question refers to the practitioner's effort to explore, discover and face the dark aspects of their own personality (Yanagita 1997: 34–35).

[31]In his work *Naikan—Theory and Cultural Relevance* (1996), Takao Murase discusses the three Naikan questions in the context of the psychological characteristics of Japanese culture and suggests that the third question exclusively represents the Japanese psychology of sin. The first two Naikan questions Murase defines as representing respectively the psychology of gratitude and that of filial piety (Murase 1996: 156–165).

[32]For further references, see the seminal work of the German Jungian psychologist Erich Neumann *The Great Mother—An Analysis of the Archetype* (1955). Neumann points out that only when we have considered "the whole scope of the basic feminine functions—the giving of life, nourishment, warmth, and protection—can we understand why the Feminine occupies such central position in human symbolism and from the very beginning bears the character of "greatness" (Neumann 1955: 43).

interpretations, including, for example, the one suggested by Takao Murase, who discusses traditional Japanese concepts of maternity such as "the self-sacrificing mother" (Murase 1996: 166–169). However, here we adhere to what founder Yoshimoto suggested on the subject. According to him, there are five main reasons why among all interpersonal relationships, Naikan places the greatest value on exploring that with mother (Yoshimoto and Miki in Baba et al. 1984: 320–322):

- *the maternal figure symbolizes the entire humankind*—as psychologist Masami Kusunoki points out, we have been one body with our mother over the nine months before birth and during that time she has been our environment, our whole world (Kusunoki 1980: 5). The mother "is a total environment, a "mother universe", and the infant is but a small part of this immense and exciting unit" (McDougall 1989: 32); since mother is the very first person that we have contact with, she is "the most crucial Alter" (Lebra 1976: 206) and the relationship with her plays a key role in the formation of our personality. As such, this relationship speaks volumes of the way we relate to others and also of the quality of our interpersonal relationships. However, the Naikan practitioner should try to explore their relationship with their mother not from the perspective of their dependence on her as her child, but from the perspective of a relationship between two independent individuals.
- *doing Naikan about one's mother paves the way to experiencing the essence of Naikan*—there are many examples when while doing Naikan about their mother, practitioners intensively experience their own sinfulness and other people's love. This experience is considered to possess great therapeutic power. Undoubtedly, it may occur while doing Naikan about one's father or partner, but in most cases it is very likely to occur when Naikan about one's mother is being practiced. Additionally, the practitioner may become aware also of traditional associations of maternity such as unconditional love, care, and forgiveness that manifest themselves through other persons, too (Miki 1976: 275).
- *doing Naikan about one's mother is a basic training in looking at oneself*—no matter the purpose the practitioner does Naikan for, they should start doing Naikan first about their mother. If they start doing Naikan first about the person whom they are experiencing troubles with, or about the problem they want to solve, it will not be a real Naikan but only an attempt for self-reflection, i.e., it would be a process which follows the external form of Naikan, but would still be obstructed by anxiety, self-defenses, and negative feelings toward the person or problem in question. As a matter of principle, mother is the one who has done a lot for us over a long period in our lives and to whom we have caused many troubles and difficulties, but have done or given almost nothing in return. Having realized this truth, it becomes easier to put ourselves in other people's shoes and understand their feelings objectively without coloring them with our own emotions. As Miki

summarizes, it is exactly the capacity to "reverse roles" with others that helps us distance ourselves from the biased Ego-perspective and gain an objective understanding based on real facts (Miki 1990: 68–69).Therefore, after successfully finishing Naikan about their mother, the practitioner may proceed to the person they are experiencing troubles with, because they have already prepared the ground, i.e., they have realized their own sinfulness and others' love and support. Through this rule, a function, which we term the Naikan *mirroring function* (see Fig. 6.1 in Sect. 6.2.2.1), emerges to help the practitioner objectively assess the problem from the perspective of their own imperfections.

- *the practitioner should repeat Naikan about their mother*—usually within the first two or three days of the practice the self-reflection is not yet deep enough; but as the days advance the practitioner should repeat the Naikan about their mother again, twice or even three times after doing Naikan about other significant figures in their life.
- *Japanese culture traditionally places emphasis on the mother image*—Naikan matches the Japanese psyche and the Japanese can therefore practice it relatively easily and without resistance. As Kawai points out, if the maternal principle is divided into a positive, embracing and nurturing aspect, and a negative, devouring and killing aspect, then the first one is rather strongly represented in Japanese culture where the mother image is attached an absolute value (Kawai 2009: 141). On the other hand, since the maternal figure is universal for all human beings, in its essence Naikan rises above all cultural boundaries (Yoshimoto and Miki in Baba et al. 1984: 322): "from the Naikan perspective, even a person abandoned from birth would still have something to feel grateful for towards his or her mother, just for the fact that they were taken care of in the womb and protected until birth; for that alone, such a person would still owe a debt impossible to pay back, namely his or her life. The function that image of the mother plays in Naikan is therefore not by any means limited to Japan" (Ozawa-de Silva 2006: 133).

To recapitulate, since mother is the "bridge" that connects the individual with others and the world, doing Naikan about her becomes the basis for the entire practice. If it proceeds smoothly, then so will do the Naikan about other people, too (Kusunoki 1983: 142–143).

- The interviewer joins their palms as if in prayer and bows a total of four times for each and every interview—this ritual-like procedural frame, which solemnifies the atmosphere and which to the external observer may seem unnecessarily convoluted, can be observed in no other psychotherapeutic approach—neither Western nor Eastern. In fact, Yoshimoto introduced this practice as a symbol of his reverence toward the Buddhahood that lies dormant in every Naikan practitioner (Ikemi, as cited in Nagashima 2004: 46; see footnote 22). He even used to say that "the voice of the Naikan practitioner is a voice from Heaven" and often ate with gratitude the leftovers of his practitioners' meals (Shimizu 1999: 80). This rule reflects Yoshimoto's personality and makes humility one of Naikan's most distinctive features—both externally, as manifested in gestures and conduct, and internally, as a psychological experience. From a psychological perspective this ritual-like procedural frame functions in a way similar to that of the *existential grounding* function of Naikan, i.e., showing respect to the practitioner and the recollections they report, no matter how shameful, confirms their existence and the uniqueness of their experience.[33] It can further provide the practitioner with a sense of safety and hope for a positive change. If the interviewer leaves the equal therapist–client relationship and puts themselves in the superior position of a healer, they would eventually block the entire Naikan process and contribute to the development of dependence on the interviewer. This would be especially valid in cases of practitioners who tend to excessively search emotional support from others. Needless to say, dependence on the practitioner on behalf of the interviewer should also not be eliminated as one of the possible pitfalls. This key point is directly related to the next one.

- The interviewer does not analyze or interpret what the practitioner reports nor do they provide comments or advice—they just listen carefully and at the end of each interview thank the client for their cooperation. The interviewer should talk and behave in the humblest possible, nonjudgmental and receptive way, while making sure that the client "is following instructions and reflecting successfully on the topics" (Murase in Lebra and Lebra 1974: 389). In Yanagita's words, the interviewer should always assume a servant-like attitude (Yanagita 1995: 67); they should be like a midwife who simply assists the birth of the new personality, but the entire process nevertheless remains in the hands of the practitioner and their own "capacity to give birth." This explains so as to why Naikan is defined as a nondirective approach, in which the practitioner is being freed from concerns such as "Am I right?" or "How do I look to the interviewer?" (Shimizu 1999: 79). On a symbolic plane, the principle of noninterference and of keeping psychological distance is manifested in the bowing figure of the interviewer, who simply opens the folding screen, but always remains on the other side of the imaginary border. If we render this ritualistic behavior through Jungian-tinted terminology, the interviewer bows in front of the mystic *death–rebirth* process, which occurs inside the vessel-like space contoured by the folding screen—the interviewer is allowed to observe and perhaps stand in awe of this process, but never to interfere in.

How could this mystic process be translated into the language of contemporary psychology so that Naikan's otherwise unquestionable therapeutic achievements can be validated? Having presented the method's key factors that form its therapeutic structure—external and internal—we can now proceed to search for a possible answer.

[33]As Takie Sugiyama Lebra points out, "one can imagine how disarming this gestural humility and politeness might be to a prison inmate" (Lebra 1976: 213).

6.2.2 Naikan Therapeutic Functions in the Light of the Body–Mind Interconnectedness

Even a brief review of the literature on Naikan therapy reveals an astonishingly broad scope of applications of this method—both clinical and non-clinical—for example in the field of dependencies on alcohol, drugs, and gambling; school truancy; marital and professional conflicts; domestic violence; depression; psychosomatic diseases; and terminal care. There is an array of case studies and research focused on the theorization of the method's efficaciousness as a psychotherapy.

Throughout Naikan's transformation from a religious practice through rehabilitation method for prisoners to psychotherapy, founder Yoshimoto continued to say that "Naikan is Naikan" (Ozawa-de Silva 2006: 164). Although during the later years he did not oppose the method's clinical application and even held lectures among the academia, he never cast aside the spiritual legacy of his firsthand *mishirabe* experience: in addition to the three Naikan themes, it was not unusual for Yoshimoto to ask his clients questions such as "If you die right now where will you/your spirit go?" (see footnote 10) and "For what purpose were you born? Do you live in accordance with that purpose?" (Yoshimoto 2004: 10, 19).

If we return to the history of *mishirabe*, we will remember that its essence is contained in the first of these questions, "If you die right now where will you go?," i.e., the *mishirabe* practitioner's main task was to cultivate readiness to face their own death at any moment, both physically by abstaining from sustenance and sleep, and metaphorically—by pondering over what would happen to them after they die. Additionally, during the years Yoshimoto made statements such as "Naikan means to contemplate death" and "Those who mislead themselves that there is tomorrow will very likely spend today in vain" (Yoshimoto 2004: 6, 18). He also often encouraged his clients by saying, "Do Naikan while constantly thinking of death" (Kusano 2001a: 8; Kusano 2001b: 1) and "Concentrate on Naikan each second because we never know when we are going to die" (Ozawa-de Silva 2006: 29).[34]

Although Yoshimoto's attitude to death did not survive in the contemporary Naikan practice, it still exists figuratively as a distant echo of *mishirabe* in the method's structure earlier described. Considering this, we assume that the therapeutic functions of Naikan should be searched for exactly in the way how concepts of death manifest themselves in Naikan.

[34]In addition to the similarities between Ishin Yoshimoto and Shinran that we already discussed, a striking similarity between their statements, too, could be found: "The heart that thinks there is a tomorrow is as transient as the cherry blossom, for is there not the midnight wind?" (Shinran, as cited in Reischauer 1970: 108).

6.2.2.1 The Process of Symbolic *Death-Rebirth-Reconnection*

Apart from a few articles,[35] the theme of death and its role within the Naikan practice is rarely mentioned in the Naikan-related studies and, to the best of our knowledge, no in-depth research has been carried out in the field so far. The issue is mostly discussed in articles on Naikan's introduction and application in terminal care practice (Maeshiro 2005: 213–223), but only from the perspective of approaching death, which results from an incurable disease.

It is therefore well justified to begin with what the Naikan specialist Takahiro Takemoto observed in his capacity of medical doctor. When attending to a number of patients at their deathbeds, Takemoto noticed that when patients realized they were about to die, they often reflected sincerely on their past and attempted to explore what life they had led—whether they had hurt somebody or whether they regretted something. When they were about to die, many of the patients, being surrounded by their families, would utter final words like "Thank you very much for everything" and "Take care for those after me" (Takemoto 1994: 1). On the other hand, Takemoto continues, deathbed reflections and repentance come too late. Rather, we should do them at least once in the middle of our lives and Naikan practice provides an opportunity for exactly this kind of self-exploration (ibid.); it is, as Yoshimoto explains, what Naikan is all about (Yoshimoto 1977: 7). Indeed, if we consider only the physical atmosphere required for intensive Naikan practice, we will notice some striking similarities between it and deathbed experiences: as previously described, the Naikan client sits quietly on the floor surrounded by a folding screen; they are not allowed to leave the walled-off space, except when they go to the restroom or bathroom, neither are they allowed to talk to anyone except the interviewer. With any external stimuli and unnecessary physical movements being blocked, the narrow space behind the folding screen becomes the client's whole world over one whole week, fostering the client's capacity to explore their past carefully and in detail.

However, and this is very important in Naikan, the practitioner does not simply recollect their past and reports random pieces of their life story, but they are required to do this through the prism of the three questions alone. Reflecting on one's past in such a way provides a solid structure that helps the practitioner acknowledge two existential conditions pertinent to all human beings. These conditions form the very essence of the Naikanistic philosophy, namely "the human

[35]For example, "Naikan as Mourning Work" (Takino 1980; Takino in Kawahara 1998), "Naikan and Medicine" (Takemoto 1994), "Thanatology and Naikan" (Kusano 2001a), and "The Theme of Death and Rebirth in the Naikan Process" (Kusano 2001b). In recent years, "catholic Naikan meditation" emerged as a mourning work method targeting Christians in Japan. This meditation was introduced by Naosato Fujiwara, a Catholic priest and head of *Kokoro-no-Ihori* Naikan Meditation Centre in Osaka. "The focus of Catholic Naikan upon the dead comes first from Fujiwara's initial experience of Naikan, which was a meditation on his relationship with his dead father" (Kazuyoshi in Harding et al. 2015:170). The goal of this practice "is to engage in a shamanistic exercise in a place where one artificially experiences death" (Kazuyoshi in Harding et al. 2015:171).

being is fundamentally selfish and guilty, yet at the same time favored with unmeasured benevolence from others" (Murase in Lebra and Lebra 1974: 388).[36] If put in psychoanalytic terms, this would mean the practitioner simultaneously realizes their *guilty self* and their *loved self* (Kusano 2001a: 7).

The practice of thoroughly recollecting one's past in order to strike balance of one's deed is, as already mentioned, exactly what many people do on their deathbeds or, as the American philosopher Carl Becker reports, when near-death experiences occur (Becker 1992: 20). Deathbed experiences are unique existential situations abound in retrospection, introspection, and "a more focused effort to determine "the things that really matter" than had been attempted hitherto" (Scarre in Kellehear 2009: 160). The near-death time is a time when people can finally afford to be honest with themselves, having no further need for self-deception or for casting a blind eye upon uncomfortable facts. Now they can "play their own critics, stepping temporarily out of the protagonist's role and examining their own motives, acts, achievements, and failures with more or less objectivity" (Scarre in Kellehear 2009: 158). This description is reminiscent of the deathbed *haiku*-poem by the 19th-century Zen Buddhist monk Ryōkan:

> Now it reveals its hidden side
>
> And now the other—thus it falls
>
> An autumn leaf[37]

On the verge of death, not only do we all become equal like falling autumn leaves, but this is the time when our whole life story is revealed the way it is; there is nothing left for us to hide.

Returning to Naikan therapy, we will notice that in fact this is what every Naikan practitioner does, too. There is nothing left for them to hide in the silent emptiness behind the folding screen. They recognize everything they have received, given in return, and all the troubles they have ever caused simply the way they are—not the way the practitioner subjectively interprets them. After the prolonged birth pangs of honest retrospection, the practitioner is being born to the naked truth about themselves and the way they relate to others and the world. This truth makes them, as it is the case with many dying people, more humble, forgiving, and grateful.

Therefore, experiencing death while alive could teach us to be careful as to how to spend the limited time we are given and to refrain from everything that threatens to poison it. In this case, the specific behavior observed among many death-row inmates could be an appropriate illustration: death-row inmates lead extremely fulfilling life in prison—they write poetry, draw pictures, and participate in various activities, in sharp contrast to their life-sentenced counterparts who tend to be apathetic and indifferent (Kusano 2001a: 6; Ishii 1999: 193–194). Such a behavior suggests that the constant recalling of our transient nature has the potential to add

[36]Let us remember that these were the two pillars of *Jōdo Shinshū* as initially formulated by the influential Chinese Buddhist writer Shandao in the 7th century.

[37]「裏を見せ　表を見せて　散る紅葉」(translated by Yoel Hoffmann in Hoffmann 1986: 268).

meaning to life as a one-time unique chance, and inspire us to make the most out of it: "we live so that when we die we shall have lived as if death were our daily guide. We are taught to make death an inlay in the buckle of life, to incorporate *all* of our life in each day of our life, so that we live fully and well. When a contemporary Zen monk was asked why the great Japanese Zen master Dogen wrote so stridently and repetitively about the nearness of death, the monk replied, "Dogen wants us to enjoy life" (Fleischman 1989: 241). Although "not everyone can be paradoxically spurred forward" (ibid.), such a point of view on death does not degrade, but, on the contrary, it augments further the value of life; it replaces the fear of death with death awareness, which inspires us to lead a full life. In this sense, "although the *physicality of death destroys us, the idea of death saves us*" (Yalom 2008: 33).

If interpreted in the same vein, the intensive Naikan practice could then be defined as a unique opportunity to experience symbolically our own death in the midst of life, that is, to be honest with ourselves and reconsider our behavior, rearrange our personal relationships, and reset our whole life before it is too late. Albeit figurative, the presence of death within the Naikan practice appears to function exactly in this direction—it disarms our desire for justifying ourselves and our past deeds, and makes our preconceived images flake away; for it is not an exception that exactly these desires and self-images entangle us in illusions and obscure the truth so that our relationships and even our health are brought to ruins.

All of the above explains why the third Naikan question, i.e., "What troubles/difficulties have I caused to…?" becomes central for the entire practice. As previously discussed, founder of *Jōdo Shinshū*, Shinran, interpreted sin as devoid of "substance in itself, and is but the shadow of our illusion" (Nakamura 2002: 85). We are born and live in the darkness of ignorance (Yoshimoto 1977: 7), which hinders us from understanding that not the sin/trouble itself is what matters, but its effect upon others and the world (Chervenkova 2012: 78). Therefore, Naikan urges us not only to rationally admit our misdeeds, but also to transform our attitude toward them, i.e., to realize the effect of our behavior as being deeply interconnected with others and the world. However, in order to achieve such a level of awareness, we need to leave the narrow shell of our Ego—such a tough process seems to be possible only if we first become fully aware of our own finitude. On the other hand, death is the only life event we cannot experience directly while we are alive. As the Japanese philosopher Hisao Nishimuta points out, we know about death only from the perspective of bystanders of others' deaths, and this fact likely reinforces our fond delusion that death is by no means related to us (Nishimuta 2009: 17). Even though intellectually we know the reality of finitude and death, "emotionally we reject them with fear and loathing, and we would rather say that they did not exist" (Cook in Callicott and Ames 1989: 221–222).

Considering all of the characteristics of the Naikan setting, we can conclude that it provides a favorable opportunity for the client to sense and internalize in a healthy way their own mortality—*mujōkan*. Spending almost 15 hours a day in thorough self-reflection with almost no bodily movements, the Naikan practitioner resembles a person on their deathbed. At the same time, the silent walled-off space behind the folding screen with the client sitting motionlessly inside resembles a mother's womb. The symbolism of the Naikanistic setting is reminiscent of the ancient rites of incubation—*incubatio* (see footnote 6 in Sect. 4.2). Similarly to them, in Naikan therapy the client is mentally "incubated" so as to be reborn to a new state of consciousness and, as a result, be able to reset their life (Chervenkova 2013: 40). This new state of mind manifests itself in shifting one's understanding from the Ego-biased perspective to the *sub specie aeternitatis* perspective, where the individual is born again to oneness and "his isolation and his sense of being a "stranger" in this world are once and for all overcome" (Faber 1998: 93). That is how the Naikan practitioner is reconnected, but not in some social sense alone, but also in the sense of very basic and primal oneness: the practitioner experiences their own existence not as something alien to that of all humankind, the world, and even the Universe, but as an intrinsic part of them.

How is the Naikan practitioner given a chance for subsequent symbolic rebirth and reconnection so that to experience such a primal oneness? What if during a week of tough practice the narrow space behind the folding screen turns symbolically into a coffin instead of a womb? In search for an answer, we will discuss more details of the specific process of the Naikan self-reflection.

As previously mentioned, the retrospective process in Naikan unfolds within a preset framework and rules, always starting from reflecting on the client's relationship with their mother. The successful accomplishment of Naikan about one's mother is usually considered a positive sign for the whole practice. Unsurprisingly, the mother image in Naikan therapy becomes representative for the nurturing aspects of life (*tariki*); hence reconciliation with her would be tantamount to reconciliation with the whole world. Once the client realizes that (i) their mother gave them the invaluable gift of life and (ii) their whole life up to now has been possible thanks to all the people they received care and support from, the client's Ego-biased perspective is likely to transform into a flexible understanding of the ubiquitous interconnectedness this world exists upon. From such a perspective, the client's perception, too, undergoes certain changes. These we term *Naikan dimensions of change*, namely

→ altered perception of the self (as part of the whole),[38]
→ altered perception of others and the world
→ altered perception of the problem/disease (see Fig. 9.1 in Sect. 9.1)

Each of these dimensions of change, or all of them in their entirety could manifest themselves on two planes. As mentioned previously in relation to the term *naikan* (see Sect. 6.1.6.), these are the personal and interpersonal plane, and the transpersonal plane. The first one refers to personal well-being and social compatibility—with the understanding gained through Naikan, one can become more

---

[38]It is important to mention that in Japanese the word for "self, oneself" is *jibun* (自分), which literally means "my part (of the whole)." This word is probably derived from *shizen-no-bunshin* 「自然の分身」 (Noguchi 2003: iv), which means "I am the same as Nature, Nature is the same as me".

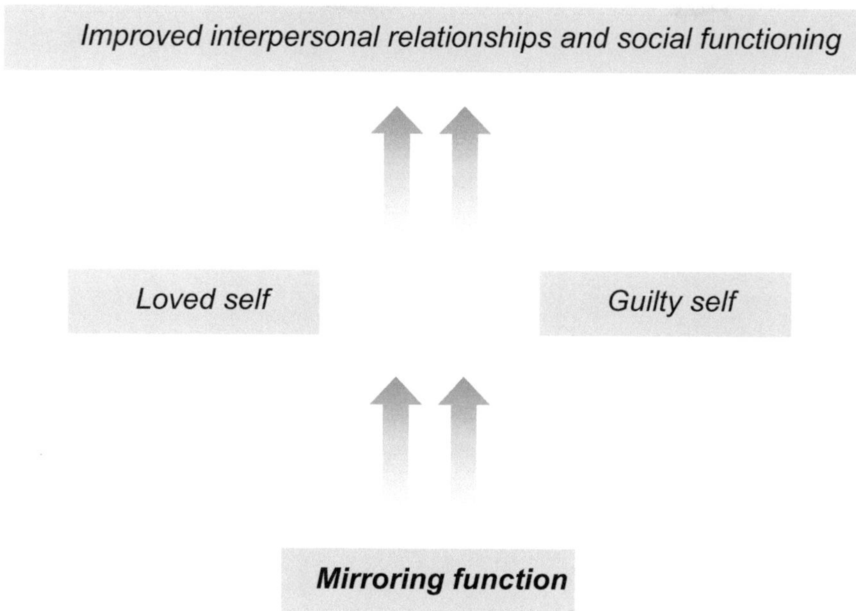

Fig. 6.1 Naikan's mirroring function and its effects (reprinted with permission from Chervenkova 2014: 128)

humble, more caring, and respectful toward others and Nature, and lead conflict-free life based on healthy interpersonal relationships. In this case, we can agree with Lebra's definition of Naikan as "moral rehabilitation" (see footnote 23) and acknowledge the method's efficacy in the field of school truancy, juvenile delinquency, marital and professional conflicts, and drug, alcohol, and gambling addictions. This is the level where the Naikan's *mirroring function* manifests itself. Looking at themselves in the mirror of their relationship with others, primarily with their mother, the practitioner understands that they have constantly been taken care of despite the problems they had caused. In other words, as previously mentioned, they recognize their *guilty self* and their *loved self*. This process is likely to foster improved interpersonal relationships and social functioning (Fig. 6.1).

The second plane refers to mutual connectedness that transcends the individual-society dichotomy: Naikan calls for the practitioner to go beyond the intellectual grasp and common sense morality to a *lived experience* of the world as one of constant interfusion where no act can have but an effect on the whole.[39]

[39]In Hinduism, this worldview is figuratively depicted as the jewel net of Indra—a wondrous net hung in the heavenly abode of the great god Indra. "If we now arbitrarily select one of these jewels for inspection and look closely at it, we will discover that in its polished surface there are reflected *all* the other jewels in the net, infinite in number. Not only that, but each of the jewels reflected in this one jewel is also reflecting all the other jewels, so that there is an infinite reflecting process

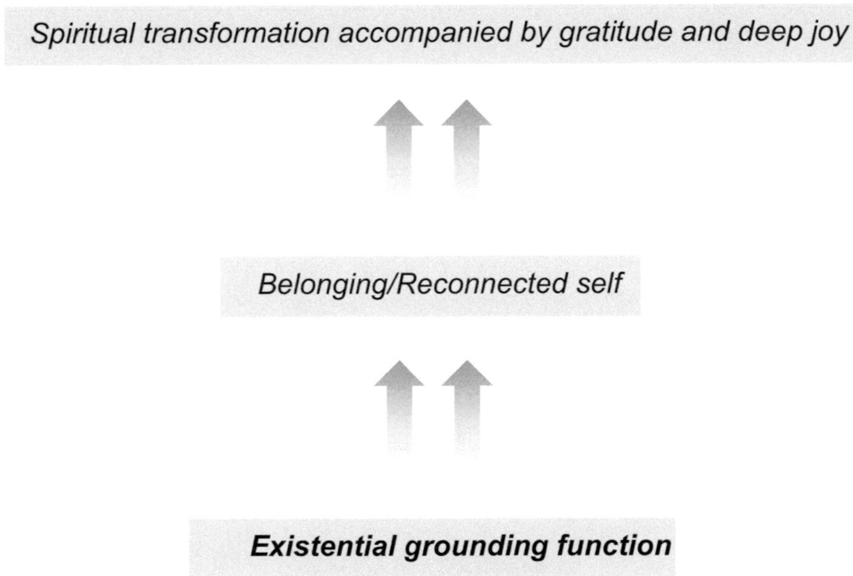

Fig. 6.2 Naikan's existential grounding function (reprinted with permission from Chervenkova 2014: 129)

The development of such a holistic worldview may evoke deep joy and gratitude—not those triggered by some external stimuli, but inner joy and gratitude that arise from giving up the Ego and *realizing*, i.e., *making real* on a daily basis, ourselves as part of the miracle of Life. In other words, we die symbolically for our past and our old selves to be reborn in a world of interdependence where we can recognize ourselves as *belonging (reconnected) selves*. On this level, a function that we described as *existential grounding* manifests itself (Fig. 6.2).

Thus, if the first plane refers to a kind of moral and social rehabilitation, the second one is the level of overall transformation—social, physical, and spiritual—which is fueled by a profound process of symbolic death and subsequent rebirth; and while the transformation that occurs on the first level may lead to improved social functioning, the deeper death-and-rebirth-like transformation could be held "responsible," we suggest, for the improvement or even complete cure of an array of diseases, as a large number of both Naikan practitioners and interviewers report. Therefore, we agree with the Naikan specialist Isao Takino that Naikan's most powerful therapeutic tool is the process of symbolically facing one's own death (Takino in Kawahara 1998: 178).

(Footnote 39 continued)

occurring" (Cook in Callicott and Ames 1989: 214). This is a relationship of "simultaneous *mutual identity* and *mutual intercausality*" (ibid.).

Now we have come to understand how *Jōdo Shinshū*'s three pillars, namely the Other-power (*tariki*), selflessness (*muga*), and sinfulness (*zange*), as well as one of the most important and influential Japanese values—*mujōkan*—underlie the process of symbolic *death-rebirth-reconnection* in Naikan therapy to form a basis for the method's key therapeutic functions to manifest themselves. The physical setting and stringent rules required for the intensive Naikan practice are *sine qua non* for this symbolic process to unfold successfully. The first step of this process is stepping across the threshold of daily routine to that of seclusion and silence. Exactly this step reflects Naikan's evolvement out of *mishirabe* and corresponds to the practice's essence as a "preparation for death" (Ozawa-de Silva 2006: 27). Similarly to the ancient rites of *incubatio*, the Naikan practitioner, too, is left all alone not only physically—they may wish for human communication, but all they find is more and more of their own solitude; even the only possible communication during the practice—that with the interviewer—is limited to reporting briefly the answers to the three questions. With the interviewer not responding, but only bowing ritualistically, the entire communication is taken out of the human world's "ordinariness" to a new state where "extraordinary" healing is likely to occur.

6.2.2.2 Naikan's Benefits to the Body

We should remember that, paradoxically, Naikan therapy do not consider healing as an end in itself. Healing appears much too limited a concept, and symptoms and diseases are never addressed directly in the Naikanistic context. Rather, Naikan therapy tries to take its clients beyond the health-sickness dichotomy while helping them polish their skills in reversing roles with others and thus realize the multi-faceted miracle of existence. Once this task is completed, healing occurs as a natural effect of the newly-acquired holistic point of view—it is this awareness that is pursued, rather than self-centered mental and physical health *per se*.

Despite Ishin Yoshimoto's initial opposition to the acknowledgement of Naikan's therapeutic effect on physical diseases, such an effect has been reported by hundreds of intensive Naikan practitioners. Positive outcomes are observed and reported by both clients and interviewers: the practitioner feels their whole body is light and at the same time full of energy; they do not get tired and do not need as much time for sleep; do not become sick and if they eventually do, they recover relatively quickly; chronic conditions such as arthritis, stuttering, high blood pressure, urticarial symptoms, liver cirrhosis, and an array of neurotic symptoms disappear before long (Takeda in Sato 1972: 227).

In the Japanese-language literature on Naikan, there are many reports on intriguing cases of physical illnesses being alleviated or completely cured by Naikan practice. These include the remarkable improvement of a 38-year-old woman's asthma and facial eczema that she had had for 10 years (Ikemi in Sato 1972: 299–300); the complete healing of a 34-year-old woman suffering for over 10 years of psychogenic vomiting (Ichijo et al. 1991); the case of a 53-year-old alcohol addict suffering from generalized alopecia who quit abusing alcohol and whose hair started growing (Matsushita and Nakamura 1992); the significant improvement of a 15-year-old girl's severe atopic dermatitis (Yamauchi and Ichii in Kawahara 1998: 107); the healing of a 61-year-old woman diagnosed with psychogenic pain disorder with severe muscle aches throughout the body that painkillers could not alleviate (Miki and Miki 2009); a female in her 20s completely recovering from a severe eating disorder (Miki and Miki 2011); and even the astonishing case of cervical cancer completely cured within a few weeks (Nakano in Ishii 2011: 79–81), etc. Such outcomes are astonishing, considering that at first glance Naikan is totally irrelevant to issues concerning body and physical health—it seems that Naikan even disregards the body, confining it to a secluded narrow space with all possible bodily movements curbed to a minimum. As "the final chapter of many people's life narratives is short on action but strong on reflection" (Scarre in Kellehear 2009: 158), so is the Naikan practice: instead of escaping the problem through talking or through some other activity, Naikan forces the person to stay where the problem is. "One cannot go anywhere, because there is nowhere to go. One must confront the issue" (Ozawa-de Silva 2006: 34).

Undoubtedly, seclusion and physical stillness "facilitate interior stillness, alertness, and calm" (Laird 2011: 16), but they also bring on "increased awareness of bodily sensations" (Reynolds 1980: 111). As the American theologian Martin Laird points out about the practice of contemplation, it "begins with our attention and our bodies" (Laird 2011: 15); and so does Naikan, too. Albiet not directly, Naikan is informed by the Eastern body–mind theory. As we specified in Part II (see footnote 7 in Sect. 4.2), according to this theory, body and mind cannot be distinguished from each other; they are even perceived as the same entity: *shinshin-ichinyo* (心身一如) or *nini-funi* (二而不二), i.e., "one is two, two is one; two sides of the same coin" (Ichikawa et al. 1977: 183), for which reason "any treatment of the body cannot be separated from psychological and spiritual dimensions" (Sheikh et al. 1996: xxi). The ancient medical texts of Japan postulate that the remedy for every disease should be considered from the standpoint of the relation between the patient's form/flesh (形•肉体) and will/mind (志•精神) (Shinmura 2006: 13). This concept is reflected on a linguistic level with phrases such as *yamai-wa-ki-kara* (病は気から), which means that diseases originate in the mind, implying that despite the lack of scientific validation the East has already solved the key issue of the psychosomatic medicine (Masunaga in Sato 1972: 110). Moreover, if we go back to the Naikan's predecessor—*mishirabe*—and consider the meaning that the Japanese put into the word *mi* (again see footnote 7 in Sect. 4.2), we understand that although matters of physical diseases or well-being appear irrelevant to Naikan, in fact they are deeply related with each other. Taking as evidence cases of chronic illnesses cured or showing significant improvement after intensive Naikan practice, we suggest the following explanation, which is based on the above-mentioned key therapeutic functions of Naikan, the *mirroring function* and the *existential grounding function*:

- Through the Naikan's *mirroring function*, i.e., seeing themselves mirrored in others and in their relationship with them, the practitioner sees their own imperfections and may thus gain insights about their disease, too. That is, they may remember what life they led back at the time they became ill, whether they experienced any interpersonal conflicts or faced challenges at work, how they responded them, etc. If we agree that every disease originates in the mind, then it means that any "unprocessed" emotions of our past function as a nuclear fuel waste—buried, but still hazardous—bound to emerge sooner or later on physical level in the form of a disease. Therefore, although in Naikan healing is not an end in itself, through the process of reconstructing their past and seeing their relations with others in a new light, the practitioner has the chance to "dissolve" those "hazardous" emotions of their past, which were perhaps related to the onset of their disease.
- Through the Naikan's *existential grounding function*, i.e., recognizing oneself as an integral part of the whole, the self starts to function in a reformulated network of relationships. The focus of this network is not the self anymore, but its relation with others and the Other-power (*tariki*). That is how the practitioner's awareness regarding their own existence shifts naturally from "I am who live" to "I am who *is* lived".[40] It is exactly the focus shift, we suggest, that helps the practitioner reconcile with the world and, as a result, regain the natural harmony between their body and mind. Once restored, this harmony eventually fosters the alleviation or cure of physiological symptoms as well.

Considering the indirect physical benefits of the Naikan practice, one may suggest that practicing Naikan toward one's own body, i.e., answering the three Naikan questions in regard to the way the client has treated their body in the past—*shintai-naikan* (身体内観)—might be reasonable. Indeed, *shintai-naikan* has proven efficacious by some cases of chronic diseases such as arthritis being cured. When the practitioner explores their past in this way, they may realize that their life hitherto would not have been possible had not their body served them (Ichimaru in Kawahara et al. 1999: 97–100). As a result, they may develop what the Naikan specialist Noriaki Kouguchi formulates as "gratitude toward one's body and viscera", which stimulates the bodily functions and is perhaps related to the alleviation or even cure of physical symptoms; moreover, the *shintai-naikan* may help the client nurture their gratitude also toward their parents and ancestors—one of the key purposes of the orthodox Naikan (Kouguchi in Miki et al. 2007: 197).

On the other hand, not all Naikan specialists entertain the *shintai-naikan* concept because it misdirects the vector of one's reflection and attention toward the self and

---

[40]This process appears somewhat similar to that of "self-emptying" of one's will, known as *kenosis* in the Christian theology. It is summarized in the Apostle Paul's words "I am crucified with Christ: nevertheless I live; yet not I, but Christ liveth in me" (Galatians 2: 20). We find this similarity interesting to mention in the context of Naikan therapy especially if we take into account that many Naikan clients "start to use passive expressions such as *ikasareteiru* ("being lived"), *aisareteiru* ("being loved") and *kizukasetemorau* ("being led to sudden insight")" (Ozawa-de Silva 2006: 10–11).

blurs the required focus on one's interpersonal relationships.[41] In the next section we elucidate further this issue in Naikan therapy through a brief comparison with the Freudian psychoanalysis.

6.3 Naikan Therapy and Freudian Psychoanalysis—A Brief Comparison

In our attempt to further understand what makes Naikan a distinctive Japanese psychotherapy, it would be well justified to compare it with non-Japanese approaches. Naikan can be interpreted in the light of and compared with Western approaches such as cognitive-behavioral therapy, family and brief psychotherapy, dream analysis, etc. (see the introduction of Sect. 6.2). However, here we focus on the parallel between Naikan and Freudian psychoanalysis, considering not only the key role which psychoanalysis played in the development of the Western psychology, but also the fact that one of the pioneers who brought Naikan to the scientific scene in Japan was the Freudian psychiatrist Rokurō Ishida (see Sect. 6.1.4.3). As previously mentioned, in his clinical practice Ishida applied psychoanalytic techniques in combination with Naikan and reported positive outcomes for the treatment of neurosis and psychosomatic diseases (Ishida in Okumura et al. 1972: 87).

The ultimate goal of every psychotherapeutic approach could be summarized in "helping the client solve their psychological and psychosomatic problems, gain self-knowledge and eventually attain personal growth in a sheltered non-daily environment." Such a goal is usually tinted by the personality of the founder of the approach and also by the theoretical framework the method is based upon. In the case of Naikan, however, no particular scientific theory can be discovered behind it —only a centuries-old spiritual tradition, which, as previously explained, was transformed into psychotherapy over the past 40–50 years owing to the firsthand religious experience of a Buddhist priest, Rev. Ishin Yoshimoto.

In Table 6.3 we present a comparison between some key points in Naikan therapy and Freudian psychoanalysis, starting with the physical environment. This comparison allows us to conclude that except for the retrospection and exploration of one's own past and the focus on the key figures in one's life, hardly are there other commonalities between the two approaches: although both of them abide by strict rules and require efforts of putting one's memories of past into words, their ultimate goals are by no means similar. As Nagayama and Shimizu summarize, the psychoanalytic retrospection is *external*, i.e., it deals predominantly with the

[41]In private communication with Junko Miki, Director of Nara Naikan Training Center (May 2011).

Table 6.3 A brief comparison between Naikan therapy and Freudian psychoanalysis (partly summarized from Yamamoto in Okumura et al. 1972: 73–76; Kitami in Baba et al. 1990: 241–262; Ichimaru in Kawahara et al. 1999: 32–46; Krech 2002: 197–205; Chervenkova 2013: 43)

	Freudian psychoanalysis	**Naikan therapy**
Where	Counseling room	Naikan training center
Who	One analyst/therapist: one analysand/client	Several interviewers: several practitioners
Body posture	The client lies down on a sofa	The client sits on the floor surrounded by a folding screen
Frequency	Sessions of 50 to 60 min, one to five times a week	Five-minute interviews on every 2 hours from 6 am to 9 pm (a total of 7–8 interviews a day)
Therapy duration	May be life-long	One-week intensive practice, followed up by daily Naikan practice
*	*	*
Cultural background	European culture; Greek mythology; Judaism	Japanese culture; *Jōdo Shinshū* Buddhism and the austere religious practice of *mishirabe*
Philosophical and theoretical background	All inner conflicts stem from the tense opposition between Eros (life instinct) and Thanatos (death instinct); Oedipus complex theory	All inner conflicts stem from the individual's innate ignorance and desires of their Ego, which dim their real Buddha-nature
Founders	Sigmund Freud (1856–1939) an Austrian-born neurologist and psychiatrist of Jewish origin	Ishin Yoshimoto (1916–1988) a Japanese *Jōdo Shinshū* priest
*	*	*
Key therapeutic tools	Free associations (however, the client has to report all of them to the therapist)	Three well-structured themes (however, the client chooses themselves which of the memories to report to the interviewer)
Part of the client/practitioner's past elucidated	Explores the ways the client has been hurt, mistreated and traumatized, i.e., the focus falls primarily on *negative emotions*	Explores the ways the practitioner has been cared for and the ways they have responded, i.e., the focus falls on *real facts*
Locus of control	During therapy, the client may often blame others for their problems	During the practice, the practitioner learns to take responsibility for their own conduct and the problems they have caused to others
Role of the therapist/interviewer (1)	The therapist confirms the client's previous experience	The interviewer supports the practitioner so that the practitioner can reverse their roles with others and, in so doing, better understand how others have felt and what they have experienced as a result of the practitioner's behavior
Role of the therapist/interviewer (2)	The therapist analyzes and interprets the client's memories, dreams, and free associations	The interviewer never analyzes what the practitioner reports; they only listen, offering a structured framework for the reflection process[a]

(continued)

Table 6.3 (continued)

	Freudian psychoanalysis	**Naikan therapy**
Therapist/interviewer—client/practitioner relationship (1)	The therapist places themselves in a superior position even literally, i.e., during the session they sit on a chair while the client is lying on the sofa	The interviewer keeps a humble attitude—during the interview they sit in front of the practitioner; also, before and after every interview they joins their palms as if in prayer and bow
Therapist/interviewer—client/practitioner relationship (2)	The therapist assumes a paternalistic attitude toward the client	The interviewer assumes both paternalistic and maternal attitude toward the practitioner: they remain strict during the interviews, but at the same time provide for the practitioner's physical comfort (prepare food, bathtub, etc.)[b]
Key points of the therapeutic process	Transference and countertransference are part of the therapeutic process; they are considered signs of progress. Also, the psycho-emotional catharsis is believed to allow emotional energy discharge and hence to alleviate the pressure that causes the problem	The Naikan setting is difficult to provide conditions for the occurrence of transference and countertransference and hence, for attachment to the interviewer. The focus is shifted from the therapist–client relationship to the practitioner's interpersonal relationships and their own attempt to redefine them. During this process, emotional catharsis may naturally occur, but it is not an end in itself
General attitude toward silence and isolation/seclusion	The time and space of the psychoanalytic session are non-ordinary, yet silence and sense of isolation are most often considered defense mechanisms	Silence and seclusion are intrinsic parts of the entire Naikan setting and therapeutic process
General attitude toward the body–mind concept	Body is considered to serve the pleasure principle; strong emphasis on sexuality	Unity of body and mind
Ultimate goals	Strengthening the Ego and enlarging its organization: "Where Id was, there Ego shall be"	Conquering the Ego and self-centeredness: "Where Ego was, there enlightenment/Buddha nature shall be"
Results	Undergoing psychoanalysis, the client improves their self-esteem	Doing Naikan, the practitioner comes away with a more accurate self-image, and develops appreciation and gratitude toward others and the world

[a]As founder Yoshimoto stated "The practitioner has not come to listen to my talks, but to practice Naikan themselves. I am the one who only listens and follows them" (as cited by Miki in Kawahara et al. 1999: 186)

[b]Commenting Yoshimoto's life story, Teruaki Maeshiro and Mieko Hariki draw parallels between Jungian psychology and Naikan, and suggest that both are strongly influenced by the maternal principle in contrast to the paternalistic Freudian approach (Maeshiro and Hariki 1994: 50–51)

client's resentments against others, while the Naikan retrospection is *internal* for it deals with real facts related to how the client themselves behaved toward others (Nagayama and Shimizu 2006: 308).[42] It means that the two appraoches' view on human nature, too, is fundamentally different—while psychoanalysis focuses on the individual and strives to confirm their dominant role, Naikan considers the individual placed within a network of interdependencies. In other words, the center of the psychoanalytic mandala is occupied by the individual *per se* and their inner world—sometimes at the expense of the reality they share with others; by contrast, the Naikanistic mandala has no center, but, as in the wondrous jewel net of Indra (see footnote 39), all of its parts owe their existence to relations of interdependence where no room for superiority or inferiority is left. For this reason, during the Naikan practice the interviewer may appear rather cold and distanced—this is a way to help the practitioner see the unbiased truth about the mutual reality they share, not the subjective truth as seen through the prism of their own fluctuating emotions. It does not mean that Naikan "denies the value of our emotions" (Krech 2002: 198) or belittles them at the expense of some vague supreme truth; it simply uses real facts as a tool for gaining profound self-knowledge based on the understanding of the common human nature that surpasses all social and cultural boundaries.

That is how the terms "sense of guilt" and "attachment" widely used in the psychoanalytic context, in Naikan are broadened to gaining insights about "one's innate sin" and "others' constant love and support." As with other emotions, Naikan does not deny the fact that we have experienced pain or have been hurt, but it does not focus on them alone. Rather, it helps us "view that pain in the larger context of the love and care others gave us" (Krech 2002: 200), because "the care and love received were just as real as the abuse" (ibid.). In the end, "any effort to seek the truth about our past must attempt to paint an accurate picture that includes everything, not just the pain" (ibid.). Such a broad viewpoint underlies the whole process of redefinition of one's past, making Naikan a challenging therapy. On the other hand, precisely because of these characteristics, Naikan can be considered, Miki suggests, a "shortcut" to insights that can be gained through years of psychoanalytic treatment.[43]

6.4 Conclusion

Over the process of Naikan's transformation out of *mishirabe*, founder Ishin Yoshimoto used to state that the approach had nothing to do with religion. However, in its essence Naikan remains deeply religious considering that when the

[42]More common points could be found between Naikan therapy and the Kleinian psychoanalysis, which includes such concepts as the good mother, envy, reparation (atonement), and sense of guilt, all of them considered pillars of the early childhood development. For further references on this comparison, see Kitami in Baba et al. (1990: 241–248).

[43]In private communication with Junko Miki, Director of Nara Naikan Training Center (May 2011).

practitioner retreats into a prolonged silence and self-reflection they may gain insight into their primordial interconnectedness with others and the world.[44] Surprisingly, however, Naikan is not interested in others—what kind of people they are, how nice or unfairly they have behaved toward us, etc. The answer to these questions Naikan considers based upon the quicksand of our own delusive mental constructs about others. Rather, Naikan is interested in the practitioner as the protagonist of their own unique life story. Thus, although the accent in the three questions seems to be put on the self—namely "What has…done for *me*?," "What have *I* done for him/her?," "What troubles have *I* caused?"—it is in fact only a part of the wider context of interdependent relationships.

As the Japanese-born American anthropologist Chikako Ozawa-de Silva points out, "most clients start Naikan with unquestioned confidence in the objectivity and factuality of their life stories. Gradually, however, clients start to see how their autobiographies are subjective and biased by their rigid perspectives on others, and they often start realizing that their autobiographical narratives are self-made constructs, subjective attempts to make sense of events and the actions of others. Through gradual and often painful stages, practitioners realize their utter dependence on other people, to the extent that their sense of being a self-made person collapses. Then, for the first time, the clients are able to see others, such as their mothers, as autonomous independent subjects, distinct from their previous expectations about how those people should be; and correspondingly, the clients begin to truly appreciate them" (Ozawa-de Silva 2007: 430). Thus, the root cause of suffering should not be sought in external conditions or in other people, but rather in one's own mind and conduct.

In the end, Naikan appears to be an approach through which culture-bound values and concepts such as these of seclusion and silence, the sense of impermanence (*mujōkan*), and the all-embracing grace (*tariki*) have been naturally turned into therapeutic tools without, however, the initial purposeful goal for healing. Naikan functions more as a way of life whose ultimate goal is the increased awareness both of oneself and the world. We all are "sick persons"—*byōnin*—whose conduct is driven by ignorance. For this reason, similarly to Shinran, Ishin Yoshimoto encouraged people to encounter their own shadows, suggesting that no boundaries exist between healthy and sick, good and bad people—we are all together in an ever-interdependent world: like pine trees—one of the "three friends of winter" (see Chap. 2 and Appendix II)—that owe their existence to the common ground, which nourishes their roots and helps them reach up to the skies strong and steadfast. However, in order to gain profound understanding of this matter, as in the ancient rites of *incubatio*, in Naikan therapy too we first need to seclude ourselves from the world both physically and metaphorically; to break up our old ignorance-based ties with it and pass through the hardships of the symbolic death-rebirth process so as to reconnect with the world in a more constructive and

[44]The interpretation of Naikan's religious essence (in a very broad sense of the word) we base on the etymology of the word "religion," which originates from the Latin *religare*—"to reconnect" (see Sect. 6.1.5.).

consistent way. In contrast to all talking psychotherapies, in Naikan—an archaeology of spirit, we do this job by ourselves; there is no one to analyze and interpret our life story. The symbolic process of reconnection that we perform inside of us paves the way to greater awareness and harmony, which naturally engender healing.

References

Addiss, Stephen, G. Groemer, J. Th. Rimer: Traditional Japanese Arts and Culture—An Illustrated Sourcebook, University of Hawai'i Press, 2006

Andrews, Allan A.: World Rejection and Pure Land Buddhism in Japan, Japanese Journal of Religious Studies, Vol. 4(4), Nanzan Institute for Religion and Culture, 1977

Anesaki, Masaharu: History of Japanese Religion: with Special Reference to the Social and Moral Life of the Nation, Kegan Paul, Trench, Trubner & Co, 1963

Anesaki, Masaharu: Art, Life and Nature in Japan, Tuttle (Charles E.) Co Inc, 1974

Baba, Ken'ichi, A. Fukushima, K. Ogawa, Y.Yamanaka (ed.): Depth Analysis of the Japanese Psyche—Depths of Maternity, Yuhikaku Publishing, 1984 (in Japanese)

Baba, Ken'ichi, A. Fukushima, K. Ogawa, Y.Yamanaka (ed.): Depth Analysis of the Japanese Psyche—Depths of the Japanese People, Yuhikaku Publishing, 1990 (in Japanese)

Bary, Wm. Theodore de (ed.): Introduction to Asian Civilizations: Sources of Japanese Tradition, Vol.1 (complied by Ryusaku Tsunoda, Wm. Theodore de Bary, Donald Keene), Columbia University Press, 1964

Becker, Carl: Death Experience—In Search of Near-Death Phenomena, Hozokan, 1992 (in Japanese)

Befu, Harumi: Japan: An Anthropological Introduction, Harper&Row Publishers Inc, 1971

Callicott, J.Baird, R.T. Ames (ed.): Nature in Asian Traditions of Thought—Essays in Environmental Philosophy, State University of New York Press, 1989

Chervenkova, Velizara: Application of Naikan Therapy to Bulgarians—Its Challenges and Possibilities (Comparative Study of Written Naikan to Drug-Addicted and Healthy Persons), Journal of the Japan Naikan Association, Vol. 18, Japan Naikan Assocation, 2012 (in Japanese)

Chervenkova, Velizara: A Pilgrimage toward the Self—Personal Experiences in Intensive Naikan, Annals of Educational Studies, Vol. 18, Osaka University, 2013 (in Japanese)

Chervenkova, Velizara: Rites of Incubation in the Modern World: The Symbolic Experience of *Death-Rebirth-Reconnection* in Naikan Therapy, World Cultural Psychiatry Research Review, Vol. 9(3), World Association of Cultural Psychiatry, 2014

Dobbins, James C.: Jodo Shinshu—Shin Buddhism in Medieval Japan, University of Hawai'i Press, 2002

Faber, Melvin D.: Synchronicity—C.G. Jung, Psychoanalysis and Religion, Praeger Publishers, 1998

Fleischman, Paul R.: The Healing Spirit—Case Studies in Religion and Psychotherapy, SPCK, 1989

Harding, Christopher, F. Iwaki, S. Yoshinaga (ed.): Religion and Psychotherapy in Modern Japan, Routledge, 2015

Hatano, Fumihiko: Why Is the Naikan Method Efficacious?—The Science of Self-Insight, Shinzansha Publisher, 1999 (in Japanese)

Hattori, Sawako: Considerations on Naikan and the Self Time, Proceedings of the 34th Annual Congress of the Japan Naikan Association, Japan Naikan Association, 2011 (in Japanese)

Hiekata, Tomizou: Aesthetics of the Japanese People, Waseda Publishing, 2009 (in Japanese)

Hoffmann, Yoel (transl.): Japanese Death Poems Written by Zen Monks and Haiku Poets on the Verge of Death, Tuttle Publishing, 1986

Ichijo, Nobuko, T. Kawauchi, T. Takemoto: Cure of Bilious Attacks through Naikan Therapy—A Case Report, Proceedings of the 14th Annual Congress of the Japan Naikan Association, Japan Naikan Association, 1991 (in Japanese)
Ichikawa, Hiroshi, Yamazaki Award Selection Committee: Phenomenology of Body, Kawade Shobo Shinsha, 1977 (in Japanese)
Ichikawa, Hiroshi: The Structure of *Mi*—Beyond the Body Theories, Kodansha Gakujutsu Bunko, 1993 (in Japanese)
Igarashi, Kazuo: Naikan Zen—A Possible Suggestion, Proceedings of the 14th Annual Congress of the Japan Naikan Association, Japan Naikan Association, 1991 (in Japanese)
Ihara, Shō'ichi: Naikan as Psychotherapy, Paper presented at the 24th Nakan Therapy Workshop in Kyoto ("On the Naikan Role in Psychotherapy"), October 2012, (unpublished; in Japanese)
Ishii, Akira: Self-Transformation within a Week—The Wonder of Naikan Method, Kodansha Sophia Books, 1999 (in Japanese)
Ishii, Akira: Naikan Therapy (in "Personal History and Psychotherapy"), Yasuda Life Welfare Foundation, 2000 (in Japanese)
Ishii, Akira: An Invitation to Naikan, Nishimura Kikaku Shuppan, 2011 (in Japanese)
Itsuki, Hiroyuki: Tariki: Embracing Despair, Discovering Peace, Kodansha Ltd, 2001
Itsuki, Hiroyuki: Self-Power and Other-Power, Chikuma Shobo, 2014 (in Japanese)
Iwaoka, Masashi: Searching for the Origins of Naikan Method—What Ishin Yoshimoto Meant to Say, Soei Publishing, 2002 (in Japanese)
Japan Naikan Association (ed.): Devoted to Naikan—The Life of Ishin Yoshimoto, Japan Naikan Association, 1989 (in Japanese)
Kamei, Katsu'ichiro: *Mujōkan*—Japanese Culture Research (3), Shinchosha Publishing, 1969 (in Japanese)
Kanamitsu, Toshio: Eastern Wisdom, Naikan—A Method for Soul Cleansing, Kounsha, 1985 (in Japanese)
Kaneko, Daiei: The Meaning of Salvation in the Doctrine of Pure Land Buddhism, The Eastern Buddhist—New Series, Vol.I (1), Eastern Buddhist Society, 1965
Kawahara, Ryuzo: Naikan Therapy, Shinkoh Igaku Shuppansha, 1996 (in Japanese)
Kawahara, Ryuzo (ed.): Clinical Naikan Therapy—Theory and Application, Shinkoh Igaku Shuppansha, 1998 (in Japanese)
Kawahara, Ryuzo, Y. Higashi, Y. Miki (ed.): The Essence of Psychotherapy—Considering the Naikan Therapy, Nippon Hyoron Sha, 1999 (in Japanese)
Kawai, Hayao: Introduction to Psychotherapy: Psychotherapeutic Approaches—Collection IV, Iwanami Shoten, 2009 (in Japanese)
Keel, Hee-Sung: Understanding Shinran—A Dialogical Approach, Asian Humanities Press, 1995
Kellehear, Allan (ed.): The Study of Dying—From Autonomy to Transformation, Cambridge University Press, 2009
Krech, Gregg: Naikan: Gratitude, Grace, and the Japanese Art of Self-Reflection, Stone Bridge Press, 2002
Kurita, Isamu: Reading Zen Master Hakuin—Reviving the Secrets of "Body-Mind Harmonization Method, Naikan", Shodensha Ogon Bunko, 2001 (in Japanese)
Kusanagi, Masao: Aesthetics of *Yūgen*, Hanawa Shobo, 1973 (in Japanese)
Kusano, Makoto: Thanatology and Naikan, Journal of the Japan Naikan Association, Vol.7, Japan Naikan Association, 2001a (in Japanese)
Kusano, Makoto: The Theme of Death and Rebirth in Naikan—The World of a Naikan Practitioner in Pictures, Japanese Naikan Medical Association, 2001b (in Japanese)
Kusunoki, Masami: The Mechanism of Naikan, Naikan Training Center, 1980 (in Japanese)
Kusunoki, Masami: Soul Voyage—Naikan Method, Japan Naikan Association, 1983 (in Japanese)
Laird, Martin: A Sunlit Absence—Silence, Awareness, and Contemplation, Oxford University Press, 2011
Lebra, Takie Sugiyama: Japanese Patterns of Behavior, University of Hawaii Press, 1976
Lebra, Takie Sugiyama: The Japanese Self in Cultural Logic, University of Hawaii Press, 2004

Lebra, Takie Sugiyama, W. P. Lebra (ed.): Japanese Culture and Behavior: Selected Readings, University of Hawaii Press, 1974
Machida, Soho: Renegade Monk—Honen and Japanese Pure Land Buddhism, University of California Press, 1999
Maeshiro, Teruaki: Mysteries of the Soul from the Standpoint of Clinical Psychology—A Talk on Naikan, Tokishobo, 2001 (in Japanese)
Maeshiro, Teruaki: Naikan as Psychotherapy, Tokishobo, 2005 (in Japanese)
Maeshiro, Teruaki: Naikan Therapy in Japan: Introspection as a Way of Healing—Introduction to Naikan Therapy, World of Cultural Psychiatry Research Review, Vol. 4(1), World Association of Cultural Psychiatry, 2009
Maeshiro, Teruaki: On the *Mi* in Mishirabe, retrieved from http://yamato-mahoroba.sakura.ne.jp/blog/2010/03/post-62.html, Yamato Mahoroba-no-Kai (Yamato Naikan Training Center), 2010 (in Japanese)
Maeshiro, Teruaki, M. Hariki: Ishin Yoshimoto—A Brief Life Story (part 1), Proceeedings of the 17th Annual Congress of the Japan Naikan Association, Japan Naikan Association, 1994 (in Japanese)
Maeshiro, Teruaki, M. Hariki: Ishin Yoshimoto—A Brief Life Story (part 3), Proceedings of the 18th Annual Congress of the Japan Naikan Association, Japan Naikan Association, 1995 (in Japanese)
Matsunami, Kodo (ed.): A Guide to Japanese Buddhism, Japan Buddhist Federation, 2004
Matsuo, Kenji: A History of Japanese Buddhism, Global Oriental, 2007
Matsushita, Muneji, H. Nakamura: On the Combined Application of Naikanistic Psychotherapy and Autogenic Training to Generalized Alopecia associated with Alcohol Syndrome, Proceedings of the 15th Annual Congress of the Japan Naikan Association, Japan Naikan Association, 1992 (in Japanese)
McDougall, Joyce: Theaters of the Body—A Psychoanalytic Approach to Psychosomatic Illness, W.W. Norton & Company, 1989
Miki, Junko, Y. Miki: Naikan-Based Counseling and Intensive Naikan—Cure of Five-Year Physical Pain, Journal of the Japan Naikan Association, Vol. 15, Japan Naikan Association, 2009 (in Japanese)
Miki, Yoshihiko: Introduction to Naikan Therapy—The World of Japanese Self-Exploration, Sogensha, 1976 (in Japanese)
Miki, Yoshihiko: The Meaning of "Standing in the Other Person's Shoes", Proceedings of the 13th Annual Congress of the Japan Naikan Association, Japan Naikan Association, 1990 (in Japanese)
Miki, Yoshihiko, J. Miki: Naikan Work—Healing the Anxiety and Becoming Happy, Futami Shobo, 1998 (in Japanese)
Miki, Yoshihiko, J. Miki: A Naikan Case Study of Young Woman Suffering from Eating Disorder, Osaka University, 2011 (unpublished; in Japanese)
Miki, Yoshihiko, K. Kuroki (co-ed.): Japanese Psychotherapies—Essence and Practice, Tokishobo, 1998 (in Japanese)
Miki, Yoshihiko, T. Maeshiro (ed.): Naikan Therapy Today—A Psychotherapy Born from Japanese Culture, Contemporary Esprit Journal, Vol. 470, Shibundo Publishing, 2006 (in Japanese)
Miki, Yoshihiko, T. Maeshiro, T. Takemoto: (ed.): Naikan Therapy, Minerva Shobo, 2007 (in Japanese)
Miyake, Tadaroku: Being Saved by Naikan—Re-experiencing Love, Bungeisha Co, 2006 (in Japanese)
Miyazaki, Tadao: What is the Origin of Naikan? (part 2), Naikan News, Vol. 12, Japan Naikan Association, 1992 (in Japanese)
Morigami, Shouyou: The Spirit of *Wabi*, *Sabi*, and *Yūgen*—A Superior Consciousness beyond the Western Philosophy, Sakura-no-Hana Shuppan, 2015 (in Japanese)
Morikawa, Keisho: The Nature of Japanese Aesthetics, Asakura Publishing, 1984 (in Japanese)

Motoyama, Yō'ichi: The Essence of Naikan—Answering Dr. Tamura's Question at the 24th Naikan Congress Symposium, Journal of the Japan Naikan Association, Vol. 8, Japan Naikan Association, 2002 (in Japanese)
Muramatsu, Motonosuke: Zen Buddhism and Naikan—Hints on Living amidst Anxiety and Conflicts, Tokishobo, 1991 (in Japanese)
Muramatsu, Motonosuke: An Invitation to "Door to Self-Discovery", Proceedings of the 18th Annual Congress of the Japan Naikan Association, Japan Naikan Association, 1995 (in Japanese)
Murase, Takao: Fundamental Issues of Naikan-Related Research, Journal of Psychotherapy, Vol. 2 (1), Japanese Psychotherapy Association, 1970 (in Japanese)
Murase, Takao: Psychotherapy and Values—An Introduction (Focusing on the Naikanistic Values), Journal of the Japan Naikan Association, Vol. 1, Japan Naikan Association, 1995 (in Japanese)
Murase, Takao: Naikan—Theory and Cultural Relevance (Clinical Psychology of the Self), Seishin Shobo, 1996 (in Japanese)
Nagashima, Masahiro: A Transformative Approach Considered from Its Origin, Proceedings of the 14th Annual Congress of the Japan Naikan Association, Japan Naikan Association, 1991 (in Japanese)
Nagashima, Masahiro: From the Standpoint of Naikan Method, Journal of the Japan Naikan Association, Vol. 10, Japan Naikan Association, 2004 (in Japanese)
Nagashima, Masahiro, M. Nagashima: Encountering Oneself through Naikan, Shunjusha Publishing, 2001 (in Japanese)
Nagayama, Kei'ichi, Y. Shimizu: Naikan Method—Theory and Practical Structure, Nippon Hyoron Sha, 2006 (in Japanese)
Nakamura, Hajime: History of Japanese Thought, Kegan Paul, 2002
Neumann, Erich: The Great Mother—An Analysis of the Archetype, Routledge & Kegan Paul, 1955
Nishimuta, Hisao: Philosophy of Death, Tokyo Tosho Publishing, 2009 (in Japanese)
Noguchi, Michizō: Human Being as a Primordial Life Form—Theory of Noguchi Gymnastics, Iwanami Shoten, 2003 (in Japanese)
Oda, Takao: Psychotherapy and the Japanese Soul—Living the Myths, Baifukan, 2005 (in Japanese)
Ohnuki-Tierney, Emiko: Illness and Culture in Contemporary Japan—An Anthropological View, Cambridge University Press, 1984
Okumura, Nikichi, K. Sato, H. Yamamoto (ed.): Naikan Therapy, Igaku-Shoin, 1972 (in Japanese)
Ozawa-de Silva, Chikako: Psychotherapy and Religion in Japan—The Japanese Introspection Practice of Naikan, Routledge, 2006
Ozawa-de Silva, Chikako: Demystifying Japanese Therapy: An Analysis of Naikan and the Ajase Complex through Buddhist Thought, Ethos (Journal of the Society for Psychological Anthropology), Vol. 35(4), The Society for Psychological Anthropology, 2007
Pilgrim, Richard B.: Buddhism and the Arts of Japan, Anima Books, 1981
Reischauer, August Karl: Studies in Japanese Buddhism, AMS Press, 1970
Reynolds, David K.: The Quiet Therapies—Japanese Pathways to Personal Growth, University of Hawaii Press, 1980
Richie, Donald: A Tractate on Japanese Aesthetics, Stone Bridge Press, 2007
Ritter, Franz: Naikan and the European Psychotherapies, Journal of the Japan Naikan Association, Vol. 8, Japan Naikan Association, 2002 (in Japanese)
Sato, Koji (ed.): Zen Psychotherapy—Naikan Method, Bunkodo, 1972 (in Japanese)
Sato, Mimasa: On the Yoshimoto-Style Naikan Method, Journal of Contemporary Esoteric Buddhism, Vol. 6, Chisan Denboin, 1993 (in Japanese)
Sengoku, Mari: Naikan Therapy and Pure Land Buddhism—The Relationship between Psychotherapy and Buddhism in the United States, Journal of the Japan Naikan Association, Vol. 11, Japan Naikan Association, 2005 (in Japanese)

Sheikh, Anees A., K.S. Sheikh, J. Achterberg (ed.): Healing East and West—Ancient Wisdom and Modern Psychology, John Wiley & Sons Inc, 1996
Shepherd, Kathleen M.: The Land and Life of Japan, Edinburgh House Press, 1937
Shimizu, Yasuhiro: Theory of Practical Naikan Interview, Journal of the Japan Naikan Association, Vol. 5, Japan Naikan Association, 1999 (in Japanese)
Shinmura, Taku (ed.): History of Japanese Medicine, Yoshikawa Kobunkan, 2006 (in Japanese)
Stanley-Baker, Joan: Japanese Art, Thames and Hudson, 1984
Suzuki, Daisetz T.: Japanese Spirituality, Iwanami Bunko, 1972 (in Japanese)
Suzuki, Daisetz T.: Japanese Spirituality (transl. Norman Waddell), Greenwood Press, 1988
Suzuki, Daisetz T.: Buddha of Infinite Light—The Teachings of Shin Buddhism, the Japanese Way of Wisdom and Compassion, Shambala Publications, 1998
Takemoto, Takahiro (ed.): Meditation Psychotherapies (Theory and Practice of Naikan Therapy), Contemporary Esprit Journal, Vol. 202, Shibundo Publishing, 1984 (in Japanese)
Takemoto, Takahiro: Compositon of Naikan Method, Proceedings of the 12th Annual Congress of the Japan Naikan Association, Japan Naikan Association, 1989 (in Japanese)
Takemoto, Takahiro: Naikan and Medicine, Ibusuki Takemoto Hospital's Naikan Training Center, 1994 (in Japanese)
Takino, Isao: Naikan as Mourning Work, Proceedings of the 3rd Annual Congress of the Japan Naikan Association, Japan Naikan Association, 1980 (in Japanese)
Tanaka, Hide: Clinical Psychology Research on the Intensive Naikan Experience—An Attempt for Interpretation of Naikan Therapy from Analytical Psychology's Viewpoint, Osaka University, 2004 (in Japanese)
Tanaka, Kyubun: Philosophizing the Japanese Aestethics—*Aware, Yūgen, Sabi, and Iki*, Seidosha, 2013 (in Japanese)
Tanni-shō: Notes Lamenting Differences (transl. Ryōsetsu Fujiwara), Ryukoku Translation Center, Rykoku University, 1962
Unno, Mark: Buddhism and Psychotherapy across Cultures—Essays on Theories and Practices, Wisdom Publications Inc, 2006
Usami, Shuue: Thank You for the Tears—From Naikan to *Fusatsu-Nembutsu*, Senkobo, 1988 (in Japanese)
Uyeda, Isao: Rites of Passage and Purification in Japanese Society: A Study of Shinto Rituals, Self-Transformation and Their Impact upon Japanese Culture, University of Oregon, 1991
Van Gennep, Aronld: Rites of Passage, University of Chicago Press, 1961
Verhagen, Peter J., H.M. Van Praag, J.J.Lopéz-Ibor Jr., et al.: Religion and Psychiatry—Beyond Boundaries, John Wiley&Sons Ltd, 2010
Yalom, Irvin D.: Staring at the Sun: Overcoming the Dread of Death, Piatkus Books, 2008
Yamakuse, Yoji: Heart and Soul of the Japanese (bilingual edition; transl. Michael A. Cooney), IBC Publishing, 2011
Yanagita, Kakusei: Naikan Practice—Training for Self-Consolidation, Inaho Shobo, 1995 (in Japanese)
Yanagita, Kakusei: Psychotherapy of Love, Naikan—A World of Joy and Calmness, Inaho Shobo, 1997 (in Japanese)
Yasuda, Noboru: The Body of the Japanese, Chikuma Shobo, 2014 (in Japanese)
Yatabe, Hidemasa: Aesthetics of Appearance—Body Work Techniques of the Japanese, Chuko Bunko, 2011 (in Japanese)
Yoshimoto, Ishin: Self-Reflection (Naikan), Yamato Gunju Kakou Ltd, 1945 (in Japanese)
Yoshimoto, Ishin: Naikan Method—Forty Years of History, Shunjusha, 1965/1989 (in Japanese)
Yoshimoto, Ishin: Naikan Method, Shunjusha, 1965/2007 (in Japanese)
Yoshimoto, Ishin: Right Up to Establishing Naikan Therapy, Journal of Psychotherapy, Vol. 2(1), Japanese Psychotherapy Association, 1970 (in Japanese)
Yoshimoto, Ishin: A Talk on Naikan, Yasuragi Journal (appendix), Jikohakken-no-Kai, 1977 (in Japanese)
Yoshimoto, Ishin: An Invitation to Naikan, Tokishobo, 1983 (in Japanese)

Yoshimoto, Ishin: Before and After Enlightenment—My Personal Naikan Experiences, Naikan Training Center, 1985 (in Japanese)
Yoshimoto, Ishin: Naikan Daily Calendar—Words by Ishin Yoshimoto, Jikohakken-no-Kai, 2004 (in Japanese)
Yoshimoto, Kiyonobu: *Shinobigusa*—A Life Dedicated to Naikan, Hirai Shinbikan, 1989 (in Japanese)
Yoshimoto, Masanobu, Y. Motoyama: An Interview, retrieved from https://www.aware-publishing.com/interview-20110612.html, Aware Publishing, 2011 (in Japanese)

Chapter 7
Dohsa-hou Therapy—Where Body Meets Soul

I love the idea of life pulsing through people—
blood and movement.

Martha Graham

Among the three representative Japanese psychotherapies presented in this book, Dohsa-hou is the youngest one, with a scientific history of some 50 years. As already discussed in Sect. 4.2, Dohsa-hou emerged in Japan congruent with the global tendencies in the psychological and psychotherapeutic world of "introducing" the body and de-tabooing the possibility of physical contact between therapist and client. Despite this, in contrast to Morita therapy and Naikan therapy, which have to some extent spread in Western Europe and America, Dohsa-hou is yet to gain popularity beyond Japan and some other Asian countries such as India, Malaysia, Thailand, and Iran. Moreover, apart from a few articles,[1] the English-language literature on Dohsa-hou is yet very scarce and the approach remains confined exclusively to the professional circles in Japan.

In the next chapter we present Dohsa-hou's history, development and theoretical background, and explain the importance of bodily movement and nonverbal communication as key therapeutic tools in this approach.

7.1 Life Is Movement, Movement Is Life

Dohsa-hou and its therapeutic tools are based on one simple truth about life: no living creature exists without moving and changing a whit; and so is it for everything else in the Universe as we know it—from the waxing and waning of the Moon to the growth and shrinkage of the tiniest cell. Movement and change are the utmost expressions of life and are essential to its continuation. Human beings make no exception to this basic law of life: we constantly express movement through our

[1]For example, Naruse (1992b), Harizuka (2006), Ghanimi (2007), Bangayan and Imura (2009), and Chervenkova and Imura (2012).

V. Chervenkova, *Japanese Psychotherapies*,
DOI 10.1007/978-981-10-3126-7_7

bodies and body is our one and only means for expressing movement—body is "your first and last garment; it is what you enter life in and what you depart life with" (Graham 1991: 7). Then it is in *movement* where body and mind intersect. As the American occupational therapist and movement artist Bonnie Bainbridge Cohen notes, human body can be likened to sand: "it's difficult to study the wind, but if you watch the sand patterns form and disappear and re-emerge, then you can follow the patterns of the wind, or, in this case, the mind" (as cited in Hartley 1995: xxiv).

Indeed, through movement or the lack of such we can gain deeper understanding of the body-mind interconnectedness; we can gain more clarity as to why, for example, patients with catatonic schizophrenia hold an awkward rigid posture and remain in a stuporous state for hours although there is no physiological dysfunction to prevent them from moving; and why, on the other hand, children with cerebral palsy overcome the physiological dysfunction and start moving their limbs. In fact, it was the astonishing case of a young patient with cerebral palsy moving his paralyzed arm under hypnosis that sparked the development of Dohsa-hou as an original Japanese psycho-rehabilitative therapy based on a completely new understanding of human bodily movements.

7.1.1 Sailing Uncharted Seas—Gosaku Naruse's Path to Dohsa-hou

Although many Japanese scientists were involved in successful experimental research on concepts of bodily movements, the pioneer and founder of Dohsa-hou is considered Gosaku Naruse. Naruse was born in Gifu prefecture in 1924. He graduated from an elite military school and later, when Japan was on the verge of its defeat in World War II, he joined the army for a while. Later on, his observations and personal experiences of that time inspired his research interest in the specificities of human body posture as represented, for example, in military commands such as "Attention! Eyes front!" (Naruse 1992a: 74).

Naruse majored in Psychology at the Tokyo Bunrika University. After he graduated in 1950, he began carrying out research in the field of hypnosis. Later, he underwent training analysis under Heisaku Kosawa, Professor at Tohoku University who had studied at the Vienna Psychoanalytic Institute and had developed the original theory of the Ajase complex. Despite the important experience, psychoanalytic concepts and interpretations did not satisfy Naruse's scientific curiosity and he began studying behavioral therapy, Jacob Moreno's psychodrama and Milton Erikson's interviewing approach. In parallel, he deepened further his research in the field of hypnosis (Naruse in Miki and Kuroki 1998: 128–129), to become the leading researcher of psychological hypnosis in postwar Japan.

In 1964 Naruse came across a report from a facility for children with disabilities in Saitama prefecture, where a 16-year-old boy suffering from cerebral palsy had managed to lift his palsied right arm to fully upright position under hypnosis. This astonishing case was considered the first successful example through which the cerebral palsy and hypnosis research met (Naruse 1998: 14). However, although the boy reported an improvement in the condition of his arm after waking up from the hypnosis, he nevertheless relapsed to the prehypnotic state of stiffness and immobility. Over the course of his research thus prompted, Naruse came to observe children with cerebral palsy during their sleep and confirmed the same phenomenon: their body postures looked relaxed and they moved their limbs relatively freely while, for example, turning in their sleep; but once they woke up, repeating such movements appeared to be impossible.

All these observations made Naruse and his co-researches wonder what actually happened during the hypnotic/sleep states so that, for example, an arm that had been immovable since the child's neonatal age started moving freely? How a motor impairment could be improved if the cause was solely physiological? (Naruse 1998: 17) Referring to the experimental research inspired by the above-described case, Naruse came to the conclusion that although the results achieved during a hypnotic state were temporary and could not be maintained after the client woke up, they suggested that there had to be something else beyond the mere brain functions that made the body move.

This hypothesis brought Naruse to a new horizon where he had to face the popular scientific fallacy that the bodily movements a newborn infant performed were mere mechanical biophysiological phenomena, which occured in response to external stimuli, but could not speak of the infant's mental activities. Such a biased viewpoint Naruse considers the root of all misconceptions not in contemporary psychology alone, but also in the general understanding of the depths of human nature and existence (Naruse 1998: 129–130). Rather, we better entertain a broader point of view and become aware that "a newborn infant moves because *movement is who and what she is*. Movement is what she does and what is making her" (LaMothe 2015: 119); that "if body mirrors the mind, then the mind's state and "movements" too produce certain responses in the body" (Chervenkova and Imura 2012: 36). This relation is clearly manifested in what is known as facial and bodily expression, for example, the bright appearance and the smooth movements when one feels joy and happiness. The mind therefore could be defined as the "engine" that steers body in a certain direction and "shapes" it in one posture or another. This means that the human body and its movements cannot be separated from the mind and considered outside of the psychological framework as mere physiological units; that each and every bodily movement is underpinned by a certain psychological process because our body "is not opposed to our intelligence, to our feelings, to our soul. It includes them and shelters them. By becoming aware of our body we give ourselves access to our entire being—for body and spirit, mental and physical, and even strength and weakness, represent not our duality but our unity" (Bertherat and Bernstein 1989: xi).

7.1.1.1 Dohsa—"To Create a Movement"

Understanding the body-mind unity not as a desk theory but as a real phenomenon that manifests itself directly in any of the activities—mental or physical—that human beings perform (Naruse 2007: 20) made Naruse conclude that, indeed, life is all about movement (Naruse 2007: 24); that movement is the essence of life and a definite proof that one is alive (Naruse 2000: 11–12). Therefore, movement has a deep existential meaning: the individual is constantly searching for a meaningful response to reality and this response is realized through movements united into one coherent network of creative activities. If we take our daily life and its components as an example, we will see that from waking up, washing our face, having breakfast, going to work, and talking with people to going back home and falling asleep—all activities that we perform are realized through the mediation of a certain movement. In sleep, too, numerous movements are performed within our bodies, for example, the eyeball movements, blood circulation, etc. Even the expression of emotions is preceded by a subtle physical tension, which prepares the ground for the emotion to be realized, that is, the body mediates the change between the current state and the state typical of this emotion (Naruse 2007: 24–25).

Considering all of the above, Naruse assumed that if movements were changed, both mind and body would change, thus proposing a new viewpoint toward the bodily movements distinct from the basic physiology principles that considered mainly the activities of the muscle-skeleton and the nervous systems. Basing his arguments on his observations of children with cerebral palsy under and after hypnotic/sleep state, he proposed that "although the child's disabilities might be caused by a physiological dysfunction, their disabilities would be influenced by certain psychological activities" (Naruse, as cited in Harizuka 2006).

With the advancement of his research, Naruse gradually summarized his assumptions and observations into a holistic approach that combines psychic activities with bodily movements and called it *dohsa-hou* (動作法)—"a way to act out; a way to perform an action, behavior or bodily movement; a way to "create a movement"[2] The name itself conveys the idea that when a certain movement is first projected on the screen of the mind, i.e., *internalized* from the realm of the abstract, then it could be performed through the body, i.e., *externalized*. In other words, what "creates" the movement is nothing but the self; hence, every physical movement is a psychological phenomenon *per se* (Naruse 1998: 46–47). Starting from this basic concept, Naruse summarized three key stages whose succession makes this process of externalization possible:

- *Intention*, i.e., the psychological mode that precedes any motor action—for example, if we want to do a handshake we first need to "picture" the movement in our mind and then stretch out our hand to the other person. The intention to do so is the psychological aspect of the movement thanks to which the movement is realized. According to Naruse, it is the misdirected intention that is to be

[2]The word *dohsa*—"movement; motion"—combines the characters signifying the verbs "to move" (動) and "to create" (作), hence "to create a movement" is one of the possible translations. In order to preserve the recognizability of the original signifiers, in this case alone we adhere to the already-adopted transliteration *dohsa* instead of *dōsa*, and *hou* instead of *hō* as it should be in accordance to the rule we apply elsewhere in the text for Japanese words with long vowels.

blamed for the condition of people with cerebral palsy and other similar impairments, considering that most of these people have all the physical "equipment"—nerves, muscles, and bones—needed for the performance of certain movements (Naruse 1998: 45). The concept of intention, no matter if intention is proper or misdirected from the standpoint of an external observer, is the key to understanding any movement and the psychological background it is based upon. As the Dohsa-hou specialist Mitsuyo Tsuru points out, awkward movement, feeble posture, or stiff body often indicate certain mental problems; they reflect one's "mental scene" (Tsuru 1992: 160).

- *Striving*, i.e., the mode of experiencing one's own self-activity—once having pictured the image of the movement in their mind, the client needs to put an effort on the realization of the image until *image* and *movement* become one. This process is controlled and synthesized by the self, which Naruse defines as a "management and coordination mechanism" (主体者という管理調整機構) (Naruse 1998: 59). This "mechanism" is responsible for the pure experience of any self-activity, for example "I am walking now," i.e., "It is *me* who is walking now." For this reason, striving is above all a subjective phenomenon and as such it can influence one's overall self-activity and condition, onset of diseases included. According to Tsuru, diseases set in when the individual experiences undesirable modes of self-activity, that is, the self attempts to perform a desirable mode of experience, but in vain (Tsuru 1992: 160). In Dohsa-hou, where difficult movement might be any movement that a healthy person considers ordinary, striving becomes synonymous to "conscious." It is exactly the process of making the movements conscious, i.e., controlled by the self in its role of a "management and coordination mechanism," and as such this process becomes one of the major foci of attention over the treatment course (Naruse 1998: 156). "To make conscious" here means tapping one's innate, yet dormant abilities, for which reason Naruse likens this process to the attainment of the *arugamama*-based state of mind in Morita therapy (Naruse 2007: 19) (see Sect. 5.2.4).
- *Bodily movement*, i.e., performing the desirable mode of self-experience—the succession of intention and striving results in the performance of the desirable bodily movement. This is a real-time conscious experience, which Naruse calls *motion experience* (動作体験) (Naruse 1998: 59). In terms of the degree of awareness of the movement, motion experience can be distinguished from two other types of bodily movements, namely (i) when our body is moved by something or someone else, that is, we experience the movement of our body in a passive way; and (ii) when performing a bodily movement without any intention, that is, under hypnotic state or in case of some diseases when we experience automatic movements beyond self-control (adapted from Harizuka 2006). In this sense, most of the movements in our daily life we perform unconsciously, which means that both the intention and striving that precede them are unconscious too; but when it comes to performing a difficult movement, for which end a special body awareness and concentration are required, then this process is conscious, that is, the mental energy released at the *striving*

stage fuels the realization of the motion on physical level at the *bodily movement* stage (Ohno and Murata 1993: 22).

Through their own *motion experience* and the therapist's support, the client can become aware of their inappropriate movements, distinguishing between them and the new proper movements; then strive to change the inappropriate movements to desirable ones, and, as a result, acquire better control over themselves and improve both their mental and physical condition. The Fig. 7.1 below presents the process of motion experience as comprising both psychological and physiological elements, and the constant feedback between them.

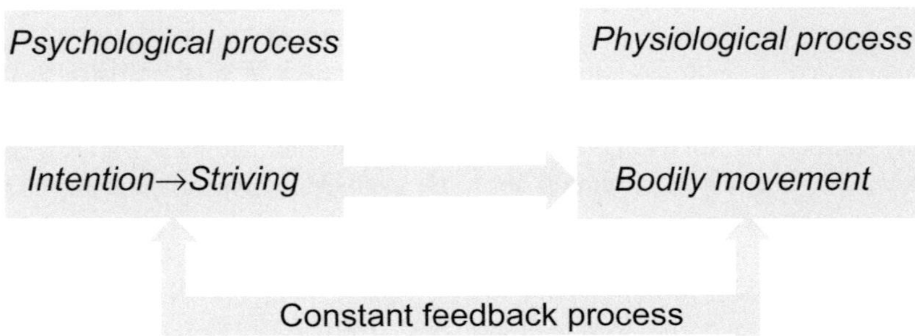

Fig. 7.1 The process of motion experience in Dohsa-hou formed by the succession of the three key stages *intention-striving-bodily movement* (adapted from Naruse 2000: 19; Harizuka 2006)

7.1.1.2 Who Can Benefit from Dohsa-hou?

As previously mentioned, Dohsa-hou emerged within the cerebral palsy research circles and at the initial stage of its development its relation with hypnosis was rather strong. Astonished to witness how under hypnosis children with cerebral palsy moved their otherwise paralyzed limbs, Gosaku Naruse and his research team were eager to discover the psychological factors that determined the accomplishment of bodily movements, i.e., to sail the uncharted seas called "psychological explanation of the motor actions."

Initially, the application of Dohsa-hou was aimed mainly at the improvement of motor impairments and spasticity of children with cerebral palsy. Their rehabilitation was carried out on the premises that (i) most of the children can move, but not in accordance with the way they want because their motion experience as a psychological process is immature or misdirected, and (ii) this psychological process can be learned and the motor dysfunction can thus be overcome (Kouno 2013: 94). The positive outcomes of the work with such children not only gave hope to patients and their families, but also allowed psychology and pedagogy to enter the field of cerebral palsy treatment, which until that point had been dominated by somatic medicine, physiology, and physiological rehabilitation. By so doing, Dohsa-hou managed to overcome the limitations of these fields, which consider children with cerebral palsy doomed because their condition results from an incurable brain damage, and to reveal that brain damage and motor impairment are not inextricably linked or at least that the cause of the physical impairment is not solely limited to the physiological damage (Ohno and Murata 1993: 6–7).

During that time, i.e., the late 1960s, Dohsa-hou was popularly known as an approach for psychological rehabilitation under the name of "motion exercise"—*dohsa-kunren* (動作訓練). Even though later on the name changed to Dohsa-hou, the method retained its strong educational aspect as one of its major premises as described earlier: if we consider any bodily movement a psychological phenomenon, then proper movement can be learned and improper movement and bodily posture can be corrected in a natural way. With such a notion on physical movement, at the beginning of the 1980s Dohsa-hou broadened its scope of application to children with autism and hyperactivity disorders, as well as to those with Down syndrome and severe intellectual disabilities. The method proved efficacious in helping them not only to improve their awkward body postures, but also to stabilize their emotions and adopt more appropriate behavioral patterns in daily life (Imura 2012: 6). Such positive outcomes allowed Dohsa-hou to enter also the field of clinical psychology by proving the relation between bodily movements and behavior, i.e., improved physical movements foster behavioral enhancement (Ohno and Murata 1993: 9).

Later on, Dohsa-hou was found beneficial also to patients with schizophrenia. According to Tsuru's observations, most of these patients share a typical body posture: either too rigid or too loose, with rounded shoulders and their chin thrust forward. If their posture is improved, Tsuru hypothesized, the patients' self-control and social behavior, too, may improve (Tsuru 2007: 58). Indeed, as a result of the Dohsa-hou sessions, the patients' facial expression and bodily movements became more vital, they started going outside more often for shopping and other daily life activities, and even their auditory hallucinations—or at least the patients' preoccupation with them—diminished (Tsuru 2007: 57–80). Other researchers reported decreased sense of depersonalization and increased "feeling herself in her body" in a female client with schizophrenia (Takamatsu 1992: 172).

With all these positive outcomes, the application scope of Dohsa-hou over the recent years broadened further to patients with anxiety, neurotic disorders, and depression, and even to cases of truancy from school (Ohba 1992: 179; Naruse in Miki and Kuroki 1998: 127). Additionally, Dohsa-hou was shown to be efficacious in the treatment of posttraumatic stress disorder, for example, after natural disasters such as the Great Hanshin Earthquake in Kobe in 1995 (Tominaga et al. 1995).[3] The method is further applied in the fields of counseling psychology and psychotherapy, whose clients may not suffer physical impairments, but in most of the cases they find it difficult to perform certain movements, for example, because of stiff neck or shoulders. The process of striving to perform an appropriate movement, which fosters higher awareness of oneself and of one's relation with the world, correlates to certain

[3]In all such cases, the method is referred to as Clinical Dohsa-hou (臨床動作法).

essential insights that the clients gain over the psychotherapeutic course (Naruse 1992b: 5).[4] Outside of the clinical setting, Dohsa-hou proves efficacious as a means of stress-relief in daily life for healthy persons or as a method for motor skills improvement among sportsmen (Naruse 1992b: 4–5; Hoshino 1992: 187–193)[5]. Remarkable positive outcomes are yielded also in the elderly care field, with clients stabilizing their postures and bettering their lifestyle (Naruse 1998: 167). In recent years, cases of dancers and actors who have found Dohsa-hou beneficial for their physical training drew attention. Such reports promise to open a new page in the development of Dohsa-hou (Naruse 2007: 112).

Nowadays the term "psychological rehabilitation" (心理リハビリテーション) is used in Japan to signify the comprehensive approach, which focuses on individual Dohsa-hou sessions that alternate with group recreation activities, play therapy, and daily life-related trainings (Ohno and Murata 1993: 10). The Japanese psychological rehabilitation should be properly distinguished from the rehabilitation psychology, which emerged in the United States in the 1950s out of research on the psychological challenges that occur over the course of physiological rehabilitation through massage, electrotherapy, or exercises offered to individuals with physical disabilities caused by disease or an accident (Hosaka 1996: 38). Considered one of the fastest growing fields in applied psychology today, rehabilitation psychology "focuses on the study and application of psychological knowledge and skills on behalf of individuals with disabilities and chronic health conditions in order to maximize health and welfare, independence and choice, functional abilities and social role participation across lifespan" (Scherer, as cited in Kennedy 2012: 15). Although the Dohsa-hou-based psychological rehabilitation strives for all such positive outcomes, its *terminus a quo* is the physical impairment seen within the context of the patient's "mental climate," whereas in cases of clients with mental disorders their condition is addressed through their bodily movements and postures. By thus undertaking the challenging task to tackle simultaneously issues of both body and mind, Dohsa-hou uses bodily movement as its key notion to shed further light on the body-mind interconnectedness.

7.1.2 Dohsa-hou's Key Therapeutic Tools

One of Dohsa-hou's distinctive features is that it emerged from the researchers' direct clinical experience, not from already extant theoretical frameworks (Naruse 1992b: 5). As such, the approach provides a fresh viewpoint and methodology which are new even to the clinical psychology circles in Japan. Yet some aspects of

---

[4]In this case, the method is referred to as Dohsa-therapy (動作療法).

[5]In this case, the method is referred to as health Dohsa-hou (健康動作法) and sports Dohsa-hou. (スポーツ動作法), respectively. However, for convenience, all the applications of Dohsa-hou are generally termed "Clinical Dohsa-hou" (Naruse in Miki and Kuroki 1998: 128).

the method could be recognized—albeit not as obviously as in Morita therapy and Naikan therapy—as specificities of Japanese culture and mentality.

7.1.2.1 Relax, Relax, and Relax!

As previously mentioned, Gosaku Naruse's research was inspired by the case of the boy with cerebral palsy moving his palsied arm under hypnosis. At that time Naruse collaborated with physicians and specialists in the education of children with physical and/or mental impairments. His collaborators drew his attention to one particular trait common for the most of these children, namely very high levels of muscle tension and spasticity (Naruse 1998: 17–18). The electromyography experiments of Naruse's co-researches proved that when a child with cerebral palsy was hypnotized, these levels amazingly fell to normal rates. However, once the hypnotic session was over, the child usually relapsed to their previous condition of hypertension and spasticity. Naruse called this type of tension *unnatural tension* (不当緊張) (Naruse 2001: 32) and considered it an important determinant of the physical impairment rather than the brain damage alone.

Although typical for children with cerebral palsy, unnatural tension can be observed even in healthy individuals because it is not limited to muscles alone, but is related also to one's mentality and lifestyle: as a result of one's idiosyncrasies, or of stress and other negative circumstances, unnatural tension may accumulate in certain body areas and pull one's body off its central axis of support. If prolonged, this tension may become chronic and may gradually distort one's proper bodily movements and posture. However, unnatural tension is rather difficult to notice by the person suffering from it (ibid.), much more so for children with cerebral palsy. As the positive outcomes of hypnotic sessions were temporary, Naruse got determined to search for new ways other than hypnosis to alleviate or even eliminate the muscular hypertension in these children. That is how he came to the concept of relaxation.

"Designed to reduce psychological and physiological tension while simultaneously promoting greater awareness of bodily sensations and responses" (Kennedy 2012: 306), "relaxation is one of the most frequently used methods for treating psychological and physical problems. There are many relaxation methods such as autogenic training, muscular relaxation, and biofeedback" (Fujino 2012: 388). In the sphere of muscular relaxation, the most widespread methods include massage, acupuncture, and application of muscle relaxant agents, ointments, or tranquilizers. Although the positive outcomes of these methods could not and should not be ignored, once their effect is over, most of the patients relapse to their morbid condition (Naurse 2001: 7). In the end, the effect of such a relaxation is similar to that induced by hypnosis, i.e., temporary. Therefore, Naruse speculated that another type of relaxation should be possible—a relaxation, which does not rely on external stimuli, but which results from the conscious effort of the individual concerned. He called this type of relaxation *self-induced relaxation* (自己弛緩) (Naruse 2001: 29–30) and considered it opposite to the widely applied methods for relaxation, because its object is not the tension itself as a physical phenomenon, but the mental effort at relaxing. This effort naturally results in lowered muscular tension (Naruse 2001: 8). In his years-long research of children with cerebral palsy, Naruse observed that when the children managed to properly relax their palsied limbs, a proper movement followed (Naruse 1998: 78). Self-induced relaxation, Naruse thus summarized, is an activity innate to every human being because the self "governs" the body as an entity, which relates to and functions in the external world (Naruse 1988: 39).

As such, this relaxation is a subject to learning through one's own experience and can be mastered through repetitive exercises (Ohno and Murata 1993: 72). This learning process requires clients to identify which tension is inappropriate and then strive to eliminate it. Over this process, the client has to encounter directly their own self because the designer of the unnatural tension is no one else but the self and therefore the self is also the one to deal with it (Naruse 2001: 30). However, the self that strives toward relaxation and the one that sustains the tension often "compete" with each other, leading the individual to a dead end. That is, when the client intends to perform a certain movement, the process of *intension-striving-performance* (see Fig. 7.1 in Sect. 7.1.1.1) cannot unfold smoothly because of this internal conflict and the client is very likely to fail as a result of physical pain, or fear and anxiety, or loss of vigor, or all. For this reason, a mere muscular relaxation cannot be expected to do much in the process of overcoming this problem. Rather, the client needs to "tune" themselves in such a way as to figure out what hampers their intention to perform a particular action and in so doing to attempt to transform the subconscious attitude that allows the inner conflict to arise (Naruse 2001: 30–31). The client therefore needs courage and strength because they have to detach themselves psychologically from their immediate surroundings, "meet" with their own body, "listen" to its voice, and *experience* what it means to relax on one's own; it is a kind of "mixing" with one's own body (Naruse 2007: 131).

At this stage the term *o-makase* (お任せ)—"to leave," "to entrust"—is often used to signify a specific attitude that the client needs to develop: while attempting to relax, i.e., to overcome the inner conflict between their relaxing and their tensed self, the client has to entrust entirely their body to the trainer's hands. The trainer, in turn, does not need to make the trainee's body submit to their hands, but only guide the trainee in the process of self-discovery and increasing body awareness. This is a very important therapeutic experience because it requires the client to "break" all hitherto posture and movement patterns (Shigehashi 1994: 15); to "throw away" their Ego and face their "naked" self the way it is (Naruse in Miki and Kuroki 1998: 135). As such, the *o-makase* experience often evokes disquietedness or can even be frightening for some clients, especially for those with autism.[6] In order to curb such feelings and produce trustworthiness, the trainer has to adopt a stable posture and instruct the trainee accurately. Considering the need of building a trust relationship, the *o-makase* experience, hence relaxation, is a significant part of the therapeutic process especially for children with autism and hyperactivity disordes (Shigehashi 1994: 15).

[6]In private communication with Hideaki Naohara, Associate Professor at Aichi Shukutoku University and a Dohsa-hou supervisor (August 2013).

The main relaxation techniques, most of which the patient usually performs while lying down on their back or side, are based on the so-called *unit movements* (単位動作). These include twisting and stretching of key body areas such as neck, shoulders and torso, arms, elbows, hip joints, knee joints, legs, and ankles—all of them are points where the accumulation of unnatural tension is most easily recognizable (Naruse 1998: 93). The presence or absence of unnatural tension in these areas is responsible for the formation of the individual posture, which in Dohsa-hou is referred to as *body dynamics* (see Schema A.1 in Appendix III). The accumulation of unnatural tension—or of *concomitant tension*[7]—in these areas distorts the innate proper body posture and is often to be blamed for an array of physical ailments such as stiff shoulders, lumbar pains, backaches, scoliosis, clubfoot, and even hallux valgus. Therefore, if the unnatural tension is relieved with the help of self-induced relaxation, not only will the physical ailment or pain diminish or be eliminated, but also the movements in that particular area will become suppler. Observing the process of significant improvement in many cases during his long-term research, Naruse came to the conclusion that although all the above-mentioned ailments could easily be mistaken for purely physiological problems, in fact they reflect the patient's "mental climate" (Naruse 1998: 93–94).

The application of the Dohsa-hou relaxation techniques in most cases result in a sensation of lightness and warmth; one's bodily movements become more vigorous and the posture is visibly improved; a sense of well-being is written all over one's face. Behavioral changes include calming down and increased concentration levels, whereas hyperactive and impulsive actions diminish significantly (Imura 2012: 8). Relaxation functions as an indispensable requirement for the next therapeutic tool—*tate-kei*—because it prepares the ground for "shaping" the desirable posture after the inappropriate one has been "broken" through the mutual efforts of the client and therapist.

7.1.2.2 *Tate-kei*—In Dialogue with Gravity

In contrast to the previous key therapeutic tool—that of relaxation—where the client performs the tasks while lying on their back or side, the *tate-kei* (タテ系) group of tasks aims at bringing the client up to the vertical position.[8] These tasks

[7]Concomitant tension (随伴緊張) is a type of unnatural tension engendered by the individual's effort to perform a certain movement, but the effort results in the simultaneous performance also of other, irrelevant movements. For example, when a child with cerebral palsy stretches out their arm to take an object, they also bend their neck or lift their shoulder (Ohno and Murata 1993: 24).

[8]*Tate* (縦) means "vertical". The character implies that the vertical dimension, which counteracts the gravity, is the one that should be "followed" (see Fig. 7.2).

The shuffle gait typical for many of the traditional Japanese performing arts (see Sect. 3.1) is used also in the avant-garde dance style *Butoh*. It is interesting that when trained in this gait, *Butoh* actors are encouraged to imagine their head, chest, back, and legs being pulled by threads in the respective directions. By so doing, actors can keep their body straight and thus walk stably and smoothly (in private communication with the Japanese *Butoh* dancer and choreographer Norihito Ishii, May 2017).

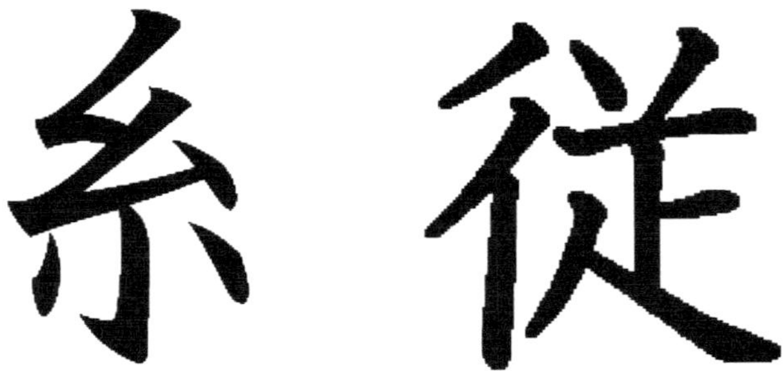

Fig. 7.2 The character for "vertical" (縦) is comprised of the characters for "thread, cord" (left) and "to follow" (right), hence "vertical" is the "thread to follow" (Henshall 1998: 281)

are related to four key postures—sitting cross-legged or on one's heels, kneeling, standing upright, and walking—any of which addresses the inner force that keeps human body vertical against gravity. In Dohsa-hou, the efforts aimed at adopting the respective posture help the client to re-experience this force and, by withstanding it, to develop a more conscious attitude toward both their bodily movements and the surrounding environment (Ohno and Murata 1993: 221).

During his research of children with cerebral palsy, Naruse noticed that children follow certain movement patterns, which result in stereotyped postures. It means that the children's proper response to gravity is impaired. In cases of healthy individuals, the key areas that form one's body dynamics should be equally balanced around a straight imaginary axis from the tip of head to the toes. By contrast, children with cerebral palsy are not able to keep their body axis vertical or at least not to the necessary extent. In other words, they are not "baptized" in gravity (Naruse 2007: 132). Therefore, Naruse assumed that if children practice exercises directly related to their response to the gravity force, they may soon develop the abilities needed for adopting the right posture. The ultimate goal of the *tate-kei* group therefore is to "bring back" all the distorted areas to their natural positions in relation to this central axis while keeping the latter straight—this is the so-called "shaping" of the body axis—*jiku-zukuri* (軸作り). In other words, the *tate-kei* group of tasks is not aimed at changing the stereotyped incorrect posture itself, but at developing a correct response to gravity by focusing on the correct position of the body axis. Once this goal is achieved, the unnatural posture transforms naturally into a proper and visibly more relaxed one.

Although the tasks of the *tate-kei* group are united by the concept of *jiku-zukuri* and the client's proper response to gravity, they can be considered separately in terms of the respective body posture adopted:

- *Sitting on the floor* is the primary posture for human beings to keep their bodies vertical against gravity. In early child development, this is the first posture that infant adopts by themselves to keep their body upright and experience for the first time the vertical dimension of the world. Additionally, as the educational psychologist Akira Onda suggests, sitting posture is typical for most of the

Eastern cultures where it signifies repose, concentration, and even meditation, but also readiness to act at any moment. Sitting is therefore an intermediate stage between lying posture, which signifies total rest, and upright position, which is usually related to activity (Onda in Naruse 1992a: 46).

- *Rising*, which includes kneeling and standing upright, is the next body posture considered essential for the early child development. It is not only the first time when the infant experiences the gravity force to the fullest, but also when they experience the way their body relates to it and attempts to withstand it. Such an experience fosters their physiological and psychological independence. Consequently, Tsuru points out, the child verifies their existence in this world, but not in the sense that the world allows them to enter into it but quite the contrary: the child opens up themselves so that the world may become part of their world, i.e., the two worlds—internal and external—harmonize with each other (Tsuru in Naruse 1992a: 57).
- *Walking* tests one's ability to stand properly on one's feet and press them firmly on the ground while moving from one point to another, be it forward or backward. Walking can also be considered an antithesis of relaxation, for which stillness in the horizontal dimension is of great importance. What is essential here is not only the individual's proper "relation" with the ground while shaping their body around a straight imaginary axis, but also the proper bodyweight distribution on one's legs (Naruse 2009: 196–197) when taking a step. Psychologically, keeping the body balanced and moving smoothly mean that first inner balance is attained and it is then externalized through the body. Such an experience, Tsuru points out, strengthens one's self-confidence (Tsuru in Naruse 1992a: 63) and confirms one's existence as a *living* creature (Tsuru in Naruse 1992a: 65).

Depending on each individual case, Dohsa-hou's *tate-kei* exercises can be applied separately or in combination. For example, for a bed-ridden child with cerebral palsy the consecutive achievement of each of the four key postures—from sitting through kneeling and standing upright to taking a step forward—is essential so that the child may start their "dialogue" with gravity and experience the world as three dimensional (Naruse 1992a: 75). Psychologically, *tate-kei* helps children experience how it feels to stand against gravity as a result of their own conscious effort here and now, considering that Dohsa-hou fosters the process of moving from supine or sitting posture to an upright one and maintaining it predominantly through one's own efforts. And for a client who can walk but whose neck or torso postures are incorrect, sitting may be beneficial, whereas for those with incorrect lower back posture kneeling is recommended. Standing upright is considered appropriate for those with patellar luxation and weak ankles or for those who have difficulties to step firmly on the ground; and mastering the correct walking is for those who experience difficulty in keeping their balance or for those whose gait lacks stability (Naruse 1998: 80).

Although the content of the psychological effort in Dohsa-hou remains difficult to identify, it often manifests itself as a self-affirmative experience. Many

Dohsa-hou clients verbalize the results of their efforts as "I feel better," "I see the world is brighter now," "I feel my body is lighter now," etc. (Naruse 1998: 96–97; Naruse 2001: 156). Such an experience likely improves the relation between one's body and the surrounding space; the concentration levels increase and a proactive attitude is taken (Imura 2012: 23; Ohno and Murata 1993: 122–123, 221). "As far as *tate-kei* is aimed at the developmental support of children with disabilities, some people doubt if this is an attempt to put them into the frame of the healthy people. However, if we observe children who try to stand up or to walk—even if they fail to do it properly—their faces beaming with joy, we cannot but agree that on a genetic level every human being strives to respond to the gravity force through a proper body posture" (Imura 2016: 11). In contrast to lying down, which makes "our boundaries less differentiated, standing up intensifes our excitement and deepens our awareness, our self-feeling, as we recognize our selves in the sphere of gravity" (Keleman 1975: 19). Indeed, the horizontal dimension represents the idea of disconnecting oneself from life and being passive, whereas the vertical one is related to the individual's proactive attitude toward life (Naruse 2007: 133). Moreover, adopting vertical posture is based on an innate pattern common to all human beings —sick or healthy—and the task of Dohsa-hou is to draw this pattern out and put it under the control of the self. When the body axis lacks balance and stability, then the entire posture becomes feeble, and, as a result, standing upright and stepping forward become difficult (Naruse 2007: 134). This inevitably causes psychological problems, too, for example feelings of inadequacy and insecurity. Therefore, no matter whether the client is a child with disability or a healthy athlete, taking the proper vertical posture likely paves the way to positive psychological changes as well (Ohno and Murata 1993: 122).

7.1.2.3 Communication

As Doha-hou was initially addressed primarily to children with cerebral palsy, the majority of whom suffered also from intellectual disabilities, nonverbal communication has remained its essentials. Verbal communication, in turn, is limited to instructing trainees during the therapeutic session and to providing positive feedback to further motivate them; it serves as a mere auxiliary tool (Naruse 1998: 126–127), giving preference to eye contacts, facial expressions, and especially to touches that trainer and trainee exchange.[9] This characteristic places Dohsa-hou in sharp contrast to many other psychotherapeutic approaches, especially those from the West. Although long associated with healing in most cultures—Eastern and Western—"touch has been eschewed by most schools of psychotherapy that are not strictly "body-oriented" (Horton et al. 1995: 443). As "Freud's prohibition against

[9]Although up to here we used terms such as "therapist", "client" and "patient", we introduce now the original Dohsa-hou terms "trainer" and "trainee". The terms "supporter/aid provider" (援助者) and "aid recipient" (被援助者) are sometimes used instead.

"gratifying" patients with touch has permeated the mainstream of psychotherapy," "little attention has been given to clinically appropriate touch in therapy" (ibid.).

Despite this widespread taboo, however, in recent years more and more attention is being paid to the significance and potential efficaciousness of touch in the context of psychotherapy and clinical psychology (Konno 1999: 37). A survey of touch in psychotherapy proves touch to be related to an array of positive outcomes including that it "provides a link to external reality; communicates concretely, "You are not alone"; communicates acceptance and enhances self-esteem; helps one create (model) a new mode of relating; puts the patient in better contact with bodily sensations; creates a bond, feeling of closeness, that therapist really cares; patients feels strengthened, reassured, comforted, or healed" (Horton et al. 1995: 451). In fact, such and other positive outcomes of touch have been confirmed numerous times over the research and therapeutic work with children with disabilities in Dohsa-hou. For the reasons explained at the beginning of this section, communication in Dohsa-hou relies predominantly on touch—considering that any Dohsa-hou task is first of all a *collaborative* activity between trainer and trainee, touch is the basis upon which *joint attention* between the two participants can unfold to ensure the smooth communication that such a collaborative activity requires.

To facilitate the establishment of joint attention, hence of smooth communication, Dohsa-hou uses a simple task called *ude-age* (腕挙げ)—arm lifting—which is realized when the trainer and trainee touch each other's palms. This task is often applied for breaking the ice in the trainer–trainee pair; for warming up at the beginning of a Dohsa-hou session; or for deepening the communication with children who are usually difficult to approach such as those with autism or severe intellectual disabilities. Through the *ude-age* task Dohsa-hou conveys basic notions of communication: "arms and hands are extensions of the chest," which is "the home of the heart, doorway to the sense of Self"; they are used "for reaching out and for protection" (Rosenberg 1985: 129). That is, arms and hands are the first and primary means of physical communication between the individual and the world, and this communication can be realized only through touch. Touch is an invitation for and encouragement to communicate and it is much more so in therapeutic context where, as the Dohsa-hou specialist Yoshitaka Konno emphasizes, touching the client's body already means touching their soul (Konno 2005: 9) or it means even to "enter directly into the archaic layers of the personality" (Bertherat and Bernstein 1989: 48). Although in a different context, the American physician Judith Smith corroborates that "the gestures and manipulations of the healer in therapeutic touch function as a way of communicating the healer's attitude (of love, care, and a deep desire to help)" (Smith, as cited in Montagu 1986: 407). This description corresponds to the key aspects of the *ude-age* task that can be seen if we elaborate on the process of the task accomplishment, breaking it down into several steps:

- The trainee adopts supine, seated, or kneeling position—whatever is most appropriate for their present condition; the trainer sits next to them
- Trainer and trainee touch each other's palms or shake hands; the trainer begins to give instructions and helps the trainee lift their arm with elbow stretched

- The trainer watches if the arm movement follows the correct mental vector and corrects it if necessary
- The trainer watches out if other body parts outside of arm and shoulder joints move or twist, or if arm lifting itself becomes too difficult
- The trainer monitors the speed of arm lifting—it should be neither too fast nor too slow
- The trainer observes how often the trainee makes eye contact and if its frequency and duration increase during the performance of the task
- The trainer observes the trainee's concentration levels and if they change over the performance of the task
- Whenever the trainee reaches the maximum of the movement, the trainer helps them lower their arm
- The trainer gradually diminishes their guidance and support until the trainee starts performing the task properly on their own (summarized from Ohno and Murata 1993: 42; Naruse 2005: 37–38; Imura 2012: 13; see Glossary).

Using the symbolic value of the two hands touching each other, the arm lifting task not only communicates the trainer's attitude—a key aspect of any other Dohsa-hou task—but it gives the participants a chance to share the uniqueness of each other's worlds. Especially in cases of children with severe disabilities, such an activity encourages them to leave their own worlds—in most cases dominated by loneliness and boredom—and enter the world of mutual communication and understanding. In this way, the communication they have been robbed of so far due to their disability now becomes possible; their uniqueness as human beings is affirmed and encouraged to unfold. This, in turn, provides a chance for the child to adopt a more acceptive attitude toward others and eventually show progress in their verbal development (Imura 2012: 14).

Besides *ude-age*, Dohsa-hou incorporates other communication enhancement techniques that are not necessarily aimed at improving bodily movements. "These techniques, which can be summarized with the term "communication movement techniques," include having the trainer and trainee jumping together simultaneously or touching their palms together and then moving in a certain direction, doing a seesaw on the floor, etc. Any of these can result in a mutual connection and understanding between trainer and trainee: more specifically, trainees' responses to the trainer's instructions suggest that they have understood the trainer's intentions implied through the task. For example, for children with severe intellectual disabilities, verbal communication can be very difficult, but when they respond to the trainer's handshake, they can be said to have understood the trainer's intention. This is valid also for a well-accomplished *ude-age* or seesaw task. In other words, these techniques are highly effective tools because they enable communication with children who are otherwise hard to be approached through bodily movements" (Imura 2016: 12).

Over the process of enhancing gradually their communication with others and the world, Dohsa-hou trainees tend to perform less self-destructive and impulsive behaviors—these diminish in a natural way, to be replaced by calmness and concentration. Such positive outcomes not only foster the further advancement of the therapeutic process, but they also help the trainee improve their daily life and social skills. At the same time, the trainee's integrity as an individual and the unique aspects of their personality are paid their due because the nonverbal communication in Dohsa-hou addresses trainers, too, calling them to receive their trainee emotionally rather than to analyze them; to overcome their prejudices and develop sensitiveness toward the specificities of the trainee's emotional and somatic language, and even to try to understand them through their own bodies.

Based exclusively on physical interaction, the communication process in Dohsa-hou enables trainees to experience a psychologically affective space-time, where an array of bodily movements and positions, contacts and distances, facial expressions and rhythms, playtime and strenuous work flow into each other. These turn the therapeutic mat into a fusion space where the participants in the trainer–trainee pair symbolically shorten the distance between their worlds through the mutual adjustment to each other's bodily movements. This allows us to define the communication process in Dohsa-hou as *touch-based movement-to-movement communication*—a powerful therapeutic tool in the realm where words have no voices.

*

To summarize, Dohsa-hou's three therapeutic tools—relaxation, *tate-kei*, and communication—are all related to the individual's ability to self-coordinate and also to increase their self-awareness. First, relaxation requires the trainee to take the "armor", i.e., the unnatural tension, off their hitherto body dynamics. Then the *tate-kei* tasks take the trainee to the opposite direction, where stabilization of the self and its active response in the form of a dialogue with gravity are required. Both literally and figuratively, the trainee needs to rearrange themselves in respect to their body axis, i.e., to the proper body dynamics which is innate to human beings. Finally, considering that any Dohsa-hou task is an act of collaboration between trainer and trainee who put mutual efforts to attain a desired goal, joint attention is very important to ensure not only posture improvement, but also the enhancement of the trainee's communication and social skills because without joint attention "we cannot construct and coordinate the shared social realities that comprise everyday life" (Bruner in Moore and Dunham 1995: 11–12). Indeed, regardless of any disabilities and diseases, we all share a world of interdependence, where, as Naruse points out, every one relies on moving to be alive (Naruse 2014: 173). This essential truth Dohsa-hou has adopted and applies in a sophisticated and original therapeutic way.

7.2 Beyond Words

In the previous section we discussed the three main therapeutic tools of Dohsa-hou. Now we will discuss them from the broader standpoint of some specific Japanese cultural codes that are essential for defining Dohsa-hou as original Japanese psychotherapy. Although, as previously mentioned, over the last two decades Dohsa-hou broadened its application scope enormously to fields such as psychological counseling and sports training, children and youths with disabilities remain its main target group. Dohsa-hou's orientation toward young people with disabilities is captured by the terms "trainer" and "trainee," to reveal the strong educational intent of the therapy and the importance it attaches to the concept of learning: disability could be overcome if the client practices diligently the proper movements until they replace the incorrect ones and until the proper ones become natural. In this sense, Dohsa-hou helps its clients to cultivate such *body awareness*, which "as the Latin verb "to educate," *educere*, indicates, is not a question of putting something in but drawing it out" (Graham 1991: 11) because "body awareness cannot be given, it can only be taken" (Bertherat and Bernstein 1989: 137) .

The concept of learning through personal experience would already by familiar to the reader from the other two Japanese psychotherapies discussed in the present book, Morita therapy (the *taitoku* principle) and Naikan therapy (practiced in training centers). Considering that Dohsa-hou is a nonverbal psychotherapeutic approach based on direct bodywork, however, such an experience becomes the therapy's focal point. In the next two sections we discuss the *karada-de-oboeru* principle and the intensive training camps as specific cultural aspects of Dohsa-hou.

7.2.1 *Karada-de-oboeru*: The Memory of Body

In a study on the characteristics of the Japanese worldview, the German philosopher Kurt Singer points out that the most typical Japanese arts such as tea ceremony and archery are aimed at "the realization of a sort of quasi-somnambulist degree of unconsciousness; only if the performer can rely on a pattern of senso-motoric coordination so deeply ingrained that no phase of the performance requires cerebral intervention, is true mastery attained" (Singer 1997: 67). This true mastery is preceded by the repetition of the same movement or action numerous times in a row until the new *kata* (型)—a pattern of experience or skill, which the teacher conveys to their disciple—becomes automatic; until the external model and the inner "movement" harmonize completely with each other. The purpose of such a modeling is "to transcend the normal physical limits of the body and achieve a level of skill that is on a metaphysical or spiritual plane" (De Mente 2004: 137). This is "the same principle and the same skill that one sees in master musicians, jugglers, typists and others who perform flawlessly, seemingly without conscious effort" (ibid.).

Such a pattern of learning and mastering skills appears to be deeply ingrained in Japanese culture: "early in their history the Japanese developed the belief that form had a reality on its own, and that it often took precedence over substance. They also believed that anything could be accomplished if the right kata was mentally and physically practiced long enough" (De Mente 2013: 2), for which reason "prior to the introduction of industrialization into Japan in the 1870s, virtually all Japanese, in whatever art or craft, spent most of their lives trying to achieve perfection in their fields" (De Mente 2004: 137). This is especially valid for the *Dō*-practices (see Sect. 3.2), which without exception are based on the concept of *kata*, more specifically on that of *kata-kara-hairu* (型から入る)—"to enter from the pattern" (Hoshino in Naruse 1992a: 176). For example, the physical practice of a certain *kata* in the *Nō*-theater is aimed also at "polishing" the performer's spirit, thus helping the performer harmonize their body-mind (Minamoto, as cited in Hoshino in Naruse 1992a: 178). In other words, the *kata*-based physical training is the main gate not only to mastering a certain skill, but also to attaining body-mind harmony.

This notion is enriched by another cultural concept in Japan—*karada-de-oboeru* (体で覚える)—"to memorize/learn or remember through one's body." Somewhat akin to the *taitoku* principle already explained in the context of Morita therapy (see Sect. 5.2.4), *karada-de-oboeru* is more concrete for it does not refer to experiencing in general, but to experiencing directly through one's own body so that a certain goal or level of mastery be achieved. Over the centuries, this concept has become "the underlying foundation for all of the arts and skills practiced in Japan, from such mundane things as weaving baskets and floor mats to writing" (De Mente 2004: 138).

It is exactly through the *karada-de-oboeru* principle, we suggest, that a better understanding of Dohsa-hou's therapeutic mechanisms could be gained. Similarly to the *Dō*-practices, Dohsa-hou's aim is to help its clients "enter from the pattern," i.e., the proper movement (*kata*) and "memorize" it through their body. However, before proceeding to this core process, any Dohsa-hou trainer first needs to distinguish which type of inappropriate movements their trainee performs: whether it is *unlearned movement*, which means the trainee has not learned sufficiently to strive to perform an intended movement; or it is a *mislearned movement*, which results from learning an inappropriate movement, i.e., the trainee has learned how to strive to perform an intended movement but in an incorrect way (adapted from Harizuka 2006). In either way the trainer should help the trainee learn a correct way to strive for the realization of an intended movement, that is, they should help the trainee "break" the old improper *kata* and "memorize" through their body the new proper one.

On the other hand, needless to specify, everyone differs in terms of physical and mental constitution. "Proper" in Dohsa-hou therefore does not mean that we all should move and behave in a similar manner. On the contrary, the method pays due attention to the uniqueness of every one's individuality—be they healthy people or people with disabilities. Rather than simply "learning" or "memorizing," "proper" in Dohsa-hou refers much more to one's ability to "draw out" and perform those "natural movements" (Kobayashi in Naruse 1992a: 66–67) that are innate to all humans as unquestionable signs of body-mind integrity. For this reason, the strong educational aspects of Dohsa-hou that we already emphasized on several occasions, can now be rendered more properly through the *karada-de-oboeru* cultural principle as an attempt to help the client "*remember* through their body," that is, the body (*karada*) can master whatever skill is concerned if it "remembers" (*oboeru*), i.e., draws out over the therapeutic course the natural movement and posture patterns (*kata*) that are innate to all human beings. That is why the use of therapy balls, crutches, mirrors and other such auxiliaries is not recommended in the Dohsa-hou sessions—clients should focus exclusively on this "recollection" process within their own bodies.

By thus jogging the memories of body, Dohsa-hou (i) helps its clients to transcend their habitual mindset, hence to harmonize the relation between their body and mind; and (ii) emphasizes how the process of gradual "recollection" of innate physical *kata* that all humans share fuels one's fortitude and motivation to transform, i.e., improve their present condition or, more properly, "return" to the natural movement patterns. However, in Dohsa-hou the transcendence of the habitual mindset and the development of such qualities—fortitude and motivation—are usually preceded by physical pain and discomfort, and/or by extreme mood fluctuations peculiar to certain diseases; and this process may be time-consuming and tiresome for it requires the trainee to encounter—more often in an unpleasant way—themselves. As Greene and Goodrich-Dunn aptly point out, although in a different context, "sometimes the harder the client's rational mind works to bring about change, the harder the unconscious works to defend against change" and this is "one of the greatest paradoxes of any therapeutic process—the paradox of healing" (Greene and Goodrich-Dunn 2004: 6). It is probably so because the client may unconsciously perceive the change as threatening to their *true self*, which "may be wounded if expressed or exposed to the world" (ibid.).

Even though in principle Dohsa-hou tolerates the trainee's discomforts and mood fluctuations that oftentimes accompany the therapeutic process, there are situations when the trainer is better to ignore them delicately.[10] Instead, trainers should be concerned with the trainee's ability to put these aside and concentrate on performing the proper *kata*—be it a posture or movement—that is required. In other words, the trainee has to move and position their body in ways that are *not yet spontaneous*, but are expected to become such ones through continuous and diligent *karada-de-oboeru* practice that jogs the memory of body. To "return" to one's innate naturalness therefore appears to be a superior way of overcoming a physical or psychological condition, or, at least, of learning to live with it in a constructive way which may spur on the further development of one's individuality.

7.2.2 Intensive Dohsa-hou Camps—Communal Life as Therapy

As previously explained, observations of children with cerebral palsy during and after states of hypnosis or sleep suggested to Gosaku Naruse that the so-called unnatural tension in awake state could be released through relaxation, whereby the positive but temporary effect of hypnosis can become permanent. The results of the relaxation exercises proved equal to those of the hypnotic sessions, giving great impetus to Dohsa-hou's development and bringing more and more parents and their children to seek help at Naruse's research laboratory (Naruse 1998: 26).

At the very beginning, Naruse carried out individual Dohsa-hou sessions at his laboratory, but it appeared this format was tiresome for both trainers and trainees; hence it was difficult to bring the expected outcomes. Over the course of his

---

[10]In private communication with Hiroaki Ueno, teacher at Higashi-Osaka Special-Needs School and a Dohsa-hou supervisor (October 2012).

research, Naruse also had the chance to observe the free play of children with cerebral palsy and came across the same phenomena as with hypnosis or sleep state: when vigorously involved in playing, the children moved unconsciously their otherwise paralyzed limbs. This prompted Naruse to organize intensive group trainings in which Dohsa-hou sessions alternated with play therapy and other group activities. Initially, he tried several trainings with duration of minimum three days and maximum 10 days. In the end, it appeared that one week was the optimal time needed for these sessions, being neither too short nor too long (ibid.).

From these attempts of group therapy for children with cerebral palsy, it was a short leap to sleepover Dosa-hou camps. The first camp of the kind was held in 1967 at St. Lucia Hospital in Kurume city, Fukuoka prefecture, where 30 children with cerebral palsy experienced the benefits of relaxation, trainer-trainee communication, and play therapy for a week. This camp, considered the official start of the Dohsa-hou intensive camp therapy, became a basic model according to which more than 70 camps a year are now held throughout Japan (Naruse 1998: 27). It is also considered the pillar of the camp therapy in Japan (Kushizaki et al., as cited in Yoshihara 2010: 73), which was introduced in the country not long before, in the early 1960s. Several years later, in 1973, the first 7-day/6-night camp was held at the *Yasuragi-sō* welfare village in Yasu Plateau, Fukuoka prefecture (Naruse 1998: 27) (see Appendix III). "Currently, short-term camps—4-day/3-night, 2-day/1-night, and 1-day camps—are also carried out. Most camps are held during the extended vacations of Japanese schools, although recently the number of short-term camps held outside of these vacations has been on the rise" (Teruta and Harada 2016: 79).

Considering that camps allow for a number of Dohsa-hou sessions to be held continuously, camps afford a good opportunity for trainees to deepen their self-knowledge, progress to the next level of their development and achieve more significant changes as compared to single sessions. Additionally, as most of the camps are carried out close to nature, they can provide children with healing experiences that neither their daily life nor any hospital environment can secure. On an interpersonal level, trainees can experience the magic of building interpersonal relationships and communicating with coevals, as well as with adults other than their parents and relatives; the memories that the trainees thus make may influence positively their daily life once they return to it (Yoshihara 2010: 73).

To maintain such a nurturing environment, any Dohsa-hou camp requires mutual efforts and precise allocation of duties in relation to camp planning, management, maintenance, and development. As the Dohsa-hou philosophy suggests, camp participants do not "merely participate, but each of them "creates" the camp" (Teruta and Harada 2016: 79). These participants are:

- Camp chief—this is the person with ultimate responsibility for the physical and mental well-being of all the camp participants whose number sometimes may exceed one hundred. The camp chief holds opening speeches every morning with the aim to encourage the participants and help them increase their motivation for further development (Itonaga 2008: 31).
- Camp manager—this person is responsible for the general camp planning and on-site management, from pairing trainers and trainees and accommodation of

participants to minute details such as providing sundry goods. The camp manager sees to the camp's smooth operation and always consults with the camp chief; the manager is the "pivot of the fan" (Yoshihara 2010: 74).

- Supervisors—usually they are university professors, special-need school teachers, or clinical psychologists who hold a Dohsa-hou supervisor license from the Japanese Association of Rehabilitation Psychology. In most of the cases, one supervisor heads a team of several trainer–trainee pairs, leads the trainer trainings, and provides consultations and Dohsa-hou trainings to parents/caregivers. A camp supervisor supervises the work of the trainers in their team and provides concrete help and advice on each session.
- Trainers—most often teachers from special-needs schools, welfare service workers, clinical psychologists, and researchers, trainers are those who carry out the Dohsa-hou sessions and are the main figures in charge of their trainees' progress. As such, they need to establish close relation with their trainee—a task, which requires extensive communication also outside of the session time, for example, trainers may feed and bathe the trainee. Trainers need to communicate also with the trainee's parents/caregivers in order to understand the parents' expectations regarding the development of their child and to gain knowledge about the trainee's background, personality, daily life habits, etc. (Yoshihara 2010: 75). Trainers write down records on the content of each Dohsa-hou session they hold and then report it to both supervisors and parents.
- Subtrainers—they support the trainers' work, for example, help a trainer hold their trainee in an upright position. Subtrainers are not encouraged to venture on undertaking activities other than the ones that trainers or supervisors ask them for (Itonaga 2008: 32). On the other hand, in contrast to trainers, subtrainers are not responsible for one trainee, for which reason they have the opportunity to observe the overall camp atmosphere and provide valuable feedback on it.
- Trainees—in principle, there are no restrictions regarding the trainees' age, sex, and type of disability (see Sect. 7.1.1.2), but some camps tend to specialize in, for example, children and youths with autism and intellectual impairments. Some of the long-standing camps welcome veteran trainees who have been regularly attending the camp since their childhood.
- Person in charge of group therapy—in most of the cases such a person is selected among the camp trainers. This person needs to always communicate their activities with the camp manager and arrange them in accordance with the camp theme. Besides the management of the daily group therapy sessions, they are also responsible for creating a pleasant and, at the same time, therapeutic camp atmosphere where all participants may establish close interpersonal relationships, enjoy new types of experiences, etc. (Kushizaki et al., as cited in Yoshihara 2010: 76).
- Person in charge of daily chores—as compared to the extrovert attitude the person in charge of group therapy must adopt, the one in charge of daily chores appears much more sober: they are responsible for the camp's health management, including hygiene, air-conditioning, meals, bathing, etc. These two persons—in charge of group therapy and of daily chores—complement each other (Nagano, as cited in Yoshihara 2010: 77).

- Timekeeper—if only one of the participants is late for a session or other activity, the entire camp cannot progress smoothly in accordance with its preset schedule. For this reason, the role of the timekeeper is very important. Most of the camps in Japan adopt the so-called "5-minutes-before" rule, which stipulates that all participants should always prepare themselves for starting/closing a Dohsa-hou session or other activity 5 minutes before the designated time (Itonaga 2008: 32).
- Trainees' parents/caregivers—in most of the cases they take part actively in the camp preliminaries, balance the camp's accounts, book the camp site, etc. In some camps, depending on the place, they may be responsible also for daily chores such as cooking, washing, and cleaning. During the camp's evening party, parents/caregivers disguise and perform dances or theatricals, sometimes in collaboration with the camp chief, camp manager, and supervisors.

Considering that all camp participants live together, the trainers and supervisors can observe not only the way the trainees perform the Dohsa-hou tasks during the sessions, but also how they behave in a daily life-like environment, assess their overall potential, and devise ways for their further rehabilitation. The trainees' parents/caregivers, in turn, "can temporarily detach from their daily routine, exchange information with other parents, and share each other's worries. For both them and their children, camp participation becomes a long-awaited annual event" (Teruta and Harada 2016: 78).

Although each Dohsa-hou camp has its own characteristics and specific atmosphere, which reflect the spirit of the local area and its people, the program of any camp that is accredited by the Japanese Association of Rehabilitation Psychology should stick to similar stringent schedule that all participants must observe. Such schedule is believed to help trainees regulate and, if necessary, correct their daily behavior regarding diet, sleeping, taking bath, etc. (adapted from Harizuka 2006) (see Table A.1 in Appendix III). Any camp schedule includes the following key activities:

- Dohsa-hou session—this is the core activity of any Dohsa-hou camp; training sessions of 50 or 60 minutes each are held three times a day: two times in the morning and one more time in the afternoon.
- Group therapy—in general, the majority of children with disabilities lack rich interpersonal relationships and few of them have the chance to experience group play with coevals. During the Dohsa-hou camps, they may engage in group activities such as singing, dancing, and drawing, whereby they become familiar with each other and with their trainers. Group therapy usually takes place after the nap (see Table A.1 in Appendix III).
- Group counseling and training for parents—considering that parents share certain worries about their children, psychological counseling and Dohsa-hou training are held for them once a day.
- Training for trainers—every camp includes also a training programs for trainers (1 hour a day), which consist of lectures by Dohsa-hou supervisors and practice between the trainers—usually in pairs—under the guidance of the supervisors.
- Team meetings—these meetings are held at the end of each camp day between the members of each team; one team usually consists of a supervisor, four or five trainer-trainee pairs, and one or two subtrainers.

- General meeting—this meeting is held between the camp chief, camp manager, supervisors, trainers, and subtrainers after all team meetings finish. A representative of each team reports on the Dohsa-hou sessions held within their team during the day, and discussions are held on the reported content.

All the activities that a Dohsa-hou camp is involved in show that the Dohsa-hou camp model not only belongs to camp therapy, but that it also enriches it by adding some distinctive features such as *strong hierarchism* when the camp is in "working regime" and *communal spirit* when daily life activities are performed. All camp participants take their meals together and, in some camps, sing the camp song before and after each meal; sleep in common rooms for four to ten persons; trainers bathe their trainees or at least help the trainees' mother or father with it, etc. These two features—strong hierarchism and communal spirit—makes the Dohsa-hou camp model distinctively Japanese because when it comes to education and training, "the Japanese way allows perhaps the least room for deviation or personal idiosyncracy" (Kawagoe 2013). Furthermore, considering the strong educational aspect of Dohsa-hou therapy, we can see that the intensive camps are based on predetermined form—*kata*—or the "right attitude" that everybody, no matter their roles and responsibilities, must follow while embracing the group values oriented toward one common goal: the physical and mental progress of the trainees. Only then the desired positive changes and a sustainable development become possible.

7.3 Dohsa-hou and Body-Mind Psychotherapy—A Brief Comparison

Earlier in this chapter we briefly outlined the characteristics of the Western rehabilitation psychology in order to prevent possible confusion with Dohsa-hou, which is the core activity of the psychological rehabilitation in Japan (see Sect. 7.1.1.2). Despite some common points also between Dohsa-hou and traditional neurological rehabilitation methods such as that developed by the German physiotherapists Berta and Karel Bobath, and by the Czech pediatric neurologist Václav Vojta, the Japanese approach should be properly distinguished from them, too (Naurse 1992b: 2). While both the Bobath method and Dohsa-hou agree that *pattern training* is needed for overcoming a physiological impairment, the former focuses on the so-called *reflex-inhibiting patterns*, which limit the client's abnormal movements and postures that result from a peculiar reflex activity of the central nervous system. By contrast, Dohsa-hou does not address the nervous system and its functions directly, but it suggests for *psychological activity-based patterns* that spur on physical movements innate to all human beings; these patterns are activated through the repetitive training of the proper, innate movements (Naruse 1974: 9–10).

Considering Dohsa-hou's concept of relaxation as a self-induced and self-controlled process in contrast to relaxation fostered by external stimuli, Dohsa-hou is more akin to the American physiologist Edmund Jacobson's progressive muscle relaxation and to the autogenic training developed by the German psychiatrist Johannes Schultz (Naruse 2001: 27). Additionally, in terms of the strong emphasis that Dohsa-hou puts on the body-mind interconnectedness with its *intention-striving-bodily movement* model, the method can be said to correspond in a certain, albeit indirect, way with the neuroscience concept of brain mapping, according to which tapping the so-called primary motor and visceral maps can help one perform almost any activity in a far better way: "the brain is highly interactive. Each part—each map—imprints its own unique stamp into the character of the mind's psychic churnings" (Blakeslee and Blakeslee 2008: 19)."

As Dohsa-hou has kept its original name even among non-Japanese researchers and practitioners, the meaning encoded in the combination of the characters for the word *dohsa* (see footnote 2) suggests that bodily movement can be "created" consciously and this creative process is what the approach is all about. This basic concept is akin to the philosophy of expressive movement introduced by the American music and bodywork educators Alexandra and Roger Pierce, which suggests that personal patterns of movements are aspects of one's character; that centering our physical structure close to the vertical axis along the force vector of gravity influences our psychological and physical well-being; that "education of movement transforms the whole person" (Pierce and Pierce 2002: 7) and that "looking at ourselves from the perspective of movement—of action in the most down-to-earth sense—provides a simple and accessible opportunity to ponder our natural form and then true our behavior to it so that we more accurately express who we are" (Pierce and Pierce 2002: 14).

Considering all of the above similarities with Western approaches on movement and body-mind interconnectedness, Dohsa-hou could properly be labeled "body-mind therapy," "movement therapy," or "somatic psychology." Each of these labels reflects, indeed, certain key aspects of Dohsa-hou, but only partially. To gain further understanding of these aspects of Dohsa-hou, we will proceed to a detailed comparison between it and another Western approach—Body-Mind Psychotherapy (BMP)—considering that the names of the two approaches read completely interchangeable.

Body-Mind Psychotherapy was developed by the American psychotherapist and dance therapist Susan Aposhyan in the 1980s. That was a time marked by an increasing interest in integrating body-mind techniques into psychotherapy and BMP emerged as a natural attempt "to accomplish this integration in a simple, sensible, and seamless manner, so that the techniques are not just tacked on, but fit integrally and intelligently into the theory and practice of psychotherapy" (Aposhyan 2004: ix). The basis of BMP lies in anatomy, physiology, and early motor development. It draws the foundations of its principles from Body-Mind Centering (BMC), an approach for movement reeducation and re-patterning developed in the early 1970s by the American occupational therapist and movement artist Bonnie Bainbridge Cohen. BMC includes "an in-depth and experiential study of anatomy and physiology, down to the cellular level" (Aposhyan 2004: 17), in addition to "synthesized studies of early motor development into the system of basic neurological actions that form the basis of the energetic development work in BMP" (ibid.).

Starting with founder Aposhyan's definition of BMP as "an approach to psychotherapy integrating somatic (body-based) techniques into the basic framework of psychotherapy" (Aposhyan 2004: ix), we shed light on several key notions which seemingly overlap in BMP and Dohsa-hou, but which, in the end, reveal the fundamental differences between the two approaches:

- *Self-knowledge through direct experience*—this is one of BMP's basic principles. The therapist invites the client to directly experience every aspect of themselves through exploring their body, but also by recognizing the *quality of mind* that they encounter in any particular aspect of anatomy. For example, if someone has a back problem, the therapist will teach them about all the anatomy and physiology involved. This study is not just intellectual, but the client is given the opportunity to experience, i.e., to touch, feel, visualize, and attend to each detail. The same approach could be applied to psychological problems like, for example, obsessions: the client "might examine the physiological and neurological patterns and mechanics involved" and thus "delineate the postures that support and perpetuate the state" (Aposhyan 2004: 18). However, even in this case, muscles, skeleton, skin, fluids, fat, viscera, and endocrine system remain the major domains of the client's experience.
  As previously explained, direct experience is one of Dohsa-hou's cornerstones; this is also the way Dohsa-hou trainers are being trained, i.e., by the direct sensation of their hands on the trainee's body and by taking the roles of trainees during intensive Dohsa-hou camps or workshops; hence the *karada-de-oboeru* principle applies to trainers, too. However, in Dohsa-hou direct experience opens the path to self-knowledge only within the framework of predetermined pattern—the Dohsa-hou task—and the constant repetition of its elements. That is, its system of experience is focused on striving for the successful accomplishment of a desired movement and much less on examining concrete physiological sensations.
- *Active movement reeducation*—in BMP, passive bodywork and manipulation of tissues go side by side with the client's active participation in the form of an unaided performance of a new movement or expression based on the new sensations perceived. "The body tissues are intelligent. They receive, perceive, and respond to messages given by the therapist's hands even before the conscious mind is aware of them. Then, through body movement, these new sensations can be organized consciously into healthier patterns of use and in this way are more clearly and consciously established and integrated within the body" (Hartley 1995: xxxi).
  In Dohsa-hou, too, the concept of movement reeducation plays a key role, but, similarly to the concept of direct experience, this reeducation is based on predetermined forms—*kata*—integrated into the body dynamics. That is, free and spontaneous responses are not encouraged and whenever performed, they are soon to be "brought back" to the right movement or posture.

- *Presupposed functional integrity of body and mind*—another BMP principle, body-mind integrity claims that when the individual "immerses" themselves in physiology at the level of molecular behavior, body and mind become indistinguishable. "Whatever the task or handicap, the client gets a good look at how they are using their bodies and how this use is affecting the problem. This gives the client a sense of empowerment and responsibility—moving beyond a sense of being pathological or having a fixed pathology" (Aposhyan 2004: 18).
  This key BMP point seems equivalent to Dohsa-hou's concept of body-mind interconnectedness, only the latter is not much interested in physiological functions and molecular behavior. Rather, it attempts to recognize the psychological pattern that underlies any dysfunction—be it a physiological or a mental one—and improve it by means of *mindful* bodily movements thanks to which the functional integrity between body and mind becomes palpable for the trainee themselves.
- *Interaction cycle*—this is "the basic format of BMP" (Aposhyan 2004: 86), a four-step cycle which begins with embodiment (the therapist's self-awareness that creates the appropriate therapeutic atmosphere), proceeds to identification of the client's desire and motivation, then to awareness of and feedback on the somatic response to this desire, and finally allows the response to turn into a complete sequence of bodily movements as facilitated by the therapist. This process "joins both clients' and therapists' awareness of how clients' developmental processes are manifesting in the clients' bodies at a particular moment" (ibid.).
  The interaction cycle format appears similar to Dohsa-hou's *intention-striving-bodily movement* model (see Fig. 7.1 in Sect. 7.1.1.1) in the sense that the latter, too, "tests" the process of the trainee's body-mind interaction at a given moment and explores the border between the trainee's limitations and potential. However, Dohsa-hou is doing it within a task-based framework, that is, it always pursues the performance of a concrete task, which the trainer chooses beforehand from a group of preset tasks.

Besides these differences, there are two more that should be outlined. First, as BMP emerged to serve and was integrated into the Western psychotherapeutic model, it relies exclusively on verbal communication for exchanging feedback with its clients. Therefore, as compared to Dohsa-hou, BMP appears more difficult to apply to clients with disabilities with whom verbal communication is not possible; unlike the BMP therapist, the Dohsa-hou trainer is challenged to draw conclusions only on the basis of the trainee's bodily movements. Second, BMP pays attention to the innate body intelligence and the physical contact between the therapist's hands and the client's body, whereas Dohsa-hou strives to spur on the trainee's proper mental attitude through bodily movement, and attaches great importance to the communication process and the *joint attention* within the trainer–trainee pair. Nevertheless, both Dohsa-hou and BMP agree on the idea that "*feeling* our bodies in the fullest sense of the word can help us feel our own vitality and the path toward psychological health, but it can also connect us to the rest of life that exists around us" (Aposhyan 2004: xii).

7.4 Conclusion

Some authors place Dohsa-hou under the heading of "Japanese bodyworks" together with the Noguchi Gymnastics Method[11] (Kawano in Haruki 2002: 274–275). At first glance Dohsa-hou is, indeed, a bodywork for it embraces a holistic view on the human nature and aims at improved self-awareness through movement and postural reeducation as other somatic methods, for example, Alexander technique and Feldenkrais method, do. However, the ultimate goal of Dohsa-hou is set even further: while striving to adopt the proper posture, Dohsa-hou spurs on one's *self-activity* as a psychological process, which, in turn, induces a rich variety of *experiences* colored by a vivid sense of reality (Egashira in Naruse 1992a: 44). Dohsa-hou believes that the ability to thus control one's body—referring to both relaxation and performance of proper movements—means that the individual has gained control over their mind. Although this process is difficult to comprehend from the viewpoint of the natural sciences (Ohno and Murata 1993: 218), the approach yields positive results where other bodywork methods hardly prove efficacious.

Additionally, unlike the verbal psychotherapeutic approaches, but similar to sports and performing arts, Dohsa-hou is based on *body* learning and *embodied* knowledge. Hence the phrase *karada-de-oboeru* appears to completely correspond to the method's name: the trainee masters their skills, i.e., progress in physical rehabilitation or psychotherapy—depending on the purpose Dohsa-hou is applied for—by *doing*, not by *talking*. Especially in cases of clients with disabilities, bodily movements are in fact their only means of expression, the only diagnostic tool that the trainer relies on, and the basis on which the whole therapeutic process unfolds. Dohsa-hou is therefore a very authentic approach in the sense that it remains untouched by any possible complications that verbal communication may cause; rather, it relies predominantly on body language, believing in the authenticity of physical movements, or the lack of such, as a barometer of the state of one's mind. In other words, the method uses bodily movement as a diagnostic and as a therapeutic tool and by so doing it introduces to the stage of psychotherapy not just body, but the body-mind unity; it emphasizes the importance of this unity within any therapeutic process, thus supporting the notion of the Eastern medicine that if body is in order, the mind too becomes ordered (Tanaka 2009: 69).

Finally, to the best of our knowledge, Dohsa-hou is the first approach that draws attention to and realizes the idea that psychotherapy is possible for individuals with severe psycho-motor disfunctions and/or mental retardation. Believing in everyone's

---

[11]Noguchi Gymnastics Method, popularly known as *Noguchi Taisō* (野口体操), is a complex of body-mind exercises for relaxation, physical improvement and revitalization systematized in the 1970s by Michizō Noguchi (1914–1998), Professor of Physical Education at the Tokyo University of Arts. The method was developed under the radical notion that likens human body to a water-full bag in which bones, muscles and viscera are floating (Noguchi 2002: 7). Noguchi Gymnastics is especially acclaimed by theatre, dance, and music performers.

innate ability to strive regardless of their condition, Dohsa-hou helps its clients to turn from passive recipients of help from the outside to active agents of their own transformation—physical, psychological, and social. In so doing, the approach questions, albeit indirectly, the cult of normalcy which often instills mistaken understandings of human wholeness and presumes that "disability always entails tragedy and suffering, absorbing it into a curative medical model that treats the condition as something to be overcome by the individual" (Reynolds 2008: 30). To put it metaphorically, if, by chance, a birch tree happens to grow in a pine forest, all the pines around it will consider it awkward with its snow-white bark and trembling leaves. However, it is still a tree and no worse than the others; only its form and behavior differ from that of the pine trees, but its very existence as a tree is an undeniable truth. This specific aspect of Dohsa-hou—namely, its potential to reach beyond the pale of the medical model and the cult of normalcy—is manifested through the communication and joint attention within the trainer–trainee pair: we all are living human beings who share an innate ability to strive for their own further development. However, exactly this aspect poses the question where Dohsa-hou should be located in respect to other psychotherapeutic approaches and whether it is a psychotherapy at all. As the American anthropologist Joan Cassell points out, "the extent of embodiment seems roughly parallel to the prestige system among doctors: psychiatrists are on the lowest rung; they are not considered real doctors" (Cassell 2000: 32). That is, psychiatry, psychotherapy and psychology tend to be disregarded as the least "embodied" specialties in the field of healthcare and well-being. For this reason, considering that Dohsa-hou is involved in bodywork, it may get a higher position; on the other hand, this bodywork in fact addresses the mind, which might be considered somewhat "undeserving."

Whatsoever the truth might be, Dohsa-hou is often described as "original and innovative Japanese psychotherapy" (Imura 2012: 3; Imura and Furukawa 2004: 157). Indeed, using the means of bodily movement, Dohsa-hou prompts the development of a subtle, yet profound awareness that might be likened to Zen Buddhist enlightenment (Kouno 2013: 37–39).[12] This awareness concerns the way

[12]Although Dohsa-hou is not related to any religious or spiritual traditions, what Dr. Bunko Kouno, a clinical psychologist, Dohsa-hou supervisor, and chief priest of the Fukuju-ji Zen Buddhist temple in Aichi prefecture suggests, appears rather relevant to the therapeutic essence of Dohsa-hou. We cannot discuss this comparison here, but we consider it a promising possibility for the enrichment of the body-mind unity concept and its relation to mindfulness in psychotherapy. Considering that there is no psyche without a living body, the ultimate goal of every psychotherapeutic approach—Eastern or Western, Dr. Kouno suggests, is the insight into one's own body-mind unity. Such an insight helps the individual reset their life, while accepting their disease or disability as they are (in private communication with Dr. Kouno, March 2017).

Additionally, Dohsa-hou's birth and development are not unrelated to the specificities of Japanese culture (Tsuru in Akita 2017: 43): certain cultural influences can be found in, for example, the method's concept of *kata* and the martial arts' concept of *shu-ha-ri* (守破離), which describes the stages of achieving mastery as "obey, detach, and transcend", i.e., the disciple first learns properly the *kata* with the help of their master, then they brush it up on their own, and, finally, they transcend the *kata* and start to move naturally. This concept is based on the earlier *jo-ha-kyū* (序破急) concept ("beginning, break, rapid") introduced in the Japanese arts by the *Nō*-theater master and Zen monk Zeami Motokiyo (c.1363 - c.1443) (Tsuru in Akita 2017: 40).

we are standing and breathing right now, or whether we are meeting the other person's gaze, etc., i.e., it takes us to the here-and-now reality and in so doing helps us recognize how our mental attitudes are expressed through our bodies and even shape them; how, as Naruse summarizes, our movements and posture are representative for our respond to and relationship with the surrounding environment (Naruse 1988: 153). This specific awareness, which makes us self-integrated and strong, yet flexible like bamboo trees—one of the "three friends of winter" (see Chap. 2 and Appendix III)—seems to be the most important Dohsa-hou message concerning not only the concept of body-mind unity, but also the way we exist *mindfully* as such a unity and the way we are *moving*, i.e., *living* in this world, between Earth and Sky. I move, therefore I am.

References

Akita, Iwao (ed.): Japanese Psychotherapies—A Body Compendium, Shinyosha, 2017 (in Japanese)

Aposhyan, Susan: Body-Mind Psychotherapy: Principles, Techniques, and Practical Applications, W.W. Norton & Company, 2004

Bangayan, Samantha, O. Imura: A Study of Dohsa-hou on an Adolescent with Cerebral Palsy in Japan, The Journal of Rehabilitation Psychology, Vol. 36 (1), Japanese Association of Rehabilitation Psychology, 2009

Bertherat, Thérèse, C. Bernstein: The Body Has Its Reasons—Self-Awareness Through Conscious Movement, Healing Arts Press, 1989

Blakeslee, Sandra, M. Blakeslee: The Body Has a Mind of Its Own—How Body Maps in Your Brain Help You Do (Almost) Everything Better, Random House Trade Paperback, 2008

Cassell, Joan: The Woman in the Surgeon's Body, Harvard University Press, 2000

Chervenkova, Velizara, O. Imura: The Will for Rising Up—A Case Study at a Summer Dohsa-hou Camp, The Journal of Rehabilitation Psychology, Vol. 38 (2), Japanese Association of Rehabilitation Psychology, 2012

De Mente, Boyé Lafayette: Japan's Cultural Code Words—233 Key Terms That Explain the Attitudes and Behavior of the Japanese, Tuttle Publishing, 2004

De Mente, Boyé Lafayette: Kata: The Key to Understanding and Dealing with the Japanese, Tuttle Publishing, 2013

Fujino, Haruo: Effects of Dohsa-hou Relaxation on Body Awareness and Psychological Distress, Japanese Psychological Research, Vol. 54(4), Japanese Psychological Association, 2012

Ghanimi, Farzaneh: The Study of Relation Between Dohsa-hou—A Japanese Psycho Rehabilitation Method—and Gestalt Therapy, The Journal of Rehabilitation Psychology, Vol. 34(1–2), Japanese Association of Rehabilitation Psychology, 2007

Graham, Martha: Blood Memory—An Autobiography, Doubleday, 1991

Greene, Elliot, B. Goodrich-Dunn: The Psychology of the Body, Lippincott Williams & Wilkins, 2004

Harizuka, Susumu: Historical Overview and Prospect about Practical Usage of Psychological Rehabilitation (Dohsa-Hou), Psychological Rehabilitation Homepage, retrieved from http://www.hes.kyushu-u.ac.jp/sinriha/english.html, Kyushu University, 2006

Hartley, Linda: Wisdom of the Body Moving: An Introduction to Body-Mind Centering, North Atlantic Books, 1995

Haruki, Yutaka (ed.): Somatic Psychology—Posture and Expression-Based Psychological Paradigm, Kawashima Shoten, 2002 (in Japanese)

Henshall, Kenneth G.: A Guide To Remembering Japanese Characters, Tuttle Publishing, 1998
Horton, Judith Anne, P.R.Clance, C.Sterk-Elifson, J. Emshoff: Touch in Psychotherapy: A Survey of Patient's Experience, Psychotherapy: Theory, Research, Practice, Training, Vol. 32(3), American Psychological Association, 1995
Hosaka, Takashi (ed.): Rehabilitation Psychology, Contemporary Esprit Journal, Vol. 343, Shibundo Publishing, 1996 (in Japanese)
Hoshino, Kimio: "Jiko" Control of Motor Skills and Mental Conditions by Athletes through Dohsa, The Journal of Rehabilitation Psychology—Special Edition, Vol. XVII, XVIII, XIX, Japanese Association of Rehabilitation Psychology, 1992
Imura, Osamu: Dohsa-hou and Children with Disabilities, Osaka University, 2012 (unpublished; in Japanese)
Imura, Osamu: The Birth and Development of Dohsa-hou (in "Introduction to Dohsa-hou—An Integrated Japanese Body-Mind Therapy"), Osaka University, 2016
Imura, Osamu, T. Furukawa: Development of Psychological Rehabilitation in Okinawa Prefecture —A Way for Local Contribution by University of the Ryukyus, Human Sciences Annals of University of the Ryukyus, Vol. 13, University of the Ryukyus, 2004 (in Japanese)
Itonaga, Kazufumi: Psychological Rehabilitation for Children with Disabilities, Annals of Osaka Kyoiku University, Vol. 57(1), Osaka Kyoiku University, 2008 (in Japanese)
Kawagoe, Aileen: The Intangible Curriculum of Japanese Education, retrieved from http://educationinjapan.wordpress.com/education-system-in-japan-general/the-intangible-curriculum-of-a-japanese-education, Education in Japan Community Blog, 2013
Keleman, Stanley: Your Body Speaks Its Mind, Center Press, 1975
Kennedy, Paul (ed.): The Oxford Handbook of Rehabilitation Psychology, Oxford University Press, 2012
Konno, Yoshitaka: The Significance of Touch in the Developmental Clinical Psychology, Annals of the Faculty of Education, Vol. 33, Bunkyo University, 1999 (in Japanese)
Konno, Yoshitaka: Dohsa-hou as Mutual Blending—Searching the Body-Mind Connection, Gakuensha, 2005 (in Japanese)
Kouno, Bunko (ed. Gosaku Naruse): Becoming Aware through Bodily Movements—Supportive Process in Clinical Psychology (Changing the Movements Changes both Mind and Body), Institute for Zen Studies, 2013 (in Japanese)
LaMothe, Kimerer L.: Why We Dance: A Philosophy of Bodily Becoming, Columbia University Press, 2015
Miki, Yoshihiko, K. Kuroki (co-ed.): Japanese Psychotherapies—Essence and Practice, Tokishobo, 1998 (in Japanese)
Montagu, Ashley: Touching: The Human Significance of the Skin (Third Edition), Harper & Row Publishers, 1986
Moore, Chris, P.J. Dunham (ed.): Joint Attention: Its Origins and Role in Development, Psychology Press, 1995
Naruse, Gosaku: Dohsa and Dohsa-Kunren Theory from the Standpoint of Bobath Method, Research Bulletin of Educational Psychology, Vol. 18(2), Kyushu University, 1974 (in Japanese)
Naruse, Gosaku: The Era of Image, Seishin Shobo, 1988 (in Japanese)
Naruse, Gosaku (ed.): Health and Sports Clinical Dohsa-hou, Contemporary Esprit Journal (Appendix), Shibundo Publishing, 1992a (in Japanese)
Naruse, Gosaku: Recent Development of Dohsa-hou in Japan, The Journal of Rehabilitation Psychology—Special Edition, Vol. XVII, XVIII, XIX, Japanese Association of Rehabilitation Psychology, 1992b
Naruse, Gosaku: The Wonders of Posture—Supple Body and Mind Bring Health, Kodansha Blue Backs, 1998 (in Japanese)
Naruse, Gosaku: Dohsa-hou—Theory and Methodology of A Brand New Psychotherapy, Seishin Shobo, 2000 (in Japanese)
Naruse, Gosaku: Relaxation—A Way for Releasing the Tension on One's Own, Kodansha Blue Backs, 2001 (in Japanese)

Naruse, Gosaku: Movement Excercises, Psychological Rehabilitation Research Center, 2005 (in Japanese)

Naruse, Gosaku: The Movement Mind, Seishin Shobo, 2007 (in Japanese)

Naruse, Gosaku: Body and Mind—Body-Oriented Clinical Psychology, Seishin Shobo, 2009 (in Japanese)

Naruse, Gosaku: Development of Dohsa-Therapy—Body-Mind Harmony and Revitalization, Seishin Shobo, 2014 (in Japanese)

Noguchi, Michizō: Noguchi Gymnastics—Listening to the Body, Shinjusha, 2002 (in Japanese)

Ohba, Nobue: Application of Dohsa-hou to Anxiety Neurotic Patient, The Journal of Rehabilitation Psychology—Special Edition, Vol. XVII, XVIII, XIX, Japanese Association of Rehabilitation Psychology, 1992

Ohno, Kiyoshi, S. Murata (ed.): Dohsa-hou Handbook—A Technical Introduction for Beginners, Keio Gijuku University Press, 1993 (in Japanese)

Pierce, Alexandra, R.Pierce: Expressive Movement: Posture and Action in Daily Life, Sports, And The Performing Arts, Da Capo Press, 2002

Reynolds, Thomas E.: Vulnerable Communion—A Theology of Disability and Hospitality, BrazosPress, 2008

Rosenberg, Jack Lee: Body, Self, and Soul: Sustaining Integration, Humanics Limited, 1985

Shigehashi, Shiro: Arranging the Posture, Phoenix Journal, Vol. 46, Center for Clinical Psychology and Human Development, Kyushu University, 1994 (in Japanese)

Singer, Kurt: Mirror, Sword and Jewel—A Study of Japanese Characteristics, Japan Library, 1997

Takamatsu, Kaoru: Application of Dohsa-hou to Schizophrenic Patient, The Journal of Rehabilitation Psychology—Special Edition, Vol. XVII, XVIII, XIX, Japanese Association of Rehabilitation Psychology, 1992

Tanaka, Yasuo (ed. Shuji Goto): Basics of Oriental Medicine, Nippon Jitsugyo Publishing, 2009 (in Japanese)

Teruta, Eri, S. Harada: Dohsa-hou Camps and Monthly Meetings in Japan (in "Introduction to Dohsa-hou—An Integrated Japanese Body-Mind Therapy"), Osaka University, 2016

Tominaga, Yoshiki, T. Miyoshi, K. Nakano: Body Speaking, Speaking to the Body—After the Great Hanshin-Awaji Earthquake: Practical Report on the Mental Care Provided through Dohsa-hou to Disaster Victims, The Journal of Rehabilitation Psychology, Vol. 21, Japanese Association of Rehabilitation Psychology, 1995 (in Japanese)

Tsuru, Mitsuyo: Theoretical Considerations of Dohsa-hou, The Journal of Rehabilitation Psychology—Special Edition, Vol. XVII, XVIII, XIX, Japanese Association of Rehabilitation Psychology, 1992

Tsuru, Mitsuyo: An Invitation to Clinical Dohsa-hou, Kongo Shuppan, 2007 (in Japanese)

Yoshihara, Masataka: Psychological Significance of Dohsa-hou Camps as Camp Therapy, Annals of Educational Studies, Vol. 15, Osaka University, 2010 (in Japanese)

Part IV
Into the Depths: Silence Beneficial, Silence Torturing

The penultimate part of this book discusses the practical application of the three Japanese psychotherapies—Morita, Naikan, and Dohsa-hou. We present in chronological order three respective studies in an attempt to illuminate further the essence and dynamics of these approaches.

Chapter 8
The Will to Rise—A Case Study at a Summer Dohsa-hou Camp

8.1 About this Study

The present case study was carried out within the 10th Okinawa Eima Camp held by the Japanese Association of Rehabilitation Psychology in August 2010 on the island of Ishigaki, Okinawa prefecture. The 6-day/5-night camp took place at the Okinawa Prefecture Ishigaki Youth Center, an educational facility located in a rich natural area nearby the seashore of Ishigaki. It hosted 10 trainees aged between 6 and 20, nine of whom were local residents. Each of the trainees had the characteristics of their respective conditions—for example, Down syndrome and cerebral palsy—while sharing an almost complete lack of verbal development.

8.1.1 Case Description[1]

The trainee described in the present study was a boy named Sei Tanaka, who was aged 6 years and 8 months at the time the camp was held. According to the information the trainee's mother provided during the initial interview, Sei was born after a normal pregnancy with a weight of 2,604 g. After turning 5 months old, Sei got bacterial meningitis, which caused hydrocephaly accompanied by absence seizures and brain atrophy. Additionally, at that time his hearing worsened significantly with examination results showing no responses from his left ear and a 60 dB moderate hearing loss in the right one; for this reason, at the time of the study

[1]All the descriptions presented hereafter are based on the author's daily records in her capacity of trainer. The Dohsa-hou technical terms are intentionally left untranslated, excluding when a term is introduced for the first time. For further details, see Glossary.

This case study was first published in Chervenkova, Velizara, O. Imura: The Will for Rising Up—A Case Study at a Summer Dohsa-hou Camp, The Journal of Rehabilitation Psychology, Vol. 38(2), Japanese Association of Rehabilitation Psychology, 2012.

V. Chervenkova, *Japanese Psychotherapies*,
DOI 10.1007/978-981-10-3126-7_8

Sei was using a hearing aid. Two months later, when Sei was 7 months old, he underwent a shunt operation which brought significant improvement. Nevertheless, even after his first birthday Sei was not able to keep his head upright or to sit on his own; taking and holding objects was difficult, too, as unnatural muscular tension was observed in his limbs, predominantly in his left arm. Sei's intellectual and verbal development was heavily impaired; he cried often, his facial expression was rather limited, he did not laugh at all, and seldom smiled.

8.1.2 Aims and Objectives

As reported by his mother, Sei started Dohsa-hou training at the age of 1 year and 4 months. Since then the mother has been truly devoted to her son's rehabilitation, investing efforts on doing Dohsa-hou exercises at home and on attending Dohsa-hou trainings. Considering all of the specificities of Sei's disease and present condition, the trainer set three major goals for the six-day Dohsa-hou camp, namely (i) helping Sei relax through basic Dohsa-hou warm-up and relaxation techniques such as *ude-age* (arm lifting) and *kukan-no-hineri* (twisting of the torso); (ii) helping the trainee straighten his waist and limbs so that he can perform properly *agura-zai* (sitting cross-legged on the floor) and *ritsui* (upright position); and (iii) helping Sei improve his nonverbal communication skills and enrich his facial expression through the establishment of joint attention and through the proper alternation between Dohsa-hou tasks and breaks abound with playful moments.

8.2 Six Summer Camp Days in Ishigaki—Efforts and Outcomes

In this section we present each of the days of the 10th Okinawa Eima Camp and the daily Dohsa-hou sessions in detail.

8.2.1 The Therapeutic Process

8.2.1.1 First Camp Day: Initial Interview

Although the trainer, trainee Sei, and the trainee's mother had already met before when they came for the camp, they spent one hour discussing Sei's recent condition and the most helpful exercises his mother had been practicing with him at home. They also discussed the most recent improvements the mother had noticed in Sei's bodily movements and communication skills. After the initial interview, the trainer applied basic Dohsa-hou techniques such as *ude-age* and *kukan-no-hineri* under the guidance of her supervisor. It was essential not only for warming up the trainee, but also for helping the trainer and the trainee get to know each other and establish a good therapeutic relationship. Although it was still the first camp day, Sei did not show any signs of unwillingness to practice while performing the required Dohsa-hou tasks. On the contrary, he seemed to enjoy them and smiled back several times. Probably as a result of the successful warm-up, Sei was able to perform excellent *ritsui* position with the team supervisor. Sei was relatively self-confident in standing upright with his facial expression becoming brighter. This encouraged his trainer and made her look forward to the next camp day when the full-blown morning-to-evening training was to begin.

8.2.1.2 Second Camp Day: Intensive Work Begins

First Session (09:00–10:00) In contrast to the previous day and to the surprise of the trainer, this morning Sei was sleepy and yawned quite often. The trainer therefore started the session by alternating the basic techniques of *ude-age* and *kukan-no-hineri*. Sei was not reluctant to perform them, but his bodily movements nevertheless remained rather languid. The trainer then made several breaks during which she tried to make him smile by drawing her face near his and smiling, and also by playing with his hands and fingers.

Second Session (11:30–12:30) Sei was still sleepy; the trainer applied *kukan-no-hineri* for another 2–3 times, but at a very slow pace, helping his muscles relax properly. Near the end of the session, Sei seemed refreshed and performed *ritsui* properly together with the supervisor.

Third Session (16:00–17:00) During the first 10–15 minutes of the session Sei was nervous, thus making the trainer decide not to force him doing exercises; the trainer tried to play with him instead. Soon afterward, Sei calmed down and, surprisingly, he started smiling at the unfamiliar teachers and volunteers who were sitting around the mat. Moreover, he managed to grasp the trainer's fingers while playing. The trainer felt that he is already in good shape and she attempted to apply *ritsui*; to everyone's surprise it was an excellent one. This was a moment of success, excitement, and joy for both the trainee and his trainer. From this moment on, the performance of a proper *ristui* position became the general focus of their mutual efforts. At the end of the session, when Sei saw his mother entering the room, he smiled and approached her crawling, grasped her hand and, although the floor appeared to be slippery for him, he managed to rise while she was holding him. Everyone around rejoiced at Sei's behavior, especially the trainer and Sei's mother, who hugged and kissed him.

8.2.1.3 Third Camp Day: Intensive Work Is Underway

First Session (09:00–10:00) Sei was sleepy again, but in contrast to the beginning of the second day, this morning he maintained good eye contact with the people sitting around the mat. Therefore, the trainer did not force him to immediately start doing the exercises, but dedicated the first 15 minutes to hugging him and playing with him while encouraging his nonverbal communication with the others. Later on, when the trainer felt Sei was ready, she applied *ude-age*, which Sei enjoyed very much, and then switched to *ritsui*. The trainee performed it very well with his knees, hips, and waist straightened, while waving merrily his hands and trying to touch the trainer's face. When his mother came, Sei welcomed her with a toothy smile.

Second Session (11:30–12:30) As compared to the morning session, Sei cheered up; the trainer decided to focus on the *ritsui* position. After applying simple relaxation tasks such as extension of arms and legs, the trainee not only performed a good *ritsui*, but he also put efforts on standing on his legs. As a result, in this upright position he managed to do one-two proper steps forward—a success that he enjoyed very much together with the trainer.

Third Session (16:00–17:00) Sei was in a good mood from the session's very beginning—not only did he smile, but he also laughed several times. He also maintained good eye contact with those sitting around the mat for quite a long time—around 30 s—and he rolled about on the mat completely on his own. The trainer let him enjoy these playful moments for a while and then applied *ritsui* again. At that point, Sei put proper muscular tension into his neck and legs in order to maintain the good posture. He enjoyed the group therapy that took place after the third session.

8.2.1.4 Fourth Camp Day: Positive Outcomes Emerge

First Session (09:00–10:00) In contrast to the previous early morning sessions, Sei was in a good mood and not sleepy. He seemed to have got used to the camp environment: he smiled more often and maintained good eye contact with the people sitting around the mat. During that time he performed an excellent *ritsui*, making two or three steps toward the trainer and even trying to climb on her crossed legs. Considering Sei's progress, the trainer decided to apply also *agura-zai*—at this point the trainee put proper tension in his waist and neck, thus performing a proper posture while looking straight forward.

Second Session (11:30–12:30) Sei seemed to be a little tired after the first session, but the trainer nevertheless decided to remain focused on *ritsui* and *agura-zai*, both of which Sei performed very well. When at the end of the session his mother entered the room, he managed to crawl to her place while following with his eyes the people who were coming in and going out of the room.

Third Session (16:00–17:00) Probably because Sei practiced hard during the first two sessions, he became sleepy during the third one. Additionally, and to the surprise of the trainer, he also had two absence seizures. This made the trainer more careful and sensitive in regard to the trainee's own pace of performing Dohsa-hou tasks. During this session, the trainer allowed short breaks more often and applied *ritsui* only once. Although Sei was sleepy, he performed it well again and again tried to climb on the trainer's crossed legs. Later on, during the group therapy he perked up and even managed to get on his elbows while crawling on the floor.

8.2.1.5 Fifth Camp Day: Final Daylong Efforts

First Session (09:00–10:00) During the first session of the camp's final day, Sei was sleepy, but after performing *ude-age* and *kukan-no-hineri* he became more cheerful. Nevertheless, the trainer refrained from applying intensively *ritsui* and *agura-zai* and dedicated the time left to play and short breaks while lying next to him on the floor.

Second Session (11:30–12:30) Sei was a little tired after he played with student volunteers during the break between the two sessions. Therefore, the trainer started the session with extension of the arms and legs—an activity that Sei enjoyed very much, often smiling back. During the session's second half he performed well both *ritsui* and *agura-zai* but he tried neither to walk nor to keep his head upright while adopting the respective postures.

Third Session (16:00–17:00) After the lunch break Sei looked refreshed; the trainer decided to apply *agura-zai*. Sei performed it very well with visible improvement as compared to the previous days because of the increased proper muscular tension he put into his neck and back. Moreover, he managed to maintain the *ritsui* posture for about 15–20 s in comparison to some 10 s before.

8.2.1.6 Sixth Camp Day: The Camp's Final Day

09:00–10:00 Sei came for the final training session in a relatively good shape and mood; the trainer applied *ude-age* several times, during which Sei's elbows were remarkably relaxed, followed by *ritsui*, both of which he performed well.

After the last training finished, the trainer and Sei's mother had a closing session when they discussed the outcomes of the past camp days such as the trainee's richer facial expression, and his increased ability to put proper muscular tension into his neck, back, and limbs.

8.2.2 Discussion

As previously mentioned, among the three Japanese psychotherapies subject of the present book, Dohsa-hou is probably the least known outside of Japan and some Asian countries, let alone Eastern Europe and the trainer's homeland, Bulgaria. Although, as shown in the comparative Table 4.1 (Sect. 4.2), Dohsa-hou emerged within the global trend of "introducing" the body into psychotherapeutic context, such approaches nevertheless remain exceptions in the word-dominated psychotherapeutic world where physical contact between therapist and client is taboo. It is important to remind also the conclusions that we previously made: Dohsa-hou not only "brings" body into psychotherapeutic context, but it draws the attention further to bodily movement as an unequivocal expression of the body-mind unity. Additionally, it emphasizes the importance of the nonverbal communication between trainer and trainee, their ability to share joint attention, and the unique atmosphere of communal work and life, which permeate the intensive Dohsa-hou camps.

All of these specificities manifested visibly in the present case of the 6-year-old trainee suffering from hydrocephaly—Sei—who attended the 10th Okinawa Eima Camp: as Sei's mother reported, before the time of the camp Sei has attended only one-day Dohsa-hou trainings, but it was the first time he participated in a 6-day/5-night camp. Although it was expected that attending such an intensive camp would be a challenging task for him—indeed, there were times when he was sleepy or nervous—Sei managed to accommodate relatively quickly to the camp's atmosphere and schedule. Still from the very beginning, Sei understood the tasks of *ude-age* and *kukan-no-hineri* and strived to relax properly the unnatural tension in his limbs under the trainer's guidance; at the same time, he managed to put muscular tension where needed, i.e., in body areas such as knees, hips, and waist. These efforts helped him perform successfully a proper *ritsui* position (the third session of the second camp day)—it was a miraculous moment when the trainer felt she was nothing but a prop for the tiny boy who put his own muscular tension into his knees, hips and waist, and, as a result, managed to properly rise and stand on his own; these were followed by taking one-two steps during the second session of the third camp day. Since these moments of success for both Sei and his trainer, the communication between them deepened significantly—this manifested itself in increased occasions of sharing joint attention not only during the sessions, but also during the short in-session breaks when, while lying on the floor, they looked silently into each other's eyes and smiled.

Then, on the third session of the fifth camp day, Sei not only managed to rise and stand on his own, but also to maintain the *ritsui* posture thus adopted for relatively long time of about 15–20 seconds. At that moment, he visibly demonstrated joy and satisfaction by waving his hands, smiling, and also by pronouncing certain, albeit unarticulated, sounds to express further the positive experience engendered by his own efforts.

As the camp progressed, Sei also became able to perform activities he had not done before in his daily life—for example, climbing on the trainer's or on his mother's crossed legs while being held up under his armpits. Such activities appeared simultaneously with the increased number of occasions when he made eye contact not only with the people he was familiar with—for example, his mother, trainer, and supervisor—but also with unknown people attending the camp such as specialists on a study tour or volunteers. As expected, the camp atmosphere, which differs from that of the trainees' daily lives, was very important for Sei, too, prompting his interest toward other people and helping him to improve his communication skills.

As for the daily life activities performed at the camp, the trainer helped Sei's mother with feeding him and on several occasions she did it herself. An activity performed apart from the Dohsa-hou sessions, it likely contributed further to the improvement of the communication within the trainer–trainee pair and brought forth the positive therapeutic outcomes. Other such activities included taking walks in the camp vicinity with Sei in his stroller and dancing at the camp's evening party while the trainer was carrying him in her arms; at that point, they both enjoyed the heartwarming hospitality of the local people of Ishigaki.

Around a month after the summer Dohsa-hou camp in Ishigaki, the trainer and her trainee, Sei, met again. Initially, Sei looked a little sleepy in his stroller, but when he saw the trainer he smiled, and then he started waving his hands and laughing. It was a very important sign that Sei had memorized his trainer well enough so as to recognize her even a month later. Moreover, both his facial expression and bodily movements had become more varied with obvious signs of growth that was now manifested as an unequivocal result of the intensive six-day Dohsa-hou camp. Additionally, the muscular tension he properly put in his legs and waist was now remarkable as compared to the time before the camp, thus proving that the camp goals had been successfully achieved.

8.3 Conclusion

Attending an intensive Dohsa-hou camp as a trainer is one of the key requirements for specialists who want not only to experience directly Dohsa-hou themselves, but also to tap the method's therapeutic essence. The description of the camp's overall environment shows that this essence first of all refers to the harmonious *communal life*, in most of the cases in the countryside. This specificity seems to be an indispensable requirement on whose basis only the second important condition—*the personal efforts* and *the communication within the trainer–trainee pair*—can successfully unfold.

A nonverbal approach focused precisely on the establishment of a strong trainer–trainee relationship through mutual acceptance and joint attention while performing a certain task, Dohsa-hou gives the trainer the role of a partner who strives together with the trainee on their way to rehabilitation and further growth. Through this mutual striving, Dohsa-hou provides its clients with *experiences* that they rarely, if ever at all, have the chance to taste amidst their daily lives. For example, for children such as the trainee presented in this case—Sei—who almost all the time sit in their stroller or lie down in their bed, standing on their legs, and rising through their own effort is an experience that has the potential to spur on their impaired development. Even though the conventional medicine often considers the rehabilitation of such conditions a hopeless endeavor, Dohsa-hou believes that this experience is extremely important for the trainee's both physical and mental development. This is so because such an experience reveals that there is movement—in this case study, moving from the horizontal to the vertical dimension as an activity innate to all humans; with movement, there is life. In other words, the individual, as far as they are living human beings, are not hopelessly frozen in their disease or disability—their vital energy is there, it needs only to be revived.

This process of "defrosting" seems to be one of the major tasks for any Dohsa-hou therapist, i.e., helping clients to taste through their bodily movements new experiences by practicing the imaginary right *kata* in the space between the trainer and trainee—the empty-centered structure of *ma*. As a result, clients can eventually “destroy” the old dysfunctional patterns of movement and “create” new ones, to duly integrate into their daily lives. However, as already mentioned, this process often evokes resistance or/and fear, in addition to physical pain as observed in quite many cases. The framework of an intensive Dohsa-hou camp is therefore of extreme importance as it provides sense of security to the trainer–trainee pair, whose mutual efforts are supported—both tangibly and figuratively—by all other camp members in the common space-time they share.

On the other hand, these mutual efforts do not cease once the camp is over. Quite the contrary, the end of a camp and the successfully achieved goals pave the way to setting new ones, even though the trainer and the trainee may never practice again as a pair. Similarly to the other Japanese psychotherapies, Dohsa-hou, too, could be likened to an endless road on which the travelers—trainees and their trainers—advance with small steps at a time. The case study presented in this chapter is not an exception: Sei and his trainer are still walking this road today—almost six years after the summer camp in Ishigaki (see Appendix III). They both keep on attending Dohsa-hou trainings and intensive camps even though there might be long periods when no improvement in Sei’s condition seems to take place. Even though the chances to practice again as a trainer–trainee pair are rather slim, whenever they meet, the joy of their silent but heartfelt communication is growing more and more; and so does their mutual will to rise and grow up.

Chapter 9
Tortured Bodies, Tortured Souls—A Fieldwork Research on Written Naikan with Drug Addicts

This chapter presents the first Naikan-related fieldwork research in Eastern Europe and in Bulgaria. It includes two studies carried out among drug and alcohol addicts in remission undergoing psychological and social rehabilitation at a day-care center in the capital Sofia. The studies had two major goals: (i) to research the opportunities for application of Naikan in Bulgaria and (ii) to discuss the approach's efficaciousness in the rehabilitation of addictions. These two studies are presented in detail in the next sections.[1]

While carrying out this fieldwork research and later, while discussing the results, we were mindful of professional ethics. At the same time, we wanted to avoid soulless anonymity and the medical colonization that the Indian literary theorist Gayatri Chakravorty-Spivak refers to when saying that "the master text of the medical journal article needs the suffering person, but the individuality of that suffering cannot be acknowledged" (as cited in Frank 1995: 12). We believe that we have not become colonizers and that all the participants in our research can easily recognize themselves in the text.

9.1 Study I: Changed Attitudes

Located on the border between Europe and Asia, Bulgaria is known for its rich historical heritage and bountiful nature, but also as being the European gateway of the so-called Balkan route for illicit drug trafficking. Additionally, the fall of the country's communist regime in 1989 accompanied by a wave of economic crises and all-penetrating moral and social ambiguity, marked the beginning of a long period of transition. Under these circumstances, over the past 25 years there has been an increasing trend toward drug use and abuse in the country. According to a 2015

[1]The whole fieldwork research, including also the application of written Naikan among healthy individuals, was first presented in Chervenkova (2012; 2013).

V. Chervenkova, *Japanese Psychotherapies*,
DOI 10.1007/978-981-10-3126-7_9

survey by the European School Survey Project on Alcohol and Other Drugs, Bulgarian students scored higher than the average "on lifetime use of illicit drugs other than cannabis (11% versus 5%) and lifetime use of new psychoactive substances" (ESPAD 2015). Together with Belgium, France, Latvia, Monaco, and the United Kingdom, Bulgaria was the top country in 2011 "as regards lifetime use of any illicit drug other than cannabis, with prevalence rates around 10%" (Hibell et al. 2012: 13). Additionally, a long-term survey carried out by the Bulgarian National Focal Point on Drugs and Drug Addictions shows that heroin remains the illicit drug which is most difficult to combat in the country, with more than 90% of the users seeking professional help; the number of heroin addicts is still on the rise although increasing at a slower pace compared to the mid-1990s (NFP Bulgaria 2011).

Against such a background, the number of drug rehabilitation centers, therapeutic communities, and specialized clinics, where people experiencing problems with addictive behavior and their families may seek professional help, have also been on the rise in the country. One such center hosted the two studies on Naikan therapy.

9.1.1 About This Study

Place: The present study was carried out in "Solidarity," a nongovernmental day-care center for psychological and social rehabilitation of alcohol, drug, and gambling addictions, in the Bulgarian capital of Sofia. Similar to most of the Naikan training centers in Japan, "Solidarity" is located in a quiet neighborhood and observes a stringent daily schedule. Excluding weekends and holidays, its clients should arrive every morning at 9 a.m. and be engaged in various activities until 5 p.m. Along with psychological consultations, role-play trainings, and art therapy, clients are also engaged in daily chores such as cleaning and cooking.

The center's rehabilitation approach is based on a therapeutic community model introduced to "Solidarity" by the Belgian drug rehabilitation association "Trempoline," known for its success especially in the treatment of heroin abuse. "Solidarity" further provides trainings and psychological support for the addicts' families and keeps a hotline with a wide range of information on drugs. The therapeutic program is voluntary and its optimal duration is 12 months, followed by a 6-month period of resocialization. Its activities are regularly monitored by the Bulgarian National Center for Addictions and supervised by renowned professors from the Sofia University, as well as by the president of the Belgian Federation of Therapeutic Communities and pedagogic director of "Trempoline", Ruud Bruggeman.

Time: August 2–16, 2011 (two weeks)

Method: Written Naikan—during the study's two weeks, after going back home from the day-care center, participants had to spare one to two hours on doing Naikan consecutively about their mother, father, and somebody third—a grandparent, sibling, or a close friend, and then write down what they had reflected on. On the next morning they had to submit their notes to the center's staff. The survey was carried out in three phases:

- During the survey's first phase, a presentation about Naikan therapy and the survey's aims and objectives was given to the center's director and staff. During the discussion that followed, informative English-language materials about the approach were handed out (for example, Miki 1998; 2002).
- After obtaining an approval from the center's director, Dr. Elena Nikolova, a presentation and an explanatory meeting for the clients was held. As it was holiday time, only five clients were undergoing rehabilitation in "Solidarity" at that point, compared to eight to 10 usually. Out of them, four agreed to participate in the study. They were provided with explanatory notes about the Naikan method that the author had prepared in Bulgarian.
- At the end of the second week, the participants' notes were collected. The center's tight schedule did not allow time for personal interviews, but only for a one-hour semi-structured group interview.

Participants: Table 9.1 presents the personal profiles of the four clients as of the time of the survey (August 2011). Except for participant A, who was an amphetamine addict, the other three participants were heroin addicts; except for participant D, the other three participants had undergone previous treatment before applying to "Solidarity".

9.1.2 The Written Naikan Practice

A summary of the participants' notes of their written Naikan practice and also their general impressions on the practice are presented in Table 9.2. It should be mentioned that participant B, who showed interest and motivation during the explanatory meeting, dropped out before long. Also, participants C and D reported that they found sitting in silence very difficult. During both studies, silence appeared to be one of the major challenges related to the application of Naikan to drug addicts—an important issue to be discussed in detail in Sect. 9.2.

We interpreted these results using the Naikan dimensions of change—an original model we introduce for tracking and interpreting the attitude changes that occur over the Naikan practice (see Sect. 6.2.2.1). This model begins with "gaining insight into one's sinfulness" and eventually finishes with "self-transformation," with each of the in-between dimensions functioning as signs of positive change as well (Fig. 9.1). Using this model, we analyze the Naikan practice of the participantsby referring to the content of the notes they submitted and also to that of the group interview (Table 9.3); however, we do not present the interview transcript.

9.1.3 Discussion

During the present study, we came across several challenges, the most difficult among which were (i) the participants not following the basic instructions for written Naikan and (ii) the extreme fluctuations in their attitude and motivation.

Table 9.1 Personal profiles of the four participants as of August 2011 (average age: 29 years)

	Age/Sex	Marital status and family background	Educational and professional background	Type of drug abuse	History of the dependence syndrome	Start of rehabilitation at the center
*	*	*	*	*	*	*
A	22/Male	Single; Parents divorced when A was 9 years old; Alcohol-addicted father (timeline of addiction unknown); A lives with his mother	High-school education; Unemployed	Amphetamines	Started at the age of 17; A has undergone a one-year rehabilitation at a therapeutic community, but he relapsed before long	September 2010 A's mother applied, but during the initial interview A demonstrated willingness to join the program
B	25/Female	Single; Parents divorced; Father has a mental disorder (unclear from when)	Several years ago B left university, but reenrolled in October 2010	Heroin, but from time to time uses other illicit drugs as well	Started at the age of 19; After individual consultations, she joined the center's rehabilitation program, but relapsed a month later	October 2010 (for a second time) Applied on her own
C	34/Male	C lives with his girlfriend and their two children	High-school education; Unemployed	Heroin	Started at the age of 29 after the birth of his children; C has undergone community-type treatment, but relapsed	November 2010 Applied on his own
D	35/Male	Single; D lives with his parents and elder brother	High-school education; Unemployed	Heroin	Started at the age of 25; No previous treatments	April 2011 Applied on his own

Table 9.2 Summary of the participants' written Naikan and general impressions on the practice

	Days spent on written Naikan	Number of pages submitted	Persons about whom Naikan was done	General impressions about Naikan
*	*	*	*	*
A	4 days	4 pages	Mother (unfinished)	I gained access to the positive memories of my past and re-experienced some positive emotions; the Naikan practice can be very efficacious
B	2 days (gave up on the second day)	no notes submitted	–	Initially I was highly motivated, but in fact I did not liked practicing written Naikan; I prefer to try intensive Naikan; I gained insight about some past events of my life that I understood before, but only rationally
C	2 days	2 pages	Mother (unfinished)	I got upset when I had to sit and be silent; it was difficult to remember my past; also, I was not motivated enough
D	8 days	9 pages	Mother; Father; Childhood friend (all unfinished)	It is difficult to remember the past while sitting in silence; I need to listen to music

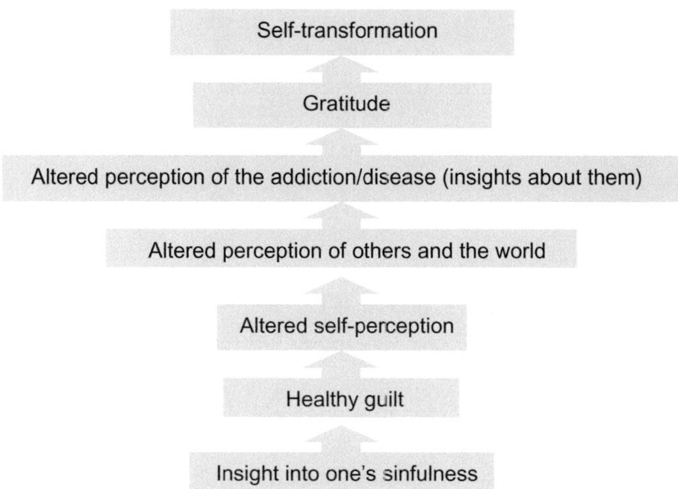

Fig. 9.1 Naikan dimensions of change start from insight into one's own sinfulness and eventually lead to self-transformation

As a result, the time the participants spent on the practice was rather insufficient and the content of their notes was sketchy. Notwithstanding these issues, the study appeared to be useful not only for this particular group of participants abusing drugs, but as a reference point for the possibilities of Naikan therapy in the field of addictions in general.

These possibilities, we suggest, can be rendered through the *Naikan dimensions of change* model. First, if we consider the characteristics of drug dependency, we may summarize that addicted people often cut themselves off mentally from others and withdraw in the world of their own desires—for example, participant D (see Table 9.3). Furthermore, a sense of dysfunction and inability to share a consensus reality with other people are also common (ibid.). However, such kind of attitude and behavior is difficult to fit in a world of interdependence. If we return to the theoretical interpretation of Naikan therapy (Sect. 6.2), we will remember that the method's roots are in the Buddhist view of the individual as being driven by ignorance because not the sin/trouble itself is what matters, but its effect upon others and the world (Chervenkova 2012: 78). This insight becomes the basis for a healthy sense of guilt. In contrast to the pathological sense of guilt, which is rarely based on real facts and only attempts to deny the very existence of the self, the healthy one originates from the realization that the individual has been provided with help and support, yet they have caused troubles to those who have helped them (Miki and Miki 1998: 123–124).

Therefore, an insight into the effects brought about by one's way of thinking and behavior naturally paves the way to gratitude and eventually to self-transformation, which may include a possibility for overcoming the addictive behavior. Even if this change is accommodated into the model's first level—the personal and interpersonal one, which may foster the improvement of one's interpersonal relationships and social functioning (see Fig. 6.1 in Sect. 6.2.2.1)—the rehabilitation of drug addictions could be fertile ground also for the transpersonal level to manifest itself. Through the next study we attempt to shed light on this possibility.

9.2 Study II: Clinical Aspects and the Therapeutic Power of Silence

According to a survey of the research trends in Naikan therapy in Japan, in recent years the research among Naikan clients with addictions topped the list, with some 8.9% of the total number of participants. Also, among the types of the Naikan method, written Naikan occupies 10.2%, ranking second after intensive Naikan that is applied at Naikan training centers across the country. On the other hand, although Naikan was first spread among prisoners and juvenile delinquents, its application in correctional institutions today occupies a mere 1.0% (Tsujita et al. 2011: 29–40). Additionally, most of the Naikan-related surveys and research are carried out in Naikan training centers, universities, and hospitals, but those at correctional

Table 9.3 Content of the written Naikan practice and the group interview based on the *Naikan dimensions of change* model

Name	Healthy guilt	Altered self-perception	Altered perception of others and the world	Altered perception of the addiction/disease (gaining insights about it)	Gratitude
*	*	*	*	*	*
A	I feel guilty about my mother having spent some $4,000 on my treatment so far	I believe I can become a more positive person; my motivation for rehabilitation increased	I started loving my mother more and more; I do not want to forget what she has done for me; I want to meet my father	I find drug addiction related to negative emotions such as sadness; using drugs, we try to bury our sense of emptiness	I am grateful for my mother's unconditional love and help
B	–	I want to get rid of my addictive behavior	–	I want to respect my parents more than I do now	My gratitude did not increase much
C	–	I want to concentrate more than I do now	Instead of sitting in silence, I prefer to go out and cycle with my children; I want to spend more time with my family	I want to get rid of my heroin addiction; I feel a strong desire to become healthy again	I felt deep gratitude when I remembered a moment of my childhood when my mother gave me a present
D	Being focused on myself, I did not recognize the problems my parents have had to face because of my behavior	I want to give up my arrogant behavior and become more patient and tolerant	I want to talk with my parents more often; I really appreciate them; I realized I am not the center of the world	Because of the addiction, I am not able to show enough respect to others	I am grateful for my father's support

institutions are extremely rare; also, to the best of our knowledge, very few, if any, Naikan-related group interviews are held in correctional institutions or addiction rehabilitation centers outside of Japan.

9.2.1 About This Study

This study presents a group interview and a discussion on Naikan as part of a follow-up study with the clients of the "Solidarity" day-care center for addiction rehabilitation in Sofia, Bulgaria. The interviewees were all the six clients of the center at that time. Of them, four participants were diagnosed with heroin addiction, one had an alcohol addiction, and one was addicted to amphetamines.

In the next section we present only the group interview and the group discussion, omitting the first and second phases of the follow-up study, namely the explanatory meeting and the content of the clients' written Naikan. Using the information from the interview, we discuss the clinical aspects and the therapeutic power of silence both of which we consider important topics in the context of Naikan therapy, especially when the method is applied in the rehabilitation of addictions. The personal experiences and valuable thoughts that the clients shared in the interview throw light both on the nature of addictions and on the wide therapeutic spectrum of Naikan therapy.

Method: Semi-structured group interview; during the interview, the interviewer used a recorder with the consent of both the clients and the center's director and staff. The clients answered one after the other and then a group discussion followed. As an aftermath of their drug abuse, most of the participants did not speak fluently enough; hence the dots throughout the text.

Time: February 22, 2012

Interview length: 40 minutes

Interviewees: All the six clients at that time (four men and two women; average age 28.6 years). Of them, two participated in Study I alone (participant C in Study I/interviewee F and participant A in Study I/interviewee H), another two participated in Study II alone (participants E and J), one participated in both studies (participant D), and one participated in neither of them (interviewee G) (see Sect. 9.1).

9.2.2 The Group Interview

Interviewer: Hello, everyone! Thank you for participating in our study! I would like to open this interview right away and ask you what are your general impressions on your two-week written Naikan practice? What did it make you think of? (*Clients start answering one after the other*)

E (*21-year-old woman; single; unemployed; addicted to heroin; art school graduate. E was the only child of her father's second marriage. Her parents divorced when she was a child. E has elder brother from her father's first marriage, but she has never met him. At the time of the study, she lived with her father. E became addicted to heroin 6 years ago and has been on methadone treatment since. In September 2011 her father took her to the "Solidarity" day-care center. E participated in Study II alone and did written Naikan only about her mother*).

(*does not speak smoothly enough*)

–It was very interesting for me. It provoked my interest…In fact, for me… Through Naikan I realized the great importance of the so-called trivial things. You understand that someone loves you; not the abstract things, but real facts…someone has prepared food for you and has fed you. These seeming trivia actually mean a lot. I like this thing about Nakian very much. It attracted my interest. These things may seem trivial, but actually they are not. I realized they are very important. Also, to become aware of these things, one has first to go deeply into their past, to "sink" there. There is no other way. I think that Naikan gives exactly this unique chance, this opportunity…But for me, doing Naikan the proper way was quite difficult…I mean you are not allowed to listen to music or do other things. But still I think I realized many things about my past. I became aware of my mother's kindness toward me. For example, why my mom bought me the toy I wanted so much when I was a child…stuff like that, you know…Well, you see, I tried hard, but it did not work out, I did not do Naikan properly (*lowers her eyes and becomes silent*). There were many people at home that time, it was noisy…(*becomes silent again*).

Interviewer: Was that the reason you gave up practicing Naikan before long?

E: Well, you see, at the very beginning I managed to write for more than one hour, but during that time many…you know, other things started coming to my mind. For example, "Right now I want to rearrange my wardrobe." But later on, I concentrated and recollected many episodes of my past.

Interviewer: However, it is difficult to say that you practiced written Naikan for the whole two weeks, isn't it?

E: Yes. It was impossible to continue after dad came back from a business trip (*silence*). And I gave up.

Interviewer: I see, E. Is there anything else you would like to say?

E: It was very interesting for me. You know…I felt it, I felt it…While I was writing, I became aware of the way my mother felt back then, her feelings (*silence*)… all those special things that she has done for me, all her good intentions, her feelings toward me, her love…To be honest, I felt great the moment I realized these. A very nice moment! I felt great when I felt it (*smiles slightly than prolonged silence follows*).

Interviewer: Thank you, E, for sharing this experience! To become aware of other people's feelings is very important, indeed. If there is anything else that you would like to share with us right now...

E: No. That's all.

Interviewer: Thank you very much! D, how was it for you?

D (*35-year-old man; single; unemployed; heroin addict. At the time of the study, D lived with his parents and 43-year-old brother. D became addicted 10 years ago. In the past, he has tried to quit his drug abuse on his own, but in April 2011 he turned up at "Solidarity" to seek professional help; D was the only one who participated in both Naikan studies*).

–Frankly speaking, I did not spend much time on the written Naikan. I wanted to complete at least the Naikan about my mother, but…You see, it is usually assumed your mom does this and that for you, she loves you and makes lots of sacrifices in the name of your well-being, etc. Well (*silence*), last time (*Study I*) it was ok, I was feeling ok, but this time I literally wallowed in negative emotions both during and after finishing the practice (*silence*). I mean…what troubles my mother has had to face because of me. At the very beginning I thought that, well, I remember most of the things I wrote the previous time, so now I wanted to dredge other memories up. In fact, the previous time I did not gain any insight. I know well all these things, you know. Through all these years since my early childhood my mom has shown her love and support and understanding to me. But if I compare this time with the previous time…somehow…a sense of guilt…you see, I felt out of place both while doing the written Naikan and after having finished it. It seemed I remembered well the things my mom has done for me over the years, but what I have done for her I hardly remembered (*in a slightly vexed voice*). The facts that were easy to remember were the troubles and difficulties I have caused her. I remembered lots of them and I had plenty to choose from (*smiles bitterly with downcast eyes*). And, I told you, even after finishing I did not feel well, physically and mentally.

Interviewer: Did you clearly feel the difference between the two times of Naikan practice?

D: Yes. The first time was ok. I felt ok (*silence*).

Interviewer: The volume of the notes you submitted this time exceeded that of the previous study, but this time, too, you wrote about one person only.

D: True.

Interviewer: Would it be right to say that this time you gave up because of the negative feelings you experienced?

D: Well…(*thinking*). You see, I did not have much time (*silence*). Well, yes, I gave up because of them (*the negative feelings*). Because of them I felt awful.

Interviewer: You know, D, I understand the way you feel, but exactly these feelings are important part of any Naikan experience. I think that you can "use" them as a basis to proceed further with your written Naikan practice.

D: I do not know (*thinking*). I think this sense of guilt is mainly toward my mother. Of my parents, she is very…she is very sensitive, very emotional. My father is more…(*silence*) kind of open-minded, whereas she often takes everything too personally. As if I have no feelings and do not care at all how she feels because of me and the things I do and say. If I do Naikan about my father, maybe it would not be that bad (*long silence*).

Interviewer: So, would you like to continue doing written Naikan even though the present study is finished?

D: Yes, yes (*smiles slightly*)

Interviewer: You mean doing Naikan about your father and one more person?

D: Well, the third person…if it is a friend…

Interviewer: It could be some other relative as well—for example, a grand-parent or a sibling; a close friend is also ok.

D: You see, when I was 13 our family moved house. I used to contact my friends of the former neighborhood, but as the time passed we lost touch. Some of them moved abroad (*prolonged silence; downcast eyes*).

Interviewer: If you wish you can continue practicing written Naikan...

D: No problem (*answers with slightly indifferent look on his face and shrugs shoulders; then suddenly becomes invigorated and continues talking*). In fact, I do not remember much of my father when I was a child. I used to be closer to my mom. He used to juggle two jobs and you could hardly see him around (*silence*)... Anyway, I think I will remember somehow.

Interviewer: Thank you. If there is anything else you would like to share...

D: (*thinking for a long time*) As I already said, this time I was constantly attacked by a sense of guilt. At the beginning of puberty, I stopped sharing my thoughts and interests with my mother. But she is a worrier, you know, a sensitive person, and she wants to know about me, she constantly asks about this and that and does not fall asleep before I get back home...Although I know it...(*long silence*) I think I did not gain any special insight during this study. The things she has done for me and my brother, especially for me, her sacrifices...I know them well. As I said before, this time I felt really awful (*long silence*).

Interviewer: Do you think that these negative feelings are related to some weak point of the Naikan method itself?

D: (*almost interrupting the interviewer*) No, definitely not! The sense of guilt (*in a loud voice*)... All the troubles I have caused her...(*suddenly becomes silent*). A lot of troubles. I should not have done that to her. This was a question of just a little effort on my part. But...back then I really did not pay any attention. I totally ignored other people's feelings and did only what I wanted. What an egotist! (*smiles bitterly with downcast eyes; then a prolonged silence follows*)

Interviewer: D, you can continue your written Naikan practice. I assume that it will open up more new vistas for you.

D: OK.

Interviewer: Thank you very much! F, this time you did not participate in the study, but if there is anything you would like to share with us...

F (*35-year-old man; unemployed; addicted to heroin. At the time of the study, F lived with his girlfriend and their two children. His parents and elder brother lived separately from him in the country. F became addicted 5 years ago, after the birth of his children; F underwent rehabilitation in a therapeutic community, but relapsed before long. In November 2010 he applied for rehabilitation in "Solidarity" on his own. F participated in Study I alone (participant C).*

–I did not participate, so I have absolutely nothing to say. Moreover, I am not interested at all (*in a frustrated tone*).

Interviewer: I see. I assume that the explanatory meeting on the follow-up Naikan study was not interesting for you at all.

F: (*almost interrupting the interviewer*) The previous time I did written Naikan, but it was very difficult for me. Sitting in silence was awful! Also, there is not enough space at home.

Interviewer: If there was enough space, would you do Naikan then? Do you think that Naikan could be of help to you?

F: Of course. When I did it the previous time, I managed to remember episodes that I had almost completely forgotten. Was it not for Naikan, I could definitely not remember them (*prolonged silence*). Among the things I have done, there were both good and bad ones.

Interviewer: Well, what then do you think about the idea of recollecting one's past? What could its point be?

F: Well…(*in a hesitant voice*). There was something that seemed like a sense of guilt, but it waned almost completely with time. When I was young, I did a lot of mistakes, but guilt I feel mostly about the things I did after my 23–24 year of age. You know, at 23 or 24 you are already an adult, a mature person, right? To learn from one's own past mistakes is the most important lesson (*becomes silent with downcast eyes*).

Interviewer: Thank you. G, how about you?

G (*33-year-old man; single; unemployed; addicted to alcohol. G's mother passed away several years ago. At the time of the study, G lived with his father and 27-year-old brother. In the past, G was addicted to heroin, but quit on his own. G has undergone rehabilitation at a therapeutic community. In December 2011 he applied to "Solidarity" on his own. G has studied Law at university, but dropped out. According to information provided by the center's staff, G demonstrated strong resistance toward practicing written Naikan; he was the only one who did not participate in either study*).

–I did not participate (*smiles derisively*).

Interviewer: I know (*everyone laughs*). Anyway, if there is anything you would like to say now…

G: No. It was interesting, but I was not motivated at all (*silence*). Still, I find the Naikan questions very interesting. They help you dredge up things that you have almost completely forgotten. That's all I can say.

Interviewer: Thank you. H, how about you?

H (*22-year-old man; single; unemployed; addicted to amphetamines. H was the only child to divorced parents. At the time of the study, he lived with his mother and her second husband. H became addicted at the age of 17 and underwent rehabilitation in a therapeutic community, but relapsed. In September 2010 his mother took him to "Solidarity." H participated in the first study alone (participant A).*

(*speaks in hesitant manner with downcast eyes almost all the time; uses many speech fillers*)

–Is it my turn? This time I did not do written Naikan. These days I am as busy as a bee. Well, I am motivated, but…(*silence*). Well, otherwise…There are things I want to say about my parents, but…There are troubles I have caused them, but I do not consider these such big troubles (*long silence*). But…they…well, they are, I mean…they bully me (*sighs deeply*). I do not know…We will see…Well, I have stolen small sums and small things from them, but back then…you know, there was almost nothing to steal, you know. I mean, if there was more, I would steal more, but…I mean, in my personal understanding I have not stolen that much. I mean… Well, that is all I can say (*prolonged silence*).

Interviewer: It seems you do not consider Naikan very useful for your current rehabilitation…

H: Yes, it seems so. It would not be that useful for me…(*downcast eyes; prolonged silence*) We'll see…I mean…(*prolonged silence*)

Interviewer: Thank you. J, how about you?

J (*26-year-old woman; married; unemployed; addicted to heroin. J was an only child. At the time of the study, her parents lived separately from her in the country;*

her husband worked abroad, while J lived with their 5-year-old son. J planned to move to her husband's place together with their child. In the past, J used to abuse heroin together with her husband. She had never sought professional help before, but she had purchased methadone on the black market in an attempt to self-medicate. In October 2011 J applied for "Solidarity"'s rehabilitation program on her own).

(*speaks relatively fluently*)

–Oh, you know, I liked this approach (*Naikan*) very much (*smiles and speaks enthusiastically*), but I did not manage to write down anything. On the other hand, over these two weeks I kept constantly the three Naikan questions in my mind. Doing so helped me a lot. Reflecting on my past, I managed to highly appreciate all the things my parents have had done for me up to now. Reflecting on my past… they (*the parents*)…they have done their best. In fact, we usually remember the bad things very well and over a long time; we remember all the troubles and difficulties the other people have caused us and always try to justify ourselves. But once you reflect on your life, on what your parents have done for you and have given you, you realize the fact that you could hardly repay them until the end of your life and it helps you see everything from a different perspective.

You know (*in a cheerful voice*), thanks to Naikan I felt deep gratitude toward my parents and it is now helping me improve my relationship with them. For example, I started talking to my father on the phone more often as compared to before and to discuss this and that with him. I communicate with him very well now and this makes me feel very happy! Usually we do not notice the so-called trivial things, but they are very important in our life. Everyday our closest people do something for us, but we ignore it and do not appreciate it because we take it for granted. Through Naikan I became aware of this truth and that is why I like the approach very much!

Interviewer: Does it mean that you would practice written Naikan from now on?

J: Yes, for sure. I will have time and space over the next several days.

Interviewer: This is wonderful! You can start with your mother, father, and one more person.

J: Yes, ok.

Interviewer: Thank you.

(*after the end of the interview a free group discussion followed*)

E: In fact, I tried to write a little about my father, but…(*sighs deeply*) you know, I can hardly forget his negativism, his behavior. It was very, very difficult. I remembered the bad things he has done…I do not know…His behavior. My father is very austere, he has a very complicated personality…(*silence*). I am not sure if I could practice properly written Naikan about my father. I was wondering how doing Naikan about a person who has caused you lots of troubles could be of help…I do not know.

Interviewer: Well, no one knows in advance, but if you try it by yourself, you will understand. One of the most important things about the Naikan practice is to stick to the three questions. As it was written in the explanatory notes I handed out two weeks ago, when doing Naikan about a person who has caused you troubles, you first need to put aside your negative emotions toward him or her for a while and just follow strictly the Naikan rules. This gives you the chance to look at the same person from a different perspective and, as a result, your mental image of him or her may change. Human personality is multi-faced and dynamic. Therefore, if through the Naikan practice you manage to see the person in question from a different perspective, then your relationship with him or her will most likely undergo positive changes, too.

E: (*listens carefully and nods*) Yes, some memories popped up…I mean, I went back…While I was reflecting on my past, I realized that my father was actually not such a bad person. I said to myself, "Hey, he is not that bad!," and I felt happy, you know. It was a very nice feeling (*smiles*).

Interviewer: This is wonderful! You experienced yourself what it means to see the same person from a different perspective and this is a very precious experience. As you know, this is the first Naikan-related study in Bulgaria and all of you are the pioneers in that field. You put efforts into going back to your past and shared such precious experiences. That is very worthy!

D: (*in an excited voice*) I am very happy that we are the pioneers in the Naikan research and practice in Bulgaria. Also, I thought that I would not be able to remember other episodes of my past than the ones I remembered during the previous study, but, interestingly, new ones popped up. That is how I realized that most of my hitherto attitudes and assumptions have been wrong. No doubt, thanks to Naikan one's attitudes can change remarkably.

Interviewer: And it also could be helpful for your rehabilitation here, at the "Solidarity".

D: Yes, of course (*thinking for a while*). Even without meeting and talking to the person directly, you can "meet" him or her again in your heart and relate to him or her. You can feel the person (*silence*). Because, as I already said, I know well the facts, but only rationally. But when you do Naikan and you go back to your memories, you can re-experience the past. For example, the moment someone has made you happy (*silence*)…your feelings at that time…(*silence*).

Interviewer: You mean you can experience these feelings again?

D: Yes, yes, exactly! Experience once again those feelings (*prolonged silence*). The joy, the surprise…Well, when you do something wrong, it is normal for your parents to scold you. But I realized that even if I have caused many troubles to my parents, yet they kept on supporting me over the years. Once you understand this truth, your motivation to become a good person increases. Well, in fact you may not change that much…maybe I will keep on going the old way…but still (*smiles bitterly and becomes silent*)…The truth somehow touches the heart.

Interviewer: As F already said, reflecting on one's own past is a good chance to learn from one's own mistakes.

D: Yes. Thanks to the rehabilitation I am undergoing here, I realized much about my life and my way of thinking, but after doing written Naikan I felt a remarkable change taking place within me. You see, I started talking with my mother. I started sharing with her the way I felt, where I would go today and whom I would meet, what time I would be back home, etc. In the past, the moment my mother asked me one of these questions, quarrel was on the way (*prolonged silence*). I considered myself an adult and hated all these stupid questions (*with a slightly angry voice*). Moreover, I myself did not know at all when I would be back home, etc. Now it is completely different. My attitude and my feelings changed a lot. For example, whenever she used to ask me "What did you eat today?," I used to get furious (*silence*). Of course, my mother did not intend to irritate me. She asked out of love and concern. And even though I completely understood her feelings, I answered her "I ate when I was hungry! It's none of your business!" (*prolonged silence ; downcast eyes*). But now even if I feel a little nervous, I answer her politely. There is a positive change for sure (*with a happy face*).

Interviewer: This is a very precious experience, indeed! Thank you for sharing it with us!

D: (*almost interrupting the interviewer*) Yes, yes! I see that my mother is much more relaxed now and this makes me very happy. In the past, the moment she entered my room, you could feel the tension in the air. My relationship with her now is completely different.

Interviewer: Thank you very much, D! These words are very suitable for wrapping up the interview. Thank you all for your cooperation!

9.2.3 Discussion

Often defined as one of the most daunting public and mental health problems of modern society, drug and alcohol addictions pose a great challenge not only to the affected individuals, but also to their families and friends. People close to drug and alcohol addicts cannot help asking, "How can he/she continue with such a destructive behavior?". The attempt to understand the nature of addictions and define the factors that likely determine it—if any specific ones can be identified—has given rise to various biological, psychosocial, and psychodynamic theories. Before embracing any of these theories, however, we need to ask one simple, but important question that goes beyond any theory and gets directly to the core of the problem: "What is the function of the addiction in the user's life?" Dismissing this question and labeling addictions mere "bad habits," "self-destruction," or "wanton behavior" would rob any therapeutic or rehabilitation process of their utmost humane dimension, turning them into a series of mechanical procedures.

Searching for the answer to this question, some researchers such as the Canadian physician Gabor Maté have arrived at the conclusion that "addictions always originate in unhappiness, even hidden. They are emotional anesthetics; they numb pain" (Maté 2013). Indeed, if we look deeper into any addiction history, we will most likely come across childhood memories of divorce, serial abandonment, severe physical and/or psychological abuse, and overall traumatizing environments. "My patients' histories,"Maté points out, "are chronicles of pain upon pain" (Maté 2011: 26). Needless to say, this is not always the case and causes cannot necessarily be related to traumatic experiences, but such experiences "appear to be associated with substance-use disorders" (Khantzian and Albanese 2008: 4). "I don't believe that any specific trauma causes chemical dependency, but there is some correlation between certain life stressors and adolescent chemical abuse," the American psychologist Laura Stamper corroborates (Stamper 1997: 11–12). "Some of these stressors include early grief or loss issues, a history of physical, sexual, or emotional abuse, neglect, learning disabilities, a history of alchohol/chemical abuse in the family. When kids get in trouble with drugs, it is because the chemical use and lifestyle meets many needs—like medicating painful feelings. However, not everyone who experiences a traumatic childhood turns to drug use, and some chemically dependent adolescents had fairly unremarkable childhoods. But, there is a common thread in the lives of children who abuse drugs: they suffer from a poor self-concept. Certain painful events have a negative influence on the formation of a young person's identity" (Stamper 1997: 12).

Indeed, traumatic experiences are likely to rob the young person of their faith in people, their sense of social belonging, and of a general sense of the meaningfulness of life. "People who have endured horrible events," the American psychiatrist Judith Herman emphasizes, "suffer predictable psychological harm. There is a spectrum of traumatic disorders, ranging from the effects of a single overwhelming event to the more complicated effects of prolonged and repeated abuse" (Herman 2015: 3). In their theory of addiction as self-medication, the American physicians Edward Khantzian and Mark Albanese point out that the addictive behavior of their patients is rarely, if ever, driven by hedonistic motives. "There is ample indication of the loneliness, depression, anxiety, and continuing effects of early trauma that affect the great majority of these "hedonistic" individuals" (Khantzian and Albanese 2008: 123). What usually makes clients resort to substance abuse is the soothing, warm "embracing" effect the substance has on their unbearable psychological suffering. Most of the patients—be they addicted to drugs or alcohol—have a history of physical, sexual, or psychological abuse, which makes living difficult and eventually leads to mood, anxiety, or dissociative disorders (Kobayashi 2012: 1098). In confirmation to this statement, a survey in the United States showed that "nearly 60% of the people serving time in state prisons for drug offense in 2007 had no history of violence or of any significant selling activity" (Maté 2011: 24). These facts suggest that drug abuse is rarely related to gaining financial or material benefits, but much more to helping users cope, albeit temporarily, with their emotional problems.

As shown in the present study, too, most of the study's participants had difficult family histories or had lived in a dysfunctional environment. These factors may explain why addicted clients value short-term pain relief over their physical and mental health, and even their lives. Considering this, it is appropriate to define two key points related to the Naikan therapy and its application in the field of addictions. First, many addicts get irritated easily, they are short-tempered, and tend to neglect other people's feelings and emotions—for example, participant D and his mother; participant J and her father: because of the needle, they often "have the needle" thus *destroying their interpersonal relationships*. Furthermore, as we summarized in Sect. 9.1.3, addicted clients tend to psychologically cut themselves off from others and withdraw in an impenetrable world of their own as if encapsulated in a thick membrane (Chervenkova 2012: 78) to keep the sharp needles of the world out and thus soothe their emotional pain. Especially in cases of clients who have started abusing substances at an early age, such a cut-off prevents them from building healthy interpersonal relationships (Koga 2011: 129), to likely result in an inability to share the reality with others. This inability, the Japanese psychiatrist Toshiaki Tadai notes, turns them into runaways and takes them to the same no-man's land inhabited also by recluses, suicides, patients with eating disorders, Internet- and game addicts, and stalkers, each of them contributing to the spread of social pathology that can simply be defined as escapism (Tadai 2005: front cover).

On the other hand, however, if we neglect the all-pervasive psychological pain so easily recognizable in the life stories of most of the addicted clients and label their addictive behavior mere weakness of will or careless escapism, we are likely to walk into the trap of inhumane and narrow-minded judgment. Therefore, as previously mentioned, we first need to understand "what kind of despair could lead someone to value short-term pain relief over life itself? And what might be the source of such despair?" (Maté 2011: 26). If schematized, this pain is what throws the addicted clients into a vicious circle as shown in Fig. 9.2. One of the possible ways for addicted patients to disentangle themselves from this circle then could be first to see the reality of the facts as they have never seen it before because of the pain and, later, because of the specificities of their addictive behavior. In this sense, Naikan and its straightforward approach toward reality is rather appropriate for addiction rehabilitation: reflecting on their past through the three Naikan questions, drug- and alcohol-addicted practitioners have the chance to realize that this world is a place not of grief, pain, and despair alone, but also of love, care, and joy. As some of the participants in the present study noted, this is the realization that "someone loves you;" "someone has prepared food for you and has fed you;" "my mother's feelings toward me, her love" (participant E); "the moment someone has made you happy" (participant D); and that "everyday our closest people do something for us" (participant J). The realization that such positive facts exist in one's past and present has a soothing effect over the psychological pain and it may also evoke, as participant J reported, deep gratitude—a feeling that cannot be produced by external stimuli alone.

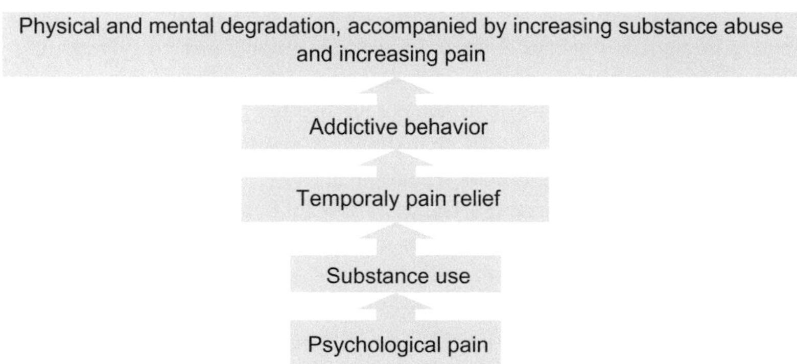

Fig. 9.2 The vicious circle of addictive behavior

That is how in the field of addictions, the Naikan's existential grounding function described in detail in Sect. 6.2.2.1, transforms into a *bridging function*, i.e., the drugs have taken the abusers to an imaginary world of temporary pain relief, whereas Naikan has the potential to take them back to the real world. However, this is not the previous world of pain, but a world where love and care do really exist; the clients can then experience that they belong to this reality—something that most addicts appear to have been unaware of.

Considering all of the above, we can conclude that Naikan therapy has a high potential in the field of drug rehabilitation: out of the six interviewees, three—E, D, and J—experienced healthy guilt, the strongest reported by participant D, and also re-experienced past moments of joy and happiness. These likely helped them improve the communication with their parents. In these cases we see how one of the toughest challenges of addictive behavior—the ruined communication and interpersonal relationships—can to a great extent be overcome through Naikan—for example, the remarkable positive change participant D reported in the communication with his mother as a result of his written Naikan practice. Furthermore, we can also conclude that the valuable insights of these participants served as a model for the remaining three participants—F, G, and H—who were rather reluctant to practice Naikan. The group interview and discussion were not mere investigative tools, but had also a therapeutic potential: as in the orthodox version of the intensive Naikan, where practitioners can hear the confessions of all others in the room and these confessions can spur on their own self-reflection, in the present group interview even the reluctant participants gained certain insights—for example, participant H ("There are troubles I have caused them").

As a second key point, the first one being the ruined interpersonal relationships, we should mention that most of the addicted clients get bored easily; they find it difficult to concentrate and to stay alone in silence—for example, participant E reported she could not concentrate and wanted to rearrange her wardrobe. Probably it was one of the major causes as to why, as previously mentioned, during the survey's written Naikan phase none of the participants followed the instructions properly and most of the notes they submitted were rather sketchy. We thus concluded that *addicts feel especially uncomfortable with silence* and this specificity poses a significant challenge for the application of Naikan therapy to addictions, considering that seclusion and silence are among the method's key features.

Although in a different context, the discussion of silence that we made in Sect. 4.1 appears to be useful for drawing conclusions about the role of silence in drug rehabilitation, too. Considering that silence is neither a mere absence of noise nor the ceasing of conversation or of some activity, it could be defined as an autonomous phenomenon similar to that of life and death; it brings all habitual activities to an end. Hence, it has the potential to serve as a bridge from a state of inner chaos and dissipation to a reordered state of being where one has the chance to reset one's life and open it up to new possibilities for a more constructive way of living. In other words, if we borrow Jungian terminology, silence may function as an *archetype of transformation*: it possesses a therapeutic meaning, but not "as if it were an energy or an instrument used to bring about certain effects" (Sardello 2008:

59); rather, "healing currents of Silence are intrinsic to Silence itself, integral to its very nature" (ibid.). Therefore, if one manages to access their symptom/addiction within silence and observe it carefully from the perspective of that state of reordered being, then they may attain a new perspective of the symptom/addiction, as well as of themselves, others, and the world (these aspects we labeled *Naikan dimensions of change*, see Sect. 6.2.2.1 and Fig. 9.1 in Sect. 9.1.2).

However, before embarking on such a promising trip, one must consider their relationship with silence. For many people who have become accustomed to the background noise as one of modern life's distinct features, silence is unsettling, unnatural, and even fearsome. Additionally, "like the Roman god Janus, silence holds two faces" (LeClaire 2009: 88) and may thus evoke polyvalent emotional responses, including experiences of darkness and oppression, expressed on individual, interpersonal and even national levels. "In a collective sense," the American Jungian analyst Henry Wilmer suggests, "we can consider the silent treatment of nations" in the form of "diplomatic frigidity, snub, social and political disdain" (Wilmer 2000: 32). Undoubtedly, immersing oneself in silence as a voluntary act and being silenced are two opposites. "To be silenced is crippling, belittling, constricting, disempowering. Chosen silence can be healing, expansive, instructive" (LeClaire 2009: 88); "being silenced, whether externally or internally, means being cut off from our genuine selves" (LeClaire 2009: 89) because "that silence is a place of nonbeing, a place of control, from which all our yearning is to escape" (Maitland 2009: 28). Receiving the silent treatment may therefore result in self-alienation and in questioning or even rejecting one's own existence. These, in turn, may aggravate to dysfunctional and pathological states. For this reason, experiencing silence the negative way—what we term here the *clinical aspects of silence*—can be added to Stamper's list of the possible risk factors for the onset of substance-use disorder.

Considering all of the above, it appears natural that drug addicts feel uncomfortable with silence: when their years-long inner noise encounters the silence "prescribed" by Naikan, they experience something unknown or even frightening, and different defenses start to emerge—for example, participants F and H, and especially G. Additionally, silence may remind drug abusers of a childhood experience of silent treatment or may become a metaphor for the social shame and stigma that are usually attached to addictive behavior. As Khantzian and Albanese point out, "the addiction lifestyle itself contributes to an ongoing pattern of trauma" (Khantzian and Albanese 2008: 61–62), the consequences of which include "emaciation; skin infections, ulcers, and scars; unkempt and run-down appearance; restlessness and anxiousness; irritability and agitation; downcast and depressed mood; distrusting and/or paranoid thinking; visual hallucinations, and hallucinations of bugs under the skin" (Khanztian and Albanese 2008: 72). In this case, too, unconscious defenses may start functioning. As shown in Fig. 9.3, sitting in silence may significantly obstruct the natural flow of the therapeutic power of silence in Naikan.

The above-mentioned archetypal essence of silence—the capacity of silence to bring the individual to deeper levels of self-reflection and transformation—represents what we name here the *therapeutic power of silence*. This capacity of silence is probably one of the most important phenomena related to Naikan to an extent that

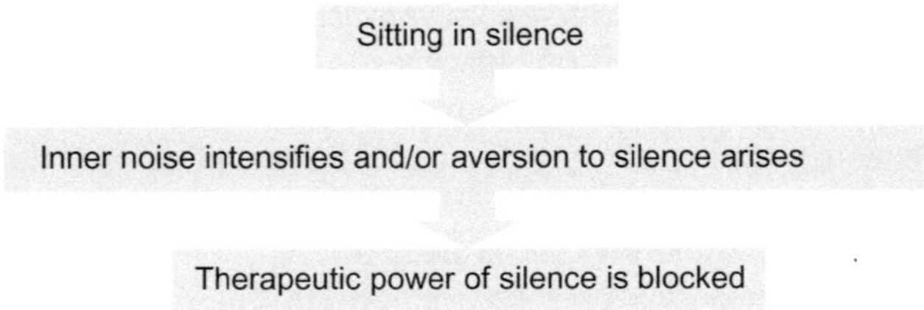

Fig. 9.3 Reluctance to sitting alone in silence in case of drug and alcohol addictions

it is tantamount to the Naikan's therapeutic power itself; hence the therapeutic power of silence could become a key point in drug- and alcohol-abuse rehabilitation. However, in order to overcome the challenge with the negative emotional response toward silence during the Naikan practice among addicts, we first need to overcome the negative attitude and associations that the phenomenon of silence itself may evoke.

As shown in the present study, the application of a two-week written Naikan practice is well justified among drug addicts in remission. However, as a result of the characteristics of addictive behavior, strict adherence to the rules of Naikan is difficult to expect (as the present research confirm). In order to overcome the practitioners' initial fears and defenses, we suggest that during the first 3–4 days of the practice, the addicts should not stay secluded in silence, but just try to keep the three Naikan themes in their mind and integrate them into their daily routine (as participant J did). As a second phase, on the fifth day the addicts may start writing down some notes regarding what they have reflected on during the day for 15–20 minutes daily. Until the final day of the practice, this phase should be gradually increased to

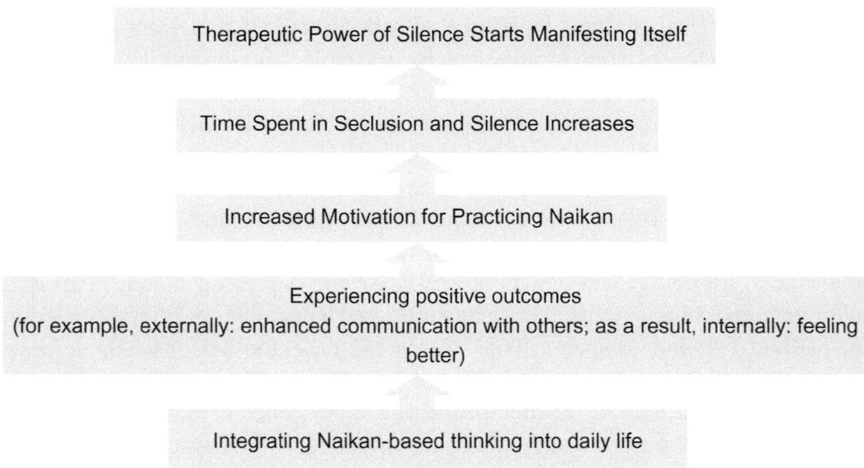

Fig. 9.4 The process of gradual integration of Naikan-based thinking into the daily routine of drug addicts in rehabilitation

hour and a half or two hours daily. Thus, with the first phase of 3–4 days serving as a smooth transition to the real practice of written Naikan, the addicts have the chance to overcome naturally their initial fears and defenses, and gain positive outcomes in their overall rehabilitation (Fig. 9.4). As it could be expected, the ultimate goal of any addiction rehabilitation is not merely quitting the substance abuse, but turning toward a more constructive way of living as compared to before (Kusano 1992: 102).

9.3 Conclusion

Considering the two Naikan studies among drug addicts in Bulgaria, Study I—practicing written Naikan, and Study II—a group interview and discussion, we suggest that silence is one of the most important issues related to any addiction rehabilitation; however, within our knowledge, this issue has not received almost any research attention so far. As previously mentioned, silence could be thought of a phenomenon of the same order as the phenomena of life and death, i.e., it cannot be controlled or produced artificially. In silence we have nowhere to hide; we are forced to see our own flaws, deepest fears, and Ego-biased assumptions about others and the world. What is very important about the silence in Naikan therapy is that in the moment of uttermost vulnerability and "nakedness," silence may give the practitioner its most wondrous boon: the harmony of integration and independence understood as being fully related to others and, at the same time, fully free in oneself. Such an experience could be described by the religion-tinted words of Naikan's founder Ishin Yoshimoto: "I felt as if I was saved after having run around the crater of an active volcano" (Yoshimoto 1965/2007: 100).

Returning to the field of addictions, we can now see that through the process of overcoming the initial resistance toward silence in Naikan and allowing silence to manifest its therapeutic power, drug and alcohol abusers may gain profound understanding about themselves and they way they relate to others and the world. This, in turn, may provide them with a chance for changing the course of their addictive behavior for the better. Being people whose tortured souls have made them torture their bodies in the name of a temporary relief, addicted clients tend to be afraid not of death, but of being alive. However, sacrificing one's body, health, and even life to the pyre of drugs, runs counter to the Naikan's baseline principles and to its ultimate goal. As we discussed in Sect. 6.1, the concept of death and of one's readiness to part with life has been considered the highest possible merit for any *mishirabe* practitioner; although rather subtly, death still permeates the Naikan practice and setting even today. What differs in the two attitudes toward death, however, is that drug abusers pay with their health and life to gain a fake reality where they tangle themselves up in dysfunctional relationships and addictive cycles; whereas Naikan's goal is to draw the practitioner to the ultimate truth about the human condition: we are sinful, yet we are loved and taken care of. If we paraphrase this statement from the standpoint of Khantzian and Albanese's self-medication hypothesis, we may have been hurt and abused, yet we have been loved and taken care of. Becoming aware of this truth, drug-addicted Naikan practitioners may allow the Naikan's existential grounding function/bridging function to manifest itself during their hours of seclusion and silence, i.e., to experience that, indeed, they belong to this world and they can share it with others in a healthy and constructive way. As a result, they may start traversing the long path from psychological destitution and the torments of their ailing bodies to hope, serenity, and freedom.

References

Chervenkova, Velizara: Application of Naikan Therapy to Bulgarians—Its Challenges and Possibilities (Comparative Study of Written Naikan to Drug-Addicted and Healthy Persons), Journal of the Japan Naikan Association, Vol. 18, Japan Naikan Association, 2012 (in Japanese)

Chervenkova, Velizara: "I can already talk with my mom and dad"—Clinical Aspects and the Therapeutic Power of Silence (A Group Interview and Discussion about Naikan Therapy with Drug-Addicted Patients in Bulgaria), Journal of the Japan Naikan Association, Vol. 19, Japan Naikan Association, 2013 (in Japanese)

European School Survey Project on Alchohol and Other Drugs (ESPAD): Bulgaria—Key Results 2015, retrieved from http://www.espad.org/country/bulgaria, ESPAD, 2015

Frank, Arthur W.: The Wounded Storyteller: Body, Illness, and Ethics, University of Chicago Press, 1995

Herman, Judith L.: Trauma and Recovery: The Aftermath of Violence—From Domestic Abuse to Political Terror, Basic Books, 2015

Hibell, Björn, U. Guttormsson, S. Ahlström, O. Balakireva, T. Bjarnason, A. Kokkevi, L. Kraus: The 2011 ESPAD Report—Substance Use Among Students in 36 European Countries, retrieved from www.espad.org/Uploads/ESPAD_reports/2011/The_2011_ESPAD_Report_FULL_2012_10_29.pdf, The European School Survey Project on Alcohol and Other Drugs, 2012

Khantzian, Edward J., Mark J. Albanese: Understanding Addiction as Self-Medication: Finding Hope Behind the Pain, Rowman & Littlefield Publishers, 2008

Kobayashi, Ohji: Understanding and Treating Alcohol and Drug Problems in Patients with Personality Disorders—Discussion from the Standpoint of Khantzian's Self-Medication Hypothesis and Faith Disorder, Clinical Psychiatry, Vol. 54 (11), Igaku-Shoin, 2012 (in Japanese)

Koga, Satoshi: Rebuilding the Personal Relationships among Alcohol Addicts in Psychodrama Setting and Support to Future Perspectives, Journal of Japanese Clinical Psychology, Vol. 29 (2), Japanese Assocation of Clinical Psychology, 2011 (in Japanese)

Kusano, Makoto: Naikan Therapy for Alcohol Dependence—On Its Mechanisms of Action, Proceedings of the 15th Annual Congress of the Japan Naikan Association, Japan Naikan Association, 1992 (in Japanese)

LeClaire, Anne D.: Listening Below the Noise—The Transformative Power of Silence, HarperCollins Publishers, 2009

Maitland, Sara: A Book of Silence—A Journey in Search of the Pleasures and Powers of Silence, Granta Books, 2009

Maté, Gabor: Why Punish Pain?—A Hit of Compassion Could Keep Drugs from Becoming a Crime Problem, YES! Magazine, Issue 58, Positive Futures Network, 2011

Maté, Gabor: Embraced by the Needle, retrieved from http://drgabormate.com/article/embraced-by-the-needle/, Dr. Gabor Maté Website, 2013

Miki, Yoshihiko (supervisor): An Invitation to Naikan (DVD), Nara Naikan Training Center, 1998

Miki, Yoshihiko: The Book about Encountering Your Heart's Treasure (transl. David Reynolds, Yuko Sakaiya), Nara Naikan Training Center, 2002
Miki, Yoshihiko, J. Miki: Naikan Work—Healing the Anxiety and Becoming Happy, Futami Shobo, 1998 (in Japanese)
NFP Bulgaria (National Focal Point on Drugs and Drug Addictions): Drug Abuse in Bulgaria, retrieved from http://nfp-drugs.bg/bg/?&itype=174&info=1046, NFP Bulgaria, 2011 (in Bulgarian)
Sardello, Robert: Silence: The Mystery of Wholeness, Goldenstone Press, 2008
Stamper, Laura: When the Drug War Hits Home: Healing the Family Torn Apart by Teenage Drug Abuse (Second Edition), Fairview Press, 1997
Tadai, Toshiaki: The Runaways—Escapism and Narcisstic Pathology, Minerva Shobo, 2005 (in Japanese)
Tsujita, Naoko, A. Morishita, T. Maeshiro: Trend Analysis of the Naikan-Related Research—A Review of General Lectures Presented at Congresses of the Japan Naikan Association, Journal of the Japan Naikan Association, Vol. 17, Japan Naikan Assocation, 2011 (in Japanese)
Wilmer, Harry: Quest for Silence, Daimon Verlag, 2000
Yoshimoto, Ishin: Naikan Method, Shunjusha, 1965/2007 (in Japanese)

Chapter 10
"Then Go and Wash Your Bowl"—Personal Experiences in Morita Therapy

This chapter presents the author's personal experience in Morita therapy over a two-week experiential hospitalization in Sansei Hospital, Kyoto, where the author was admitted to pass through all the stages required for in-hospital Morita therapy. The author spent two weeks on completely equal terms with the inpatients at that time, following the facility's stringent daily schedule and carrying out all the tasks needed for successful treatment under the guidance of the hospital director Dr. Shin'ichi Usa.

The chapter begins with a brief history of Sansei Hospital as entwined with the life story of its founder, Dr. Genyū Usa; then follows a detailed description of the author's personal experience in Morita therapy the way the approach has been applied at the hospital for more than 90 years.

10.1 Sansei Hospital—Brief History and Peculiarities[1]

Sansei Hospital (三聖病院) was established in 1922 in the precincts of Tōfuku-ji, one of the five great Zen temples of Kyoto and head temple of the Tōfuku branch of the

[1]The history of Sansei Hospital and the biographical data of its founder are summarized from Usa and Kinoshita (1987: 8–20, 191–197), Usa and Takabayashi (1987: 93–119), Usa and Kinoshita (1995: 102–103), Usa (2004: 46–50), Okamoto (2010: 51–75), and Nakayama (2014: 127–135).

Over the years, the therapeutic practices at Sansei Hospital have been subject of numerous controversies related to the application of electroconvulsive therapy by Dr. Shin'ichi Usa sometime in the past, and also to strong paternalism and lack of informed consent, none of which is originally prescribed by Morita therapy (in private communication with Prof. Shigeyoshi Okamoto, Director of Kyoto Institute of Morita Therapy, January 2016). Additionally, in contrast to Shōma Morita's wife—Hisai—neither the wife of Dr. Genyū Usa nor his son's wife provided care to the patients, thus distorting the original home-like therapeutic model and making it rather one-sided (Okamoto 2010: 58); out of reverence for Dr. Shin'ichi Usa, some people called the method "Usa therapy" instead of Morita therapy, thus projecting on Dr. Usa the image of a cult guru (Okamoto 2010: 70), etc. However, these issues are beyond the scope of this book—we present and discuss only the hospital's history and the author's personal experience with the way Morita therapy, or, more properly, its Zen Buddhist modification was applied there.

V. Chervenkova, *Japanese Psychotherapies*,
DOI 10.1007/978-981-10-3126-7_10

Rinzai Zen Buddhist school.[2] Its founder, Dr. Genyū Usa (宇佐玄雄), is considered one of Shōma Morita’s most devoted disciples (Nakayama 2014: 127).

Genyū Usa was born on April 15, 1886 in the village of Nunobiki (now Iga city) in Mie prefecture as Shizuo Nakai (中井玄雄). He was the first son of a lumber dealer family and had three siblings. Usa was contemporary of the prominent *tanka* poet Hakushū Kitahara and of the prolific composer and conductor Kōsaku Yamada, known to have formed Japan’s first philharmonic orchestra.

At the age of nine, Usa joined the monastic order of Sankei-ji, a local temple of the Rinzai school, where he adopted the family name of the temple’s chief priest Gensetsu Usa. Originally, he should undergo his religious training at the Tōfuku-ji main temple, but as the training master there was at rather advanced age, the young boy was redirected to Daitoku-ji, the head temple of the Daitoku branch of Rinzai Zen Buddhism, in Kyoto. When the training master of Daitoku-ji—Shyōin Kawashima—first met Usa, he asked him where he studied; the boy explained, to which master Kawashima replied, “Throw away that school and then come!” (Usa and Kinoshita 1995: 102–103). Master Kawashima was not against education—he simply told Usa that the abstract and theoretical thinking might be useful in the external world, but it is never so for one’s inner world; this thinking should be thrown away from one’s heart—if “imported” there, it would hinder one from attaining *satori* (ibid.).

While in junior high school, the young Usa suffered from nervous breakdown with dizziness, disrupted sleep, mysophobia, and inability to concentrate and read. As his condition aggravated, he traveled for a change of air, did mountain hiking, and even moved to a friend’s place, but to no avail. Usa eventually resorted to the family doctor of his childhood, who gave him a book and adviced him just to look at it for several minutes a day even if he did not manage to read. The doctor also asked him every day home to help with some household duties. Surprisingly, before long the young Usa became able to read again and recovered gradually to the extent that he managed to pass the supplementary exams for Waseda University with the best score. When later Usa told this episode to Shōma Morita, Morita admired what his family doctor did, saying that the doctor applied Morita therapy before it was established (Usa in Usa and Takabayashi 1987: 101–102). In Waseda University Usa studied Indian philosophy for four years, from 1904 to 1908. After graduating, he worked as a researcher at his home university; in 1910 he joined the army for several months.

In 1913 Usa underwent a rigorous Zen training at a *dōjō* of the Daitoku-ji branch and, after accomplishing the training, he was appointed chief priest of Sankei-ji—

[2]Rinzai school (臨済宗) is one of the three major Zen schools of Japanese Buddhism, together with Sōtō (曹洞宗) and Ōbaku (黄檗宗). Its basic concepts include these of the selfless/formless self and of abrupt enlightenment, *tongo* (頓悟). To help its disciples attain *tongo*, Rinzai uses methods such as shouts, *katsu* (喝), or blows delivered by the master on the disciple; question-and-answer sessions, *mondō* (問答); and meditation on paradoxical statements, *kōan* (公案). All of these are intended to precipitate a breakthrough of the normal boundaries of consciousness and awaken an insight that transcends any logical distinctions.

the temple in Mie prefecture were he was first presented as a child. However, he felt that he could not preach to all people in the same way and that he needed to know more about psychiatry (Nakayama 2014: 131); he wanted to help those suffering from mental disorders (Usa in Usa and Takabayashi 1987: 103). Despite the advice that master Kawashima of Daitoku-ji gave him in his childhood, this personal conviction led the young Usa to the Jikei University School of Medicine in Tokyo. There, in 1915 he began studying psychiatry during workdays; on weekends he traveled back to Sankei-ji to perform his priest duties. In 1919 Usa graduated successfully and started a research on nervous disorders under the guidance of Shōma Morita and Shūzō Kure; the guidance of both professors was essential in helping Usa grow as a psychiatrist (Usa in Usa and Takabayashi 1987: 106). The same year when Usa graduated from the university, Shōma Morita finalized the establishment of his therapeutic approach. Their meeting resulted in a strong master-disciple relationship that endured until the end of Morita's life in 1938.

After graduation, Usa considered returning to his life of a priest, but, at the same time, a strong desire to work as a psychiatrist and to follow the newly-developed Morita therapy emerged in his heart. Not knowing which path to choose, he headed for Kamakura where he visited Sōen Shaku, chief priest of Engaku-ji, the head temple of the Engaku branch of Rinzai Zen Buddhism.[3] To Usa's hesitation, the master replied simply, "Leave the temple" (Usa in Usa and Takabayashi 1987: 106). Meeting master Shaku was a life-changing event for the yound Usa: he got determined to advance further on his path as a psychiatrist. To this end he issued a prospectus to Tōfuku-ji for opening a clinic at the temple's precincts. "This clinic would pursue the psycho-physical health of people and help for the consolidation of a prosperous nation", he wrote in the prospectus (as cited in Usa 2004: 47). Although the temple did not intend to undertake such activities, Usa's enthusiasm won him the approval of his plan. Before long, in October 1922, Genyū Usa opened Sansei Clinic at the reception hall of Sanshō-ji (三聖寺), a branch temple of Tōfuku-ji.[4] There Usa started applying Morita therapy to patients with neurosis. At the same time, he kept on brushing up his skills as a psychiatrist—he attended lectures on Neuropsychiatry and carried out research at Kyoto Imperial University (now Kyoto University) under the guidance of Momoshige Miura and Shinkichi Imamura, both professors of Psychiatry; Prof. Imamura also supervised his therapeutic practice at the clinic.

In 1925 Shōma Morita visited the newly-established clinic where he held a lecture in front of 700 people. Later during the years, it became a tradition for Morita to stop by the clinic and hold lectures for the inpatients; the clinic was also an important source for clinical data. In 1927 Sansei Clinic was re-established in a neighboring area as Sansei Hospital with a newly-built ward with capacity for 38 patients. Genyū Usa was appointed its director and the full-fledged application of

[3]Sōen Shaku (1860–1919) was the first Zen Buddhist master to teach in the United States and the one who introduced the term *zen* to the Western world.

[4]Sanshō/Sansei literally means "three saints". The temple where the Sansei Clinic first opened was dedicated to three *bodhisattvas* of the Buddhist pantheon—Monju (文殊), Fugen (普賢), and Seishi (勢至)—hence the clinic's name and, afterward, the name of the hospital.

Morita therapy was initiated. In February of the same year Usa's only son, Shin'ichi (晋一), was born. Before long, together with Shōma Morita, Usa cured the famous playwright Hyakuzō Kurata from his obsessive disorder (see Sect. 5.1.1); as a result of the treatment, Kurata began to perceive the ringing in his ears as music (Usa and Usa 1981: 11). The next years were marked by other successful cases and the vigorous publication of books and journals. It was in October 1931 when an organization of Sansei Hospital's ex-patients was established under the name of *Sansei-kai* (三省会) and the publication of its organ—*Nature and Awareness*—was launched; the organization would held regular meetings, where Shōma Morita would deliver lectures and ex-patients would voice their personal experiences in Morita therapy. The opening ceremony, held at Tōfuku-ji, was attended by high priests. Morita delivered a speech, in which he drew a parallel between Morita therapy and *mukanjo* (無寒暑)—a concept by the 9th-century Chinese Buddhist monk Dongshan[5]; all the priests in the hall were impressed (Usa 2004: 48).

Although during the war years there were almost no patients, in 1951 the hospital was renovated and its capacity increased to 50 patients. Additionally, in August of the same year, the hospital was registered as a healthcare corporation, thus gaining its independency from Tōfuku-ji. The next year Director Genyū Usa welcomed at the hospital the German Neo-Freudian psychoanalyst Karen Horney and the Japanese Zen Buddhist scholar and philosopher Daisetz Teitarō Suzuki. They held a long talk on Morita therapy and Zen Buddhism, but when asked about the relationship between the two, Usa denied such one. However, later on Usa regretted bitterly for having done so. He wrote in his diary that he should have told Horney and Suzuki that Morita therapy and Zen Buddhism were actually the same (Okamoto 2010: 59). This meeting drew the attention of the international academic circles and the number of Western psychologists and psychiatrists visiting Sansei Hospital started increasing. Two years later, in 1954, Usa published a work titled *Shinkeishitsu Therapy through Zen*; the next year he was appointed professor at Shogen Junior College.

Genyū Usa remained devoted to his activities as hospital director and despite his denial on the relation between Zen Buddhism and Morita therapy, his background and firsthand religious experience added a distinctive touch to the approach that he applied at Sansei Hospital: similarly to Zen Buddhist practices, Usa did not rely on theoretical constructions, but prescribed his patients a simple goal-oriented lifestyle on the notion that "the Morita therapy had the same logic as Zen" (Miura and Usa in Lebra and Lebra 1974: 426). One day a woman visited Sansei Hospital, complaining of her unbearable panic attacks. "Please, help me!", she asked in a

[5]Dongshan (洞山) founded the Caodong school of Chan Buddhisim. His teachings was brought to Japan in the 13th century by Dōgen who developed them into the Sōtō school of Zen Buddhism (see footnote 2). *Mukanjo* literally means "no hot, no cold". "When it is cold, don't get fixated in the thought "It's cold!"; embrace the cold. And when it is hot don't get fixated in the thought "It's hot!"; embrace the heat. The implication is you use your subjective experience of hot or cold as a stimulus to realize it's only your ego that's having the experience. Therefore, extinguish your ego." (Ueda Sōko Tradition). Indeed, parallels can be drawn between *mukanjo* and Morita therapy's key concepts such as *toraware* and *arugamama*.

desperate voice. "Don't you understand yet?", Usa asked her softly, then put his hands on her shoulders and pushed her gently down to sit on the floor. The woman was hospitalized, completed her treatment successfully, and experienced profound positive changes in her life (Okamoto 2010: 57). Although Usa was strict with his patients, he acted out of deep love and compassion toward them—he helped them with the kitchen work, bathe together with them and sometimes even drank *sake* with those who had completed their treatment (Okamoto 2010: 56–57). "One can get cured by folding a sheet of paper or by sharpening a pencil", he guided his patients, thus bringing the non-analytical nature of Morita therapy to its utmost (Usa in Usa and Takabayashi 1987: 111).

In February 1957 Genyū Usa—the Zen Buddhist psychiatrist—passed away of cardiac asthma at the age of seventy. Immediately after his death, his son and Kyoto University's graduate of Psychiatry—Shin'ichi Usa—became the hospital's second director. At that time Shin'ichi Usa was aged only 29; he did not considered himself ready to succeed his father in running the hospital, but he had no choice: in fact, this unexpected change would secure him a Zen Buddhist-like life. "No matter if your mind is at ease or if it is anxious, you must deal with what is needed to be done right now", he would often say to his patients referring to his own experience (Usa and Kinoshita 1987: 13).

In 1961 the young hospital director was visited by Seikō Hirata, the chief priest of Tenryū-ji, the head temple of the Tenryū branch of Rinzai Zen Buddhism, in Kyoto. After observing the treatment practices at Sansei Hospital, master Hirata said that if Zen Buddhism was a flower, then Morita therapy was an artificial flower. Shin'ichi Usa was shocked to hear that; he understood that Zen transcends any rational knowledge and from that moment onward he devoted himself to applying Morita therapy even if he did not not how (Okamoto 2010: 60). Two years later, in 1963, Sansei Hospital welcomed for experiential hospitalization the founding father of Gestalt therapy, the German-born psychotherapist Frederick Perls (1893–1970), who wanted to get rid of his 40-years-long nicotine addiction.[6] Later on, foreign researchers from other countries including India, China, Switzerland, and the United States were also admitted for experiential hospitalization. As a hospital specialized in the application of a Japanese psychotherapy—Morita therapy—Sansei Hospital was visited twice by officials of the World Health Organization, in 1967 and in 1971. Although Sansei Hospital drew international attention over the years, its distinctive atmosphere contrasted visibly with that of the psychiatric facilities in contemporary Japan, most of which adopt Western practices based on medical treatment and verbal communication.

In recent years, Sansei Hospital—the hitherto oldest Morita therapy clinic in Japan—faced various difficulties, financial ones included. Because of them, at end-2014 the hospital was closed down and in January–March 2015—demolished;

[6]In the 1960s Perls became interested in Zen Buddhism: "Study some Zen in Japan. Disappointed too", he wrote in his life chronology (Perls 1969: introduction). Perls' total bed rest therapy is described by Dr. Shin'ichi Usa in his article "Ahistorical Morita Therapy" (2003).

the back then green and beautiful hospital garden is now dead under the asphalt cover of a coin parking. Despite the circumstances, Director Dr. Usa, who was aged 89 at the time of writing of this text, continues to hold the regular *Sansei-kai* meetings. Dr. Usa used to practice fervently Morita therapy until the hospital's last day of operation, keeping intact the hospital's Zen Buddhist spirit as inherited from his father—he often provided Rinzai school concepts such as *tongo* (see footnote 2) by saying that "Your very disease is your treasure" (Kawai in Usa and Kinoshita 1987: iv) and "Getting cured is always *now*. Thinking how one will get cured sometime in the future is nothing but misleading" (Okamoto 2010: 64). Besides his unflagging work as a psychiatrist, Dr. Usa is also an active archaeologist. His research on ancient tombs in Japan is highly acclaimed in the archaeological circles (Okamoto 2010: 69); his personal interest also in world art and its history was an inseparable part of the in-hospital life and treatment (see Sect. 10.2).

Some other features of the hospital which, to the best of our knowledge, are difficult to be found in any other Morita therapy clinic included:

- Instead of "clients" or "patients", the residents were called "spiritual trainees"—*shūyō-sei* (修養生) (see Sect. 3.2). They were not allowed to talk to each other —especially about their health condition—excluding situations related to their immediate work tasks and community life. Every resident in the third and fourth phases was assigned a daily duty of some sort, for example, opening the main gate early in the morning, cleaning the bathroom, etc.
- The time for waking up, taking shower, and having meal was signaled by the clap of two wooden sticks; every night at 10 o'clock the time for going to bed was signaled by striking on a wooden board. This board had the inscription "Be mindful not to waste the time of your life" (lit. "Give attention to life and death for time flies like an arrow" (「生死事大、無常迅速」), which is often hung at the entrances of Zen Buddhist temples.
- On the corridor walls and in the common room there were calligraphy and woodcarving works, some of them originally made by Shōma Morita, reading "Those who speak cannot get cured" (「しゃべる人は治りません」), "All alone amidst the communal life" (「たった一人の集団生活」), "Live without understanding" (「わからずに居る」), "Putting efforts already means that you are happy" (「努力既幸福」), "A place for truth cultivation" (「真実道場」), etc. (see Appendix I).
- Director Dr. Usa gave lectures to the inpatients three times a week, another three times weekly he held slide show presentations about world art history, and once a week the residents gathered in the common room to practice meditation, *seiza* (静坐).

All of these peculiarities did not render the hospital representative of the broader scope of Morita therapy application in contemporary Japan, i.e., predominantly as outpatient consultations at internal and psychosomatic medicine clinics and in combination with other approaches, pharmacotherapy included. From the 1980s onward, Morita therapy clinics in Japan have been on a decline. This trend became especially tangible with the 1995 closure of Kora Kōsei'in Hospital—the clinic that

Shōma Morita's disciple and successor at the Jikei University School of Medicine, Prof. Takehisa Kora, opened in Tokyo back in 1940 and headed for 55 years. The closure marked the end of a whole era of Morita therapy, urging the Morita therapy specialists to "export" the essence of the method's in-hospital treatment among outpatients (Ichikawa 2008: 84–85). Nowadays, the outpatient Morita therapy indeed uses key concepts such as *arugamama* and *toraware*, and usually begins with the concept of giving up the conventional view that clients should necessarily get rid of their symptoms. Rather, although clients cannot avail themselves of the advantages of the residential modality of treatment, they are encouraged to live as if they were healthy (Hoshino 2015: 6); they are also guided in keeping a diary, but doctor-patient communication does not rely on it (Ide and Ohbayashi 2003: 62–63) (see Appendix I). Outside of Japan, too, the "current Morita therapy represents an enriched and more complex therapeutic system than its original model" (Chen in Moodley and West 2005: 223). Besides individuals with *shinkeishitsu*, it proves efficacious also to situations in which contemporary people may find themselves, for example, "stress, pain (physical, psychological, or both) and the aftermath of trauma (physical, psychological, or both)" (Conyne 2011: 477). Other configurations of the current practice of Morita therapy include "integrative practice and psycho-education applications, emergent residential treatment and group counseling, and Internet-based education" (Ogawa 2013: 48).

There are only few hospitals left in Japan today to provide the orthodox four-stage residential mode of Morita therapy. These hospitals include the Center for Morita Therapy at the Jikei University School of Medicine in Tokyo and Mishima Morita Hospital in Mishima city, Shizuoka prefecture,[7] but neither of them has the distinctive Zen Buddhist features that Sansei Hospital had. According to Ogawa, "Tokiwadai Psychiatric Clinic was the last site where traditional Morita therapy home-care treatment took place in Japan. It was located in a crowded Tokyo district, but its inner gardens and main buildings reflected the intimate family home of Dr. and Mrs. Chihiro Fujita" (Ogawa 2013: 47); although a traditional one, neither this clinic had Zen Buddhist influences.

In the next section we present a snapshot of the Sansei Hospital's more than 90-years operation as it was seen through the author's eyes.

10.2 Two Weeks in Sansei Hospital

On the fresh Monday morning of May 20, 2013 I arrive at Sansei Hospital. Two nurses welcome me warmly and take me immediately to my room—number 3 at the end of the dusky corridor of the main (old) building. This will be my silent home for two weeks: six *tatami* straw mats, a Japanese-style desk in the corner, several metal pegs on the pale yellowish walls, and two windows looking out on the hospital's backyard. The nurses bring me bedding, hang up a black wooden plate with my name in white *katakana* letters on the sliding door and that is all. Then they gently slide and close the door. I am left all alone in emptiness and silence. Outside the windows the spring is blooming.

[7]In private communication with Prof. Shigeyoshi Okamoto, Director of Kyoto Institute of Morita Therapy (January 2016).

Then the nurses come again and ask me to the nurses station at the other end of the corridor. There I am given a blank white sheet of paper and a pencil: "You have to draw a fruit-bearing tree", they tell me smiling. Baum test.[8] I feel enthusiastic and draw for some 20 minutes: big trunk, leaves, blossoms, butterflies, flowers, and a smiling sun. Happy with having finished, I hand back the sheet to the nurses. Then the nurses give me another white sheet of paper: "One more fruit-bearing tree", they say smiling again. I am astonished. This is the first time I hear that the Baum test could be applied twice in a row. The nurses feel pity for me and suggest I should take a break: "Let's measure your blood pressure and do an electrocardiogram". The medical checkup shows nothing to worry about. After the procedures are over, I am back to the blank sheet: the second tree is thinner, its branches hide a small swallow nest with two hungry fledglings whose parents flutter around them; a Japanese-style lantern appears on the tree's right side, cherry blossoms are scattered around. After the second Baum test, I have to fill in the Yatabe-Guilford Character Test and the Five Factor Personality Questionnaire. Shortly after, Dr. Usa himself gives me a form entitled "Treatment Plan" with my name and birth date neatly filled in. In the "Diagnosis" column I read "hypochondria and anxiety".

Later on follows a tasty lunch, which one of the female residents brings to my room. After lunch she shows me the bathroom. With all the hospitalization procedures finished and having changed into my pajamas, I finally settle in the snow-white bedding (*futon*) on the floor, all alone in my room. The long-awaited trip has just begun.

The hours pass by and I realize I do not need to know what time it is; a feeling that I have arrived here long ago washes over me. I do not think about anything—I just lay in the silence … Around 10 o'clock in the evening, a nurse comes to ask me to go to Dr. Usa's consulting room. "This will be your first evening examination", she says. Not knowing what an evening examination is, I enter the room timidly. The nurse gently slides the door behind me and her steps die down in the dark corridor. In front of me, beneath the warm lighting, the 86-year-old Dr. Shin'ichi Usa sits in his white overall. He gives a deep bow to me and invites me in his extremely polite Japanese to sit on the chair across him. Then he takes out a sheet of paper with the rules of the first phase of Morita therapy—the total bed rest phase, also called "a method for returning (to one's roots)"—*kangen-hō* (還元法). The rules read as following:

- Excluding the times when you eat or go to the restroom or bathroom, you should always lie down in your *futon*.
- Conversations, reading, writing, listening to the radio, etc. are strictly prohibited.
- Snacking between meals, smoking, singing, whistling, doing handiwork, and all other activities aimed at distracting your mind from boredom are also prohibited.
- Eat according to your appetite and do not try to necessarily fall asleep if you cannot.

[8]The author's Baum test drawings are presented in Appendix I, but we do not interpret and discuss them.

- Even if many different thoughts start to gush out, do not try to get rid of them, but simply let them pass by.
- The sounds you hear, hear them as they are; the things you see, see them as they are.
- When unpleasant symptoms arise, leave them as they are.
- Always follow the instructions of the doctors and nurses, and obey strictly the treatment rules.
- Those who do not obey the treatment rules might be asked to leave the hospital.

After reading the rules to me, Dr. Usa explains that their goal and the goal of the entire first phase is to create such an environment so that the mind cannot get distracted. Another goal is wiping out the boundaries between day and night. "Total obedience", Dr. Usa explains, "is equal to healing". Deeply impressed by what I have just heard, I go to bed. The first day of the first phase is finished. Another five days lie ahead of me.

10.2.1 First Phase

Second day: I wake up by the strong sound of wooden sticks clapping. Then I hear human voices. The exact time I do not know, but it is very early in the morning, the sky is still grayish. Soon afterward I hear someone mopping the corridor in front of my room, then wiping the door of my room. Trying to perceive the sounds as they are, I manage to fall asleep somehow. A knocking on the door wakes me up again. This time this is one of the female residents who brings me breakfast: cold milk in an old-style glass bottle, two slices of bread, some margarine and jam. The knife is made of bamboo. I finish my breakfast and then fall asleep again.

As I finish the lunch I realize I do not need to sleep anymore. I have made up for all the weariness accumulated over the past hectic weeks. However, I feel sluggish, my body is somewhat heavy. I also notice that my inner perception of time has changed since yesterday. Anyway, I try not to pay attention to these sensations and follow what Dr. Usa emphasizes: "In Morita therapy it is important not think about yourself".

During the evening examination, Dr. Usa's places the paper with the rules on the small table between us and his first question is whether I obeyed the rules today. I feel as if I am being interrogated, but answer politely, "Yes, I think I did". Dr. Usa smiles and continues interviewing me while writing down his notes.

Dr. Usa's Notes: *Started biting her nails at the age of 5 after her family moved house. May be it was because of the stress. She feels ashamed of biting her nails, especially because she is a woman.*

She wants to divert herself from the isolation by sining, but there are no specific problems related to staying alone. Sometimes when she studies at home, she switches off her mobile phone and concentrates. She can stay alone at home for two or three days; likes to be among people, but also to be alone. She realizes that silence and being silent are very important. Personal perception of time is very different from the common one. She remembers episodes of her past.

Good obedience; looks calm.

Third day: Amazingly, I sleep a lot today and I also have many dreams, including one awful nightmare. I feel like I am taken out of the flow of time: I do not need to know what time it is, neither to read books or talk. When it gets darker, however, I realize that the childhood habit of biting my nails is slowly creeping back again.

Dr. Usa's Notes: *Obeying the rules has become easier. She is grateful to the person who brought her the tasty meals and to those who have prepared them. When it gets darker, the desire to bite her nails arises again. She had a nightmare. Also, in her dream she saw her father who passed away suddenly seven years ago. From time to time she remembered moments of her childhood. The lack of information is completely ok. She thought about living only here and now as if there were neither past nor future. She feels easy, not bored. She slept for quite a long time both after breakfast and lunch.*

Good obedience; good sleep and appetite.

Fourth day: Today I realize the importance of looking at the world from different perspectives—horizontal and vertical. Changing the body position changes the mind attitude. I also feel as if I did not belong to this world. I remember the writings of the Christian Desert Fathers—how it feels to be all alone in the desert …

Dr. Usa's Notes: *Various thoughts which gave her no peace came out; she feels they are difficult to bear. At the same time, she feels her body is rather relaxed. During the last one or two hours before the examination, she felt bored; remembered her late father. Noticed that the desire to bite her nails comes back when it gets dark outside, but today it was ok—it is the first time now she noticed the relation between this habit and darkness; in her daily life, she bites her nails sometimes when she feels stressed or faces a problem. No strong desire for doing something, except knitting a muffler and reading a book only for a while. No desire to clean up her room or wash clothes, neither to acquire some information from the world outside. Felt impatient for lunch.*

Good obedience and patience; no desire to talk with others; good appetite and sleep.

Fifth day: In the morning I feel a little sorry for not going back to my home country to attend the wedding ceremony of my cousin. Some strange sense of loneliness, of voluntary self-banishment from the world in a time when all close people are together and celebrate … Later during the day, I enjoy the iris flower arrangement that the other residents have put near the washbasin in the corridor. I feel my inner time flows silently toward somewhere I do not know; and it makes me feel easier. Inside myself I smile.

However, after lunch two of the female residents come to my room to help me change my bedding. As they leave, I feel embarrassed because of the thousand rules that apply to such a simple thing as changing the bedding: "You need to fold the sheets exactly this way"; "The strips should be on your right side"; "Please, be careful to put your pillow not like this, but like that" … I realize my patience and capacity to obey without asking have just been put to the test. And it seems I failed the test, because the endless inner dialogues and the feeling of embarrassment that the situation triggered did not subside until late afternoon.

Dr. Usa's Notes: *Quite relaxed, but her ears were ringing for some time. Her back ached. She considers her stay in Sansei Hospital a very precious and enriching experience. She reports that before she thought she was a nice person, but now she realized also the dark and aggressive aspects of her personality (not that her mood got darker during the day). Also, she thought about the future, what she would do when she would go back to Bulgaria—mostly optimistic and positive thoughts. She debated with herself on silence and healing, and the relation between the two.*

Sixth day: I feel relaxed and think about Dr. Usa. He resembles a monk who lives as if he did not belong to this world, but knew everything about it as if from a firsthand experience. I also realize that boredom is a synonym of ingratitude for *my time*—the most precious gift that, along with life itself, was given especially to me at birth and that I want to reciprocate for when my hour strikes; the only "field" where the seeds of my human potential can bloom and bear fruits—and I get determined to make *my time* fertile. Birth-*my time* fulfilled-death.

For lunch I have a tasty meal again, but this time it comes with a whole fried fish that stares at me from the plate with its lifeless watery eyes. I eat it somehow, but soon after this I am overwhelmed by a sense of guilt and reproach myself for fake vegetarianism. A tiny sparrow perches on the bamboo grass in front of my window and starts twittering as if to cheer me up. The silence grows more and more. I feel as if it piles up in layers, one after another. And I myself become silence.

After the lunch I go to the bathroom with one of the female residents. I do not talk to her and try to finish bathing as quickly as possible. However, she tries to talk to me, asking me if I know how to use this Japanese-style bathroom or why I should not wash my hair today. I humbly explain to her that I am still in the first phase of treatment and then become silent; but she does not give up and keeps on asking me. I leave the bathroom silently and go back to my room where I find myself indignant with this woman … Similarly to the situation with changing the bedding, now I find it difficult, if not impossible, to completely follow Dr. Usa's instructions for not paying attention to my thoughts and feelings—or at least observing and accepting them as they are—without putting them into words and searching for proper logical explanations. Furthermore, I realize how fake my own image of myself as a patient and tolerant person has been. Later in the evening, on my way back from the restroom, I pass by the room of this female resident and I realize that she has just left. In that very moment I feel sorry for my indignation with her. I realize that we should always treat people the way we treat a tender flower or a fragile vase: with drainless patience, compassion, and care.

Dr. Usa's Notes: *Strictly follows the rules and notices some inner changes. Her inner landscape became brighter. Her back did not ache. She kept silent when the female resident asked her about this and that in the bathroom. The third and the fourth day she could not wait to get to the evening examinations, wondering if she could bear the total bed rest phase until the end. She said it would be nice if we could perceive all phenomena in this world just as they are. Today she realized what it was like to live as a baby: she slept for three hours after breakfast and for another three hours after lunch. "Exactly like a baby", she says. On the other hand, she thought it would be nice if she could go outside for a little while, take a short walk, and see and smell the flowers in the garden.*

At home she usually keeps her place clean, but here she does not find it necessary to clean up, hence she does not feel the need to do it. She enjoys very much the uncluttered setting and simplicity of the Japanese-style rooms.

Dr. Usa's general conclusion: *Patient, obedient, calmed down; moods are often changing. She embraces a desire to live closer to nature, but has no other specific desires. Very good appetite (she was a little impatient for dinner), sleep is also good.*

The second phase to start as from tomorrow.

10.2.2 Second Phase

Seventh day (First Day of the Second Phase): The first day of the second phase starts with a taste of freedom. I can finally go outside in the hospital garden, see the sun and the sky, and smell the flowers. However, going outside should have a purpose, not just loitering around. Not surprisingly, the rules for the second phase are as strict as that for the first one:

- Wake up at 6:30 in the morning and go to bed at 10 in the evening (the lights are turned off at 10 o'clock).
- Spend all the daytime in the garden, being silent.
- Talks and conversations, going outside of the hospital area, smoking, snacking, reading or writing, and all other activities aimed at distracting one's mind from boredom are prohibited.
- Even if you feel drowsy, do not lie down and do not take naps. However, you can sit on the benches in the garden or squat if you want.
- During the first day, do not turn your face up to the sky and do not climb on high places.
- Do not loiter around and do not play with children if you happen to meet any. Also, do not engage in physical labor such as sweeping with a broom, etc.
- In the garden, squat here and there, look at the flowers, and observe the creeping insects. Also, do some light work such as gathering dead leaves or weeding.
- In the evening, write down your diary immediately after dinner. Then go to the workroom and try to help with some work, following the example of the fellow residents.[9]

[9]In the past, Sansei Hospital's residents used to manufacture on commission different products such as cardboard boxes for confectionery. In recent years, as there were no more orders, the residents were involved in voluntary activities such as calligraphy, drawing, knitting, *origami* paper folding, etc.

- Always follow the instructions of the doctors and nurses, and strictly obey the treatment rules.
- Lead a life in accordance with the clapping of the wooden sticks.

As from today I will not be meeting Dr. Usa for evening examinations, but we will keep on communicating through the diary in which I have to write down only what I *saw/observed* and what I *did* during the day. Questions to Dr. Usa via the diary are allowed. Also, the first time I write it, I have to share my impressions about the first phase:

Excerpts from My Diary[10]:

What impressed me during the first phase (six days):

I noticed that the desire to bite my nails appeared when it was getting dark.—*I see.*[11]

I understood (remembered?) the way a baby lives.—*Good. This is a nonverbal lively spiritual life.*

Although I slept well in the nights, I slept for surprisingly long hours also in daytime and had many dreams.—*Good.*

Withdrawing from the world, I felt the beauty of the miracle of life.—*Good.*

I understood what it means to experience the world from the horizontal and from the vertical perspective—*Good. It is nice to have different points of view toward the world.*

My inner perception for time changed significantly; it was an experience that transcended the space-time and life-death dichotomies.—*A precious experience.*

Silence was opening up like a flower bud.—*Good. It is important.*

Several times the clapping sound of the wooden sticks startled me.—*This is a new stimulus for you. Stay startled.*

I ate my meals with a feeling of gratitude.—*That's really wonderful! But having feelings about something or not does not matter at all. Acting gratefully is more important than feeling grateful.*

Diary Entry: Day First (Seventh Day of the Hospitalization) Immediately after breakfast, I went out in the garden.—*Good.* I gathered the dead leaves of the garden geranium and I cried.—*Good.* I felt as if I was throwing away all the unnecessary and unhealthy parts of my soul.—*The soul does not have good and bad parts. There is nothing to be thrown away from there.*

I observed the droplets on the lavender and the rose petals.—*Good.* A purple universe and a red universe.—*It is good that you saw the droplets as universes.*

I watched two pigeons drinking water from the puddle and two butterflies flitting around the garden.—*Good.*

---

[10] All the excerpts are translated from Japanese without any changes, except the names of some fellow residents mentioned here and there in the text; the words "male resident" and "female resident" are used instead.

[11] The sentences in Italics are comments handwritten in red by Dr. Usa directly in the diary. The residents submit their diaries every evening and receive them back the next morning to refer to the doctor's comments and answers (see Appendix I).

I hugged the maple tree.—*Good.*

I observed a big bee humming round a yellow flower; also a beetle and an ant.—*Good.*

I observed the reflection of the May sky in the pond.—*Good. In the pond, the beauty of the depths appears.*

I touched the satin-like petals of the iris flowers in the pond.—*Good. These iris flowers are called "eagle tails". The Emperor from the Kyoto Imperial Palace presented them to Tōfuku-ji temple in the 19th century.*

I observed for a long time a tiny pink flower planted in the backyard. I "shook hands" with its leaves and wept away—*Good.* I had a strong feeling that it is not me who lives, but that Life lives me.—*Good.*

Today, from morning until sunset, I observed how the light changed—for example, the green nuances in the moss and in the tree leaves.—*Good.*

From now on pay attention in all directions, try to find what concretely can be done and perform the actions one by one.

Diary Entry: Day Second (Eighth Day of the Hospitalization) Yesterday evening I was sitting in silence in my room, than I read *Kojiki*[12] for a while and went to bed around 9:30.—*Good.*

In the morning, I woke up shortly before the sound of the wooden sticks and got up at 6:30.—*Good.* After breakfast, I went out in the backyard. I noticed that the bush near the pond was all covered with dead leaves and I gathered them.—*Thank you.* Then I gathered also the dead leaves of the cyclamen and of the potted cactuses. While I was doing it, I lost track of time; I got completely absorbed in the work and became one with it.—*Wonderful!*

I found a small yellow flower on the pathway and used a paper cup as a vase to put the flower in.—*Nice art.*

I observed a beetle walking the young hydrangea leaves—a green-yellowish whirlpool.—*Good.*

I found a beautiful small stone along the pathway, took it in my palm and contemplated it.—*Good.*

I observed the graceful movements of the baby goldfish in the pond.—*Good.*

I observed a tiny insect creeping up a bamboo shoot.—*Good.*

It was a day filled with perfect silence.—*Wonderful!*

Try to find what work you can do in the evenings and do it.

→ Questions to Dr. Usa:

In the backyard there is a wooden board with the words "What you feel, feel it thoroughly" inscribed on it. What do they mean?—*It means you should not use and*

[12]At the beginning of their second phase, each inpatient was handed out a small book with excerpts from *Kojiki* (古事記)—*Records of Ancient Matters*—the oldest extant chronicle in Japan, dating from the early 8th century. Although the text in this book was in Old Japanese, the residents were encouraged to read it every morning and evening accurately, no matter if they understood the content. This task was aimed not at reading as an end in itself, but at helping one revive gradually their mental activities after getting up and calm down before going to bed.

rely on words, but just experience what you feel the way it is. If you put it in words, the experience gets blurred.

I noticed that the residents of Sansei Hospital take medicines. Why?—*They have been given these medicines at other clinics before coming here, so they should not quit. However, the real medicine in Morita therapy is considered the symptom itself.*

Diary Entry: Day Third (Ninth Day of the Hospitalization) Yesterday evening I wrote my diary after the slide show presentation about Expressionism and then I went to bed.

This morning I woke up at 6:30 and went outside after breakfast. I picked all the dead leaves from the cactuses at the entrance, and also those of the hydrangea flowers and the bushes in front of the nurses station window.—*Thank you.*

I changed the water of the yellow flower I found yesterday.—*Good job.*

I saw a small worm on the pathway and moved it away so people would not step on it.—*Good. Nice care.*

I listened to the wind and rain.—*Good.*

I observed the lively play of the sparrows in the garden and listened to their chirruping.—*Wonderful!*

→ Questions to Dr. Usa:

Do not the usual medicines suppress the so-called real medicine in Morita therapy, i.e. the symptom? Also, while taking medicaments, the residents consider themselves sick … —*Yes, medicines indeed suppress the symptoms and the residents consider themselves sick. In order to remedy this issue, we explain that taking medicines is not aimed at erasing their symptoms, but rather at helping residents live with their symptoms.*

When my father passed away suddenly, I almost did not cry nor did I put my feelings and emotions into words. Rather, I did my best to focus on what had to be done at that very moment, for example, to console my mother, arrange the funeral, etc.—*Good.* However, three weeks later, the left side of my face was struck by Bell's palsy. Everyone told me that my body got sick because I did not express my emotions related to my father's sudden death.—*Could be so.* Even now, seven years later, I do not know if they were right or not. What did I do wrong?—*It is not that you did something wrong. You have simply fallen prey to paying attention to the condition of your face.*

From tomorrow morning, start the third phase.

Rules of the third phase:

- Strictly obey the time for getting up in the morning and going to bed.
- Fifteen minutes after getting up in the morning, start cleaning up around together with all other residents.
- During daytime, try to be involved as much as possible in some activity in the garden or in the workroom.
- In the evenings, join the other residents in the workroom and work during the assigned time.

- Excluding conversations directly related to your immediate work tasks, social and other conversations are prohibited; especially talks on diseases and symptoms are strictly prohibited.
- Always attend the lectures held by the director every Wednesday, Friday, and Sunday. Submit your diary every day. On the afternoons when lectures are held, going outside is prohibited.
- Drinking alcohol and smoking is prohibited. Visitors to the hospital are allowed to smoke in the designated areas.
- Singing, whistling, listening to radio, watching TV, listening to music, playing games, etc., are prohibited, too.
- Going out and staying out overnight with no definite purpose is prohibited. Leaving the hospital and staying the night out should be reported to the hospital staff. After acquiring permission from the director, write it down in the designated book.[13]
- Keep out of the offices. Do not enter the rooms of fellow residents or the night duty room.
- If you want to skip a meal because of staying out for the night, inform staff at least 3 hours in advance. Your dinner will be kept until 6 p.m.
- Money borrowing and lending is strictly prohibited.
- Always be careful when walking down the corridor, opening and closing the doors, taking off your slippers and shoes, so as not to put others to inconvenience.
- If you want to be discharged from the hospital, you need to get an approval three days in advance.
- Always follow the instructions of the doctors and nurses.

10.2.3 Third Phase

Diary Entry: Day First of the Third Phase (Tenth Day of the Hospitalization)
Yesterday evening I wrote my diary, then helped for the preparation of the evening meditation in the workroom, read *Kojiki*, and went to bed around 10 p.m.—*Good.*

This morning I woke up at 6:30 and cleaned up the corridor together with the other residents.—*Good.*

After breakfast, I did my duties for today, i.e., cleaning up the female toilets and bringing meals to a resident in her first phase.—*Good.* Soon afterward I went out in the garden and swept the whole concrete pathway that surrounds the hospital.—*Thank you.* I felt deeply how nice it is to work.—*Good.*

[13]Residents in the fourth phase—the resocialization phase—are allowed to stay out for the night six times a month.

After I finished bathing, I felt as if being reborn.—*This is a moment that transcends time.* I was grateful for the bounty of life.—*Good. No matter toward whom or what, gratitude always represents a kind of spiritual work.*

Then I drew a picture with crayons using mainly pink and white colors.—*Good.*

Then I made a birthday card for a Japanese friend of mine and sent it.—*Good.*

Then I knitted a muffler for my academic advisor.—*Good.*

Today I ate my meals, especially the dinner, with deep gratitude.—*Good. Gratitude is the symbol of complete healing.* I feel as if my inner space has expanded.—*Wonderful!*

→ Questions to Dr. Usa:

Why are music and singing considered inappropriate in Morita therapy?—*Because they can become stimuli for the other residents and influence their inner life, hence their treatment.*

Diary Entry: Day Second of the Third Phase (Eleventh Day of the Hospitalization) Yesterday evening I folded *origami* in the workroom and knitted muffler for my advisor.—*Good.* I got very excited after Dr. Usa's impressive lecture and did not manage to fall asleep until late (10:30 p.m.)—*It is preferable to write about facts.*

This morning I got up earlier than usual (5:45), because I was on duty for opening the hospital's main gate. When I went outside at daybreak, I remembered "In spring, it is the dawn that is most beautiful"[14].—*Good.* Getting up early in the morning is so nice!—*Consciousness is cleansed.*

After cleaning up the corridor and finishing breakfast, I went outside in the garden, gathered the fallen azalea blossoms and swept all around the main gate.—*Good.*

Then in the garden I picked up some flowers with two female residents, made *ikebana* and put the arrangements here and there in the hospital.—*Good. Thank you.* It was a very nice moment!

Then I cleaned up my room, put my things in order and enjoyed the simplicity of the space around.—*Good.*

After lunch I went to the nearby florist, bought a potted yellow flower and planted it in the garden.—*Good. Thank you.* A tiny sun.—*Good.*

I also took many pictures of flowers and droplets.—*Nice art.*

→ Questions to Dr. Usa:

Is the hospitalization in Sansei Hospital possible for people with somatic diseases only or for those seeking spiritual growth?—*Yes, somatoform disorders are appropriate for Morita therapy. People who aim to develop spiritually are also welcome.*

If feelings should not be verbalized, is there any appropriate way for expressing them so as the body not to become ill?—*Yes, there is. For example, pantomime.*

[14]*Haru wa akebono* (春は曙) is one of the opening sentences of *The Pillow Book*, an 11th century Japanese classic written by court lady Sei Shōnagon.

Expression is the mind itself. However, a goal such as "the body not to become ill" is utterly irrelevant.

Diary Entry: Day Third of the Third Phase (Twelfth Day of the Hospitalization) Yesterday evening I taught one of the male residents to knit.—*Thank you.* I went to bed around 9:30 p.m.

This morning I got up at 6:30. After cleaning up the corridor and finishing my daily chore (cleaning up the entrance), I swept in front of the entrance and watered the flowers there.—*Good. Thank you for your help.*

Then I cleaned up the space around the sink in the front garden and made a flower arrangement there.—*Thank you.*

Then I observed the dragonflies over the pond and the blooming lotus in the pond, and took pictures of them.—*Good.*

After lunch I changed the water of yesterday's flower arrangements with one of the female residents.—*Thank you.* Then I picked up some white flowers from the garden and made a new arrangement, which I placed at the entrance.—*Thank you.*

Then I helped one of the residents in her first phase to change her bedding.—*Thank you.*

Both before and after having a meal, I expressed my gratitude in my heart.—*Good.*

I released a fly that had come into my room.—*Good.*

Day after day the hospital garden looks wider and wider. Every day I rediscover places I thought I knew well and I find more and more opportunities to create beauty.—*Good.* Every flower petal, butterfly and ant I watch with awe and recognize as a beautiful small universe.—*Wonderful!*

Diary Entry: Day Fourth of the Third Phase (Thirteenth Day of the Hospitalization) Yesterday evening I continued to teach knitting to one of the male residents.—*Thank you.* Then I read *Kojiki* for a while and went to bed around 9:30 p.m.

In the morning, I got up at 6:30. After cleaning up the corridor and finishing breakfast, I did my daily chore with one of the female residents (cleaning and preparing the bathroom).—*Thank you for your help.*

Then I swept around the entrance and the sink in the front yard.—*Thank you.*

I finally completed the muffler for my advisor. It was a nice moment.—*Good. He will be pleased!*

I also knitted a bracelet for one of the female residents. I will give it to her tomorrow.—*Good.*

I watered the backyard flowers and then observed the baby goldfish that the other residents moved yesterday from the bucket to the pond. I tasted freedom.—*Good.*

In the evening, I listened to the drizzle outside.

This is my last evening in Sansei Hospital. The last entry in the diary. I carry in my heart so many small universes: flowers, droplets, butterflies … and yet my heart is so light. Wide and light. Very, very wide and light. My heart is a dandelion, blue balloon, June morning sky …—*Good.*

Diary Entry: Day Fifth (Fourteenth Day of the Hospitalization and the Last One) Today is my last day here and, according to the plan, I will leave in the afternoon immediately after the Sunday lecture by Dr. Usa. Since the early morning everything is as usual except the feeling that a very precious experience is coming to an end. At the same time, I also feel that this experience will bloom inside of me sometime in the future and this feeling calms me down.

Even during my final hours here, I keep on doing what I used to do so far: I buy a flower again and plant it in the garden, observe the light that flows down the tree leaves in front of my window, and listen to the chirruping sparrows that come to greet me every day. These are not unusual things to do or observe in my daily life, but here, at Sansei Hospital, they are as if condensed—perhaps due to my own intensified ability to listen and to observe. I therefore attempt to taste them to the fullest. Later during the day, I give Bulgarian souvenirs to some of the residents. All of them get very excited about it and I receive *origami* butterflies, a sunflower, a Japanese fan, and many heartfelt smiles in return.

During the lunchtime, which is the last one to share with the residents here, I eat very slowly and listen to the sound of the wooden chopsticks. Even after finishing my meal, I remain until the last moment allowed—12:10 p.m. At the other side of the table sits one of the male residents, who sips tea and looks at his wristwatch from time to time. Everything else is just silence.

After lunch, the nurses call me to the nurses station: I have to draw twice a fruit-bearing tree again. For completely inexplicable reasons, I cannot help weeping almost all the time while drawing the first picture: as compared to two weeks ago, the tree is now plainer with blossoms transformed into apple-like fruits. The lack of countless short strokes and additional details makes the whole composition look calm and stable. The tree simply exists here and now. The second picture has a smiling sun and two birds in the upper half, while the two birdies from the pre-hospitalization picture are now "on firm ground" (see Appendix I).

After finishing the Baum tests, I take a short break and then attend Dr. Usa's Sunday lecture. He closes it by the words, "Direct your mind to the world outside, observe it carefully, and use every chance to sketch and draw". With these words inscribed deep in my heart I go back to my room, bid farewell to this simple space, take my luggage, and walk down the long corridor for the last time. Then we exchange bows and good-byes with Dr. Usa in a moment which he himself would describe as "a moment beyond time". I realize that his figure bent down with age, humility and compassion, I will always carry in my heart as a symbol of genuine humaneness and wisdom.

At the entrance, all the fellow residents gather to see me off. We take some pictures. I thank them for helping and teaching me during my stay, and then take the familiar path down to the main gate with the big white signboard reading "Sansei Hospital—Dr. Shin'ichi Usa". There I take a picture again as I did exactly two weeks ago when I walked this path in the opposite direction—toward the hospital. Everything looks the same, yet it is different as it is more meaningful and serene to me now.

After I exit the main gate with the temple-like hospital building already behind me, I dive into the evening city noise and head for the train station. At the end of the trip I feel the trip has just begun…

10.3 Conclusion

"A monk said to Jōshū, "I have just entered this monastery. I beg you to teach me." Jōshū asked, "Have you eaten your rice-gruel." "I have", replied the monk. "Then", said Jōshū, "go and wash your bowl(s)." The monk was enlightened."[15]

Thinking about her personal Morita therapy experience in Sansei Hospital, the author is difficult to find a more appropriate phrase to summarize it than "Go and wash your bowl". Leaving the interpretations of this *kōan* to the Zen Buddhist philosophers, we quote it here as a quintessence of the precious two-week experience: simply do the things that have to be done right now, perceive yourself, others and the world the way they are, and, most of all, do not overwhelm your mind with questions, especially about your health condition.

On the other hand, we are aware how difficult it is, indeed, for contemporary people to follow Jōshū's advice in the hectic course of our daily lives. Being overwhelmed with information and various stimuli from the world outside, and preoccupied with ourselves in a self-centered individualistic societies, we find it difficult to even imagine how we can simply "wash our bowls", i.e., how can we stop to pay constantly attention to ourselves and the thoughts about ourselves, and do the things that should be done—the ultimate goal of self-emptying that, Morita therapy teaches us, paves the way to both physical and mental health, and personal growth. Below we provide a possible answer to this question.

The physical environment: silence and the concept of "call for creation": The first thing that catches the attention at Sansei Hospital is the immediate physical environment: the temple-like building with its traditional Japanese tile roof, a pond with goldfish in the garden, a wooden floor corridor, and the simple beauty of the rooms carpeted with *tatami* straw mats run counter to the clinical white of the modern healthcare facilities. Also, excluding the staff's white gowns and the presence of some medical equipment such as an electrocardiograph, the overall atmosphere does not remind of a hospital in the common sense of the word. Rather, the very first impression is of a retreat where residents lead a secluded and silent life: both the atmosphere inside the hospital and outside of it, in the garden, naturally makes one keep silent. However, this is not a dead silence, but silence alive and full of meaning, which predisposes the individual placed in its bosom to listen. Embraced by such silence, people here do listen even when they talk.

---

[15]This is Case VII ("Jōshū's Bowl-Washing") of *The Gateless Gate—Mumonkan* (無門関)—a collection of 48 Zen-*kōan* (see footnote 2) compiled in the early 13th century (as translated by Reginald H. Blyth in Blyth, Reginald H.: Zen and Zen Classics, Volume Four—Mumonkan, Hokuseido Press, 1966: 81–84).

During the total bed rest phase, however, this silence could be frightening to the patient because all they can hear at this point is their inner "noise". This noise can oftentimes be deafening: long hours of daytime sleep filled with dreams are followed by midnight wake-ups flooded by complicated thoughts and childhood memories. Being deprived of the usual contact with any external stimuli that draw the attention to one direction or another, one's mind turns into a fountain from which all possible emotions and thoughts gush out in the silence. One does not know how to manage this uncontrollable process, for which reason the only solution is to leave all the thoughts and emotions pass by as they are. This is one of the key rules of the treatment's first phase.

As the days pass by and the corner has been turned (for the author that was the evening of the third day), i.e., the most intrusive thoughts, emotions, and dreams have already been "discharged", the resident seems to gradually calm down and return to a preverbal state of mind. Hence the first phase is also known as *kangen-hō*—"a method for returning (to one's roots)". In the evening of the sixth day, the author reported to Dr. Usa that she felt like a baby. This made him reduce her bed-rest phase to six days—that meant she was ready to enter the second phase, i.e., get up and go to the world outside.

During the second phase of gradual returning to the world, the author realized she had developed an inner capacity to *wait*, *listen*, and *observe*, or at least her previous capacity to do so had increased. Spending long hours in the garden, observing a single flower or simply sitting on the bench and listening to the rain was not boring at all. On the contrary, all such "inactive activities" constantly provoked the author's sense of wonder as she was discovering one after another entire universes in the tiny objects she observed or in the sounds she heard. The silence, too, was not "just silence", but it gradually started revealing itself as full of meaning and life.

As the author entered the third phase, her very first impression of the hospital garden as a rather small place was still strong; she wondered how every one of the 15–16 residents managed to find something to do every day in such a limited space. To her surprise, however, the author realized how a seemingly narrow and plain space could "grow" wider and wider. This realization helped her respond to the environment in a more proactive and constructive manner (see *Twelfth Day of the Hospitalization*). All the small "universes" during the second phase that the author used to only observe were now "calling" for her active response: the old empty plant pots in the backyard needed cleaning; the front yard sink filled with dead leaves and surrounded by dirty buckets and empty flower pots required tidying up; the azalea bushes and the potted cactuses had to be weeded; a worm on the path needed to be moved to a safer place. All these objects drew her attention, she responded to them actively, and, as a result, a positive change emerged. Obviously, these objects never "called" the attention of any one of the other residents. At the same time, the other residents were "called" by other places or situations that never "called" the author. To respond to that "call" then is the natural result of one's enhanced capacity to *listen* and to *observe/contemplate* the external world. This capacity immediately manifests itself once the hitherto obstacles that have bound it, i.e., the individual's *toraware*, are removed.

Probably for this reason, the third in-hospital phase was characterized by the author's increased awareness of the world as a source of thousands of meanings.

These she defined as *calls for creation*: calls for her to take a proactive attitude toward the world—in that case, the hospital garden. Undoubtedly, neither the world nor the hospital garden changed a whit; it was the author and her attitude toward them that had undergone transformation during the first two phases of the treatment. Such a transformation most likely resulted from (i) *"emptying" the Self* and (ii) *redirecting the attention* in a way so that more inner space was opened for a constructive interaction with the world.

The Sansei Hospital's residents led a silent, yet active life, focused on specific immediate tasks they performed every day—be these tasks part of their daily chores or voluntary activities; an active life, which required their continual creative response toward reality, leaving no opportunity for complicated thoughts about their health condition to arise. It was these actions that formed the very fabric of this silent, yet active life. Furthermore, these actions were not scattered during the day as one pleased, neither were they intended to entertain and make one feel more comfortable in order to forget one's ailments. On the contrary, the actions were part of the strict hospital discipline where meeting the immediate requirements of reality as it was—not as it had been neurotically remolded—formed the strong foothold from which residents could return to their daily life with a healthier and more constructive attitude at hand.

The metaphysical environment: again silence and the concept of "inner time": Another important aspect of the treatment in Sansei Hospital was that residents led a silent life in accordance with the natural circadian rhythm. In contrast to the total bed rest phase, whose ultimate goal is *kangen*—returning to the preverbal state of mind where no boundaries between dichotomies exist—from the second phase onward the goal was reversed to strictly following this rhythm. As it is also the case with the other two Japanese psychotherapies presented in this book, Naikan and Dohsa-hou, to follow the circadian rhythm is of extreme importance in Morita therapy, too: during her stay in Sansei Hospital, the author noticed how the strict daily schedule slowly but steadily put her inner life in order and brought it closer to a center of calmness where concerns about her condition had no place to grip. In short, an ordered physical environment directly brings forth an ordered metaphysical one.

Moreover, the day-to-day repetitiveness of certain actions at same hours—for example, the time for getting up and going to bed, having a meal, etc.—serves as a supporting point with two major functions, both essential for the treatment of neurotic disorders: first, repetitiveness *provides a specific sense of security and safety* to the residents, creating a metaphysical environment from which the world is seen no more as one of chaos and uncertainty—a vision that is not difficult for a patient with neurosis to transfer from their inner world. Second, following the rhythm *helps the residents shift their attention from their inner conflicts* to the external world where concrete tasks need to be performed. In other words, residents follow a predetermined order but, at the same time, they are responsible for maintaining it through their own attention to the performance of concrete tasks.

In the author's experience, such an ordered life led to the development of a specific time perception that we term here *inner time*. Its key feature is the recognition of the potential of every single moment to contain eternity. As previously mentioned, all the individual actions formed the very fabric of the secluded in-hospital life and their strictly timed performance provided residents with "experienced rhythms", i.e., asking questions and attempting to analyze one's condition were replaced by the pure experience of reality the way it was there and then in its rhythmic repetitiousness. It is then probable that the process of internalization of the *arugamama* principle—tasting reality the way it is—manifests itself through the individual's *call for creation* and *inner time*.

To recapitulate, the Sansei Hospital residents lived a silent, yet active and creative life in strict accordance with the circadian rhythm. The goal, as emphasized many times by the hospital director Dr. Usa, was to redirect the residents' mind to the external world, thus opening up an inner space where trust in Life the way it is —*arugamama*—would become equal to total healing.

*

I cannot determine with any certainty whether some profound inner transformation has taken place as a result of my experiential hospitalization in Sansei Hospital nor whether the symptoms of hypochondria and anxiety, which Dr. Usa wrote in my "Treatment Plan", are completely gone. After I immersed myself back in my daily life, however, I noticed several positive changes, both physical and mental: my body was more relaxed and my gait was lighter—at least over the weeks immediately after leaving the hospital; I felt the Bell's palsy side of my face was more relaxed; if I encountered the desire to bite my nails, in most of the cases I simply ignored the thought or at least prevented it from turning into a real action; amazingly for a person who used to draw abstract images with color crayons, I started sketching in pencil real objects such as trees, flowers, and vases; my interest in observing and taking pictures of small objects, especially natural ones such as flowers and insects, increased. All of these I considered manifestations of my augmented mindfulness, which likely fostered my joy of simply breathing and laughing, walking and working; of simply being alive.

When I arrived back home and realized that the long-awaited experiential hospitalization in Sansei Hospital was already in the past, I promised myself that after having finished eating I would always go and wash my bowl.

References

Conyne, Robert K. (ed.): The Oxford Handbook of Group Counseling, Oxford University Press, 2011

Hoshino, Ryo'ichi: Inpatient and Outpatient Morita Therapy at Hamamatsu University School of Medicine—20 Years of Applying Easy-to-Understand Morita Therapy, Mental News, No. 33, The Mental Health Okamoto Memorial Foundation, 2015 (in Japanese)

Ichikawa, Mitsuhiro: Outpatient Morita Therapy—An Intensive Short-Term Treatment of Neurosis, Hakuyosha Publishing, 2008 (in Japanese)

Ide, Masahiro, M. Ohbayashi: Introduction to Psychosomatic Medicine for Clinicians, NC Communications, 2003 (in Japanese)

Lebra, Takie Sugiyama, W. P. Lebra (ed.): Japanese Culture and Behavior: Selected Readings, University of Hawaii Press, 1974

Moodley, Roy, W. West (ed.): Integrating Traditional Healing Practices into Counseling and Psychotherapy—Multicultural Aspects of Counseling and Psychotherapy, Sage Publications, 2005

Nakayama, Kazuhiko: Understanding Morita Therapy through Words—A Brand New Form of Morita Therapy, Hakuyosha Publishing, 2014 (in Japanese)

Ogawa, Brian: Desire for Life: The Practitioner's Introduction to Morita Therapy for the Treatment of Anxiety Disorders, Xlibris, 2013

Okamoto, Shigeyoshi: A Study on the "Zen-Morita Therapy"—History and Development of Sansei Hospital, Interdisciplinary Journal of Social Sciences, Vol. 3 (2), The Society for Interdisciplinary Studies of Social Sciences, 2010 (in Japanese)

Perls, Frederick S.: Ego, Hunger and Aggression: The Beginning of Gestalt Therapy, Random House, 1969

Ueda Sōko Tradition (Australia), retrieved from http://www.uedateaaustralia.com/reading/%E7%84%A1%E5%AF%92%E6%9A%91-mukanjyo-no-hot-no-cold/

Usa, Genyū, S. Usa: Living with Reality, Sansei Hospital/Sansei-kai, 1981 (in Japanese)

Usa, Shin'ichi: Ahistorical Morita Therapy, Psychiatria et Neurologia Japonica, Vol. 105 (5), Japanese Society of Psychiatry and Neurology, 2003 (in Japanese)

Usa, Shin'ichi: Zen Buddhist Morita Therapy (Appendix: Hospital Diary), Sansei-kai, 2004 (in Japanese)

Usa, Shin'ichi, S. Takabayashi (ed.): Zen, Morita Therapy, Kyoto—A Collection of Commemorative Lectures on Dr. Genyū Usa's 100th Birth Anniversary, Sansei-kai, 1987 (in Japanese)

Usa, Shin'ichi, Y. Kinoshita: The World as It Is—Buddhism and Morita Therapy, Toho Shuppan, 1987 (in Japanese)

Usa, Shin'ichi, Y. Kinoshita: The World as It Is (sequel)—Similarities between Religion and Morita Therapy, Toho Shuppan, 1995 (in Japanese)

Part V
In a Nutshell

Chapter 11
Three Japanese Psychotherapies

Drawing a general conclusion on such a broad topic as the Japanese psychotherapies presented in this book—Morita, Naikan, and Dohsa-hou—is undoubtedly a challenging task because the origin, development, methodology, and scope of application of these approaches differ significantly from each other. On the other hand, their common cultural context, which we already explained on several occasions (Part II and Part III), allows us to discuss the three psychotherapies together. By so doing we can reveal one final time the authentic beauty of their Japanese "soul" and reassert their psychotherapeutic value. We therefore open this summary with the comments that the British philosopher Alan Watts makes about Eastern philosophy and relate them to the Japanese psychotherapies: these approaches are "at root, not concerned with conceptions, ideas, opinions, and forms of words at all," but rather with "a transformation of experience itself" (Watts 1953: 25). This is the canvas on which all the other peculiar elements underlying the three psychotherapies are drawn.

First, none of the three approaches *relies on words*, neither do they expect verbal communication to yield remarkable therapeutic outcomes; verbal communication is either missing or is only secondary to silence. In Morita therapy, in which the concept of seclusion and silence is brought to an extreme during the total bed rest phase, words are exchanged only for the purposes of diary keeping and brief evening examinations; in Naikan therapy, only a few words are exchanged between interviewer and practitioner with the interviewer always asking the same questions in a predetermined format and order, while the practitioner should confine themselves to providing one or two facts in response to each of the three questions—the whole interview therefore usually takes no more than 3–5 minutes; in Dohsa-hou, although the trainer's verbal instructions and feedback are desirable during the sessions, they nevertheless function as an auxiliary tool to the ultimate goal of the therapeutic process, i.e., the "creation" of the proper posture or movement. All of these seem to imply that in Japan neither the self-concept nor psychological healing is so closely

V. Chervenkova, *Japanese Psychotherapies*,
DOI 10.1007/978-981-10-3126-7_11

related to talking. That is, the construction of verbal description of the client's experience plays only an auxiliary role in these three therapies. Words just "probe" the development of the therapeutic process, but they are never meant to serve therapeutic ends.[1]

To further surprise of the Western psychotherapists, their Japanese counterparts *do not focus on the client's emotions and feelings* as they consider these quite irrelevant to the therapies' ultimate goals. Rather, only a down-to-earth attitude in combination with strict discipline are employed for the construction of a therapeutic framework that serves as a starting point from which clients can reset their life. "Strictly follow the teacher/trainer's instructions and if you do so, you may gain insight into your condition and eventually may get cured" therefore might be an appropriate slogan. In this sense, it is important to mention that across the three therapies, therapists are called *sensei* (先生), which is the common address to teachers and medical doctors in Japan even though therapists are rarely such ones. The word *sensei* is comprised of two characters, whose combination literally means "the one born before," i.e., "a predecessor, an individual who, forever a generation ahead in the age grading system, bestows upon those who come after him the key secrets of mastering a given art" (De Vos in Reynolds 1980: 127). Most of the Western psychotherapeutic approaches are culturally influenced to a certain extent, but the founder's personality and individual worldview nevertheless determine the essence of the approach. By contrast, although the Japanese psychotherapies owe their existence to bright individuals, their founders act *more as providers of deeply imbedded cultural values* and *much less as figures who develop a personal philosophy* in the form of a therapeutic approach; hence the strong opposition of the founders that their personal names should constitute the respective therapy's name.[2]

Therefore, however cold the strict discipline and inattentiveness to emotions may seem, exactly these peculiarities make the Japanese psychotherapies efficacious in restoring one's balance—both psychological and physiological—that one has lost because of one's own ignorance to go astray from the social and/or natural, and/or cosmic laws. However, this ignorance is not ascribed to the ailing individual alone, but it is considered, as we already discussed in the context of Naikan therapy, common to all humans. To paraphrase Watts, Japanese psychotherapies are interested in the transformation of states which are common to mankind as a whole and are thus psychotherapies of the "normal" man (Watts 1953: 26). They propose "to change patterns of thought and feeling which are characteristic of society as well as of the individual, though this does not amount in practice to an attempt to change society as whole" (ibid.).

[1]It is widely known that Western approaches focused upon some version of the "talking cure" appear to be less efficacious among Japanese clients. A probable explanation of this phenomenon could be related to the Japanese cultural features that we already discussed in Part II.

[2]Morita therapy is the only exception, but it was given its present name after Shōma Morita passed away (Kitanishi 1999: 183). Despite some attempts for descriptive translation based on the combination of characters of the respective words—for example, Naikan could be "introspective therapy"—the therapies retained their original names; this adds further value to their authentic Japanese nature.

Such a didactic attitude, whose specific manifestation differs in the three therapies, eventually serves *the preservation of the social harmony and wholeness*, fueled also by "the common cultural belief that the individual self is not an autonomous, separate entity, and that ideally it should be submerged in nature or the society of which it is only a part" (Lebra 1976: 231); that "the self is what to be forgotten rather than recalled and ruminated on" (Lebra 1976: 225).[3] This belief clearly manifests itself in the respective therapeutic settings of the three approaches: in Morita therapy this is the communal life from the second phase onward when the client is strongly encouraged to search for and perform activities that could benefit the whole group and, whenever possible, to perform them together with the other residents; in the Naikan therapy's orthodox version, all the practitioners stay together in a common room where the personal folding screen is difficult to prevent the others in the room from hearing one's confessions during the interviews; and in Dohsa-hou, during the intensive overnight camps everybody shares both therapeutic sessions and daily life activities to the minutest details. This "togetherness" across the three therapies is an apt example of the therapeutic applications of communal life, implying also that it is easier to share one common humanity "not when we are powerful and strong, but when we are vulnerable and weak" (Nouwen 2009: 25).

Additionally, in contrast to most of their Western counterparts, which usually take snapshots of their clients in the hermetically sealed space of the consulting room only, the Japanese psychotherapists observe their clients while they perform also daily life activities such as eating and cleaning. That is, the Japanese psychotherapies are "equipped" with both the sacred therapeutic space—the private room in Morita therapy, the folding screen in Naikan therapy, and the therapeutic mat in Dohsa-hou—and the profane space of daily routine. For this reason, in their orthodox versions the Japanese psychotherapies can be considered *home-like therapies* in the sense that both therapists and clients share the profane space of their daily life[4] within a therapeutic communal environment that transcends and enriches the usual therapist–client relationship.

Another peculiarity common to the three psychotherapies is the fact that they rarely display commitment to *any metaphysical or philosophical theory*. Despite the close relation between, for example, Naikan therapy and the Pure Land Buddhism, the therapeutic method itself is rather practical: it serves concrete purposes, while, although warmly welcomed, spiritual development that may arise as a result of the accomplished purpose is never sought after as an immediate goal. However, here we come across an intriguing paradox: being so very practical and goal-oriented, the three therapies never address directly the client's disease or impairment as a subject of treatment; much less do they discuss or analyze this condition with the client, or pursue cure at any price—neither of neurosis and obsessive disorders in

---

[3]As explained in footnote 38 in Chap. 6, the literal meaning of the Japanese word for "self"—*jibun* (自分)—is "my part (of the whole/Nature)."

[4]In private communication with Prof. Shigeyoshi Okamoto, Director of Kyoto Institute of Morita Therapy (January 2016).

Morita therapy nor of antisocial behavior or interpersonal conflicts in Naikan therapy nor of physical and/or mental impairment in Dohsa-hou. In a sense, the Japanese psychotherapies do not "sign a contract" with their clients that they will necessarily help them to get rid of their symptoms or problems. What these approaches offer is an unordinary space where clients may observe their own disharmony as manifested in their problem or disease, encounter with their true self, and, consequently, tap experiences/states that are common to all human beings: *arugamama* and *sei-no-yokubō* in Morita therapy; *tariki* and *zange* in Naikan therapy; *kata* and *karada-de-oboeru* in Dohsa-hou therapy.

This specific attitude that the three therapies share could be summarized with the term *strategic inattention—(fumon)*,[5] that is, inattention does not mean ignoring the client and their complaints, but, as Nagayama and Shimizu point out, it sets a proper mental distance between therapist and client, thus offering a clean therapeutic situation where the client's clinical condition is easier to resolve; the client's existence is accepted the way it is, no matter their condition, with maternal-like attitude (Nagayama and Shimizu 2006: 286). *Fumon* "signifies that a silence called *ma* appears by cutting off a dialogue" (Fujita 1986: 224) and the role of the therapist is therefore to "adopt this *ma* in the form of *fumon* during the treatment process" (Fujita 1986: 227). In other words, both client and therapist act as if the symptom did not exist—both of them simply entrust it to the in-between silence, *ma*. Such an attitude, the Japanese physician Itsuo Okamoto summarizes in a different context, is the very Japanese way for overcoming any suffering—that related to disease or disability included—the Japanese ensconce their troubles in the innermost recesses of their heart to an extent that it is impossible to spot any suffering judging by their speech or behavior (Okamoto 2004: 208–209). "Novelist, essayist, and playwright Yukio Mishima once likened Japan to a crucible: "There is nothing in Japan. But it is the emptiness of a crucible that absorbs everything from the outside and transforms it into something totally different. That force of transformation is Japan" (Takahashi in Iwamiya and Takaoka 2011: 432).

Instead of assuming a fighting-off attitude, the Japanese psychotherapies simply leave the transformative power of Nature to do her work: in a sense, they take refuge in the course of nature. Although the contemporary realities suggest for quite the opposite, in principle Japanese culture "never deliberately placed itself as subject in opposition to nature as object. Much more, in fact: it systematically tended to make nature its supreme referent, even its culmination" (Berque 1997: 142). The country's psychotherapies make no exception: as many of the Japanese artistic practices are "methodologies of cultivation" (Carter 2008: 14), so appear to be the Japanese psychotherapies, too. They focus on reeducation and on cultivating self-control, which may give impetus to the restoration of the natural balance between body and mind, and individual and society. At the same time, paradoxically, by doing so the Japanese psychotherapists support their clients in the process of transcending opposites such as sickness-health to thus acquire through their own

[5]An important Morita therapy concept and technique (see Sect. 5.2.3), we suggest that *fumon* applies, although in a different form and way, to Naikan and Dohsa-hou, too.

satori-like experience a comprehensive understanding of life and human condition that they can adopt and make use of in their daily life. Therefore, these approaches can be defined as *holistic ways of life*, which function as psychotherapies. Once the aim of taking the client beyond dualities is being achieved, the disorder or dysfunction is likely to dissolve naturally and the lost balance—to get restored; or at least the client has the chance to learn to live with their problem in a constructive way—a result that should not be underestimated as far as the problem's main cause, i.e., imbalance and unnaturalness, has been addressed.

Such a goal is likely to be achieved through another aspect peculiar to the three psychotherapies—that of *space-time coordination*: the methods' stringent schedules serve not as mere rules that should be followed blindly, but they structure the flow of time in accordance with the natural circadian rhythm. This rhythm predetermines the client's location and activity in every single moment, thus securing a *coordinated existence*. Additionally, the client is secluded and distanced from their daily life, and this distance contributes to their altered perception of time and also of their presence within the flow of time. The rhythmic repetition of concrete actions gives lustre even to the most mundane activities, turning them into quasi-rituals that take the individual into the here-and-now *reality*. It is interesting that clients who have undergone treatment under any of the three approaches share common impressions although the application scope of the approaches differ from each other—for example, "The world looks brighter now" (see the respective chapters in Part III). Such experiences are indicative of augmented *mindfulness* in the form of daily life awareness (Morita therapy), death awareness (Naikan therapy), and body awareness (Dohsa-hou)—they reveal that when we give up our Ego-driven interpretations of reality and immerse ourselves in it the way it is, the world appears to us in its primordial beauty as a more welcoming place to live in.

Finally, cultural differences indeed exist about how self is treated in the Japanese psychotherapies, but "it is human nature commonly shared across cultures and time that people's values are inevitably attached in the service of the ego" (Kondo 1992: 46). While many of the Western psychotherapeutic approaches aim to strengthen the Ego and confirm its position within its relationships with others and the world, the Japanese psychotherapies work toward quite the opposite: Ego should be "overcome" and "dissolved" in the common space-time that we all share; in the silence of the empty-centered structure of *ma* where all possibilities for future growth, healing included, lie dormant. Breaking the chains of this attachment to the Ego for the sake of self-transformation, which resuscitates consequently the natural balance within the body-mind unity, appears to be the ultimate goal of the three Japanese psychotherapies—a supreme art to be mastered within a lifetime.

References

Berque, Augustin: Japan—Nature, Artifice and Japanese Culture (transl. Ros Schwartz), Pilkington Press, 1997

Carter, Robert E.: The Japanese Arts and Self-Cultivation, State University of New York Press, 2008

Fujita, Chihiro: Morita Therapy—Psychotherapeutic System for Neurosis, Igaku-Shoin, 1986
Iwamiya, Takeji, K. Takaoka: Katachi (日本のかたち), PIE International, 2011
Kitanishi, Kenji: Morita Therapy, Kodansha, 1999 (in Japanese)
Kondo, Akihisa: A Zen Perspective on the Concept of Self and Human Nature, International Bulletin of Morita Therapy, Vol. 5(1–2), University of British Columbia, 1992
Lebra, Takie Sugiyama: Japanese Patterns of Behavior, University of Hawaii Press, 1976
Nagayama, Kei'ichi, Y. Shimizu: Naikan Method—Theory and Practical Structure, Nippon Hyoron Sha, 2006 (in Japanese)
Nouwen, Henri J.M.: Our Greatest Gift: A Meditation on Dying and Caring, HarperOne, 2009
Okamoto, Itsuo: A Faltering Heart—The Way the Japanese Accept and Overcome Diseases and Disabilities, Ishiyaku Publishers, 2004 (in Japanese)
Reynolds, David K.: The Quiet Therapies—Japanese Pathways to Personal Growth, University of Hawaii Press, 1980
Watts, Alan: Asian Psychology and Modern Psychiatry, The American Journal of Psychoanalysis, Vol. 13, Palgrave Macmillan, 1953

Appendix I

Morita Therapy

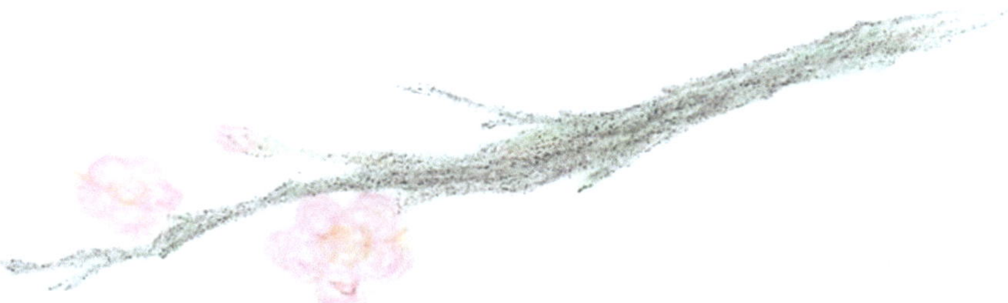

森田療法

V. Chervenkova, *Japanese Psychotherapies*,
DOI 10.1007/978-981-10-3126-7

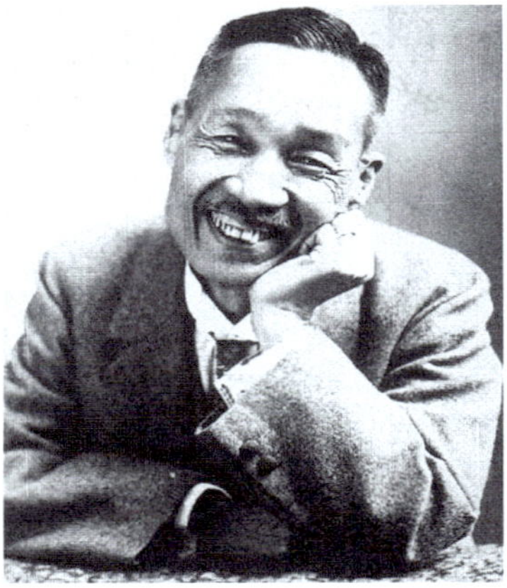

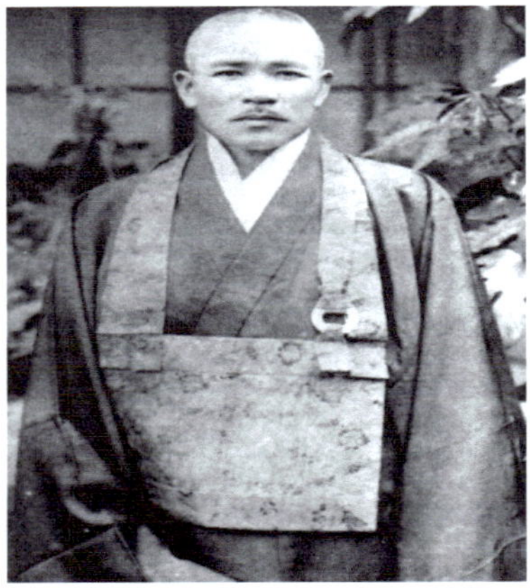

Morita therapy's founder Shōma Morita (1874–1938) in 1931 (courtesy of Hakuyosha Publishing Co); on the right: Dr. Genyū Usa (1886–1957), founder of Sansei Hospital, in his clerical garment, circa 1913 (courtesy of Dr. Shin'ichi Usa)

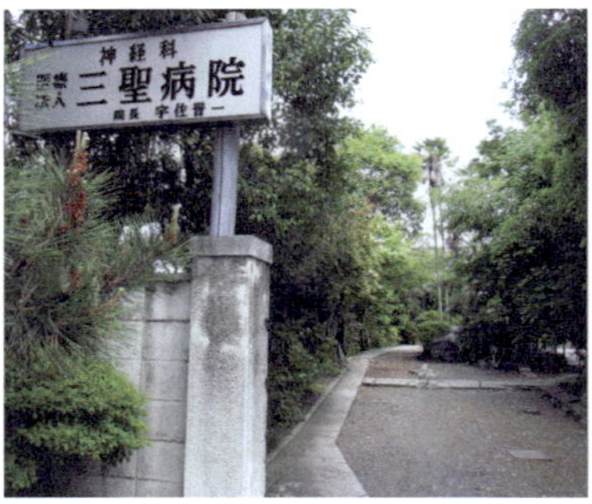

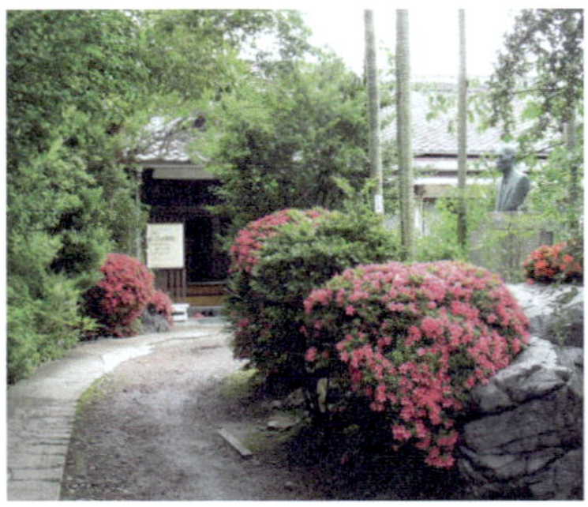

The main gate of Sansei Hospital in Kyoto's Higashiyama district. The hospital was founded in 1922 by Dr. Genyū Usa. After he passed away in 1957, his only son Dr. Shin'ichi Usa headed the hospital up until 2015 when it was closed down and demolished; on the right: the entrance to the temple-like hospital building. In the front right of it, a bust of Dr.Genyū Usa can be seen among the tress (May 2013)

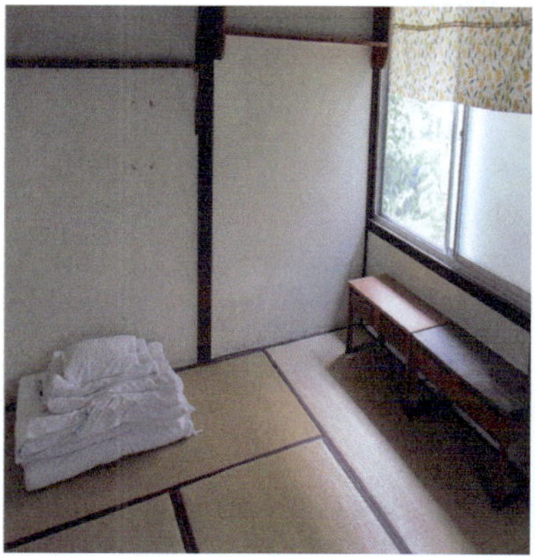

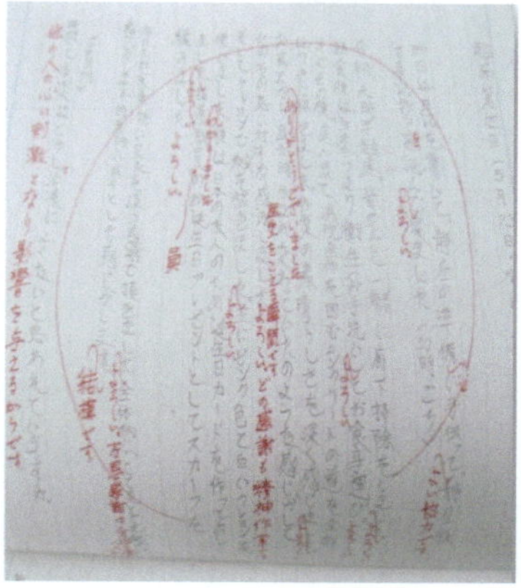

All the patients' rooms in Sansei Hospital were Japanese-style ones; on the right: an excerpt from the author's diary with Dr. Usa's comments written in red along each sentence. Writing the diary in the traditional vertical style was not a rule, but was preferable (May 2013)

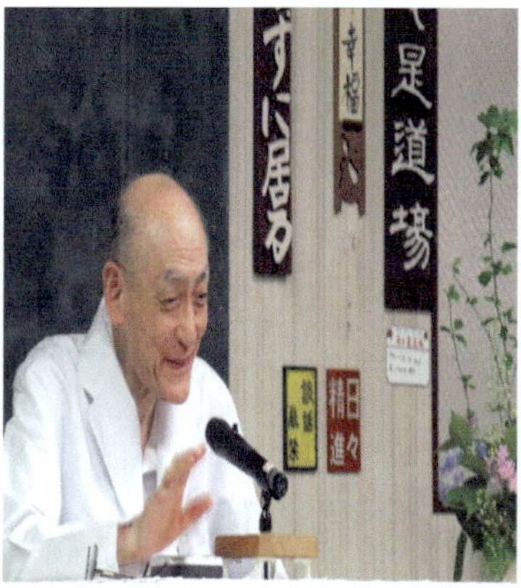

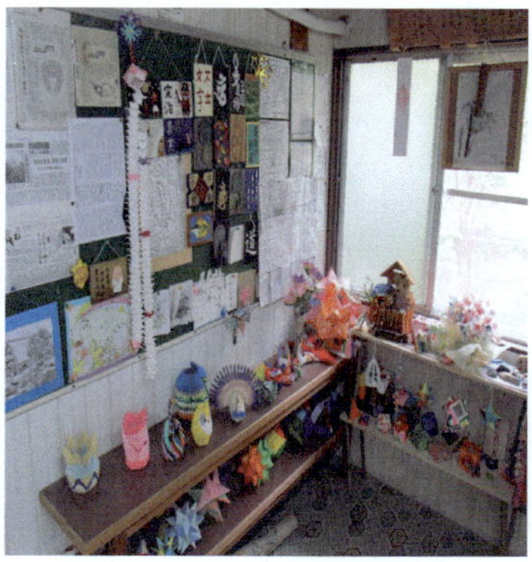

Dr. Shin'ichi Usa while lecturing in front of the inpatients at the hospital's workroom; on the right: the exhibition corner at the workroom where handiworks such as *origami* and calligraphy works, paintings and woodcarvings made by inpatients were displayed (May 2013)

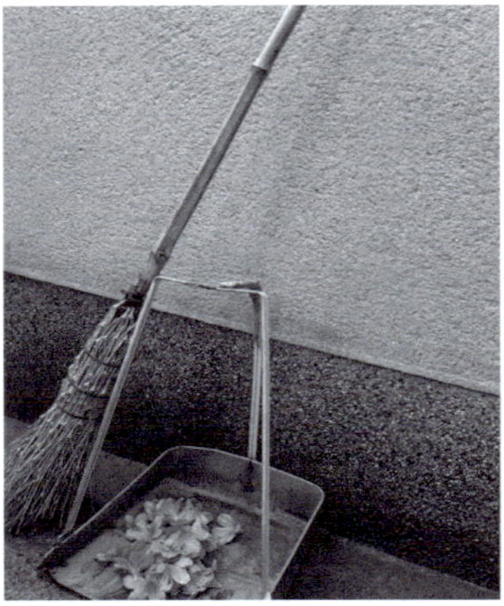

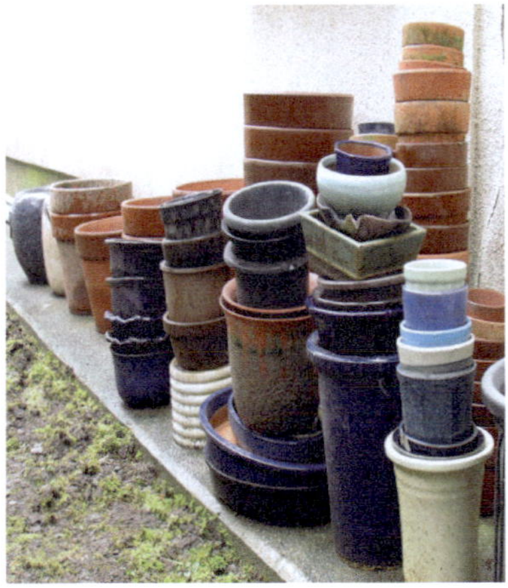

Daily life scenes from the hospital's backyard: "Putting efforts already means that you are happy" (May 2013)

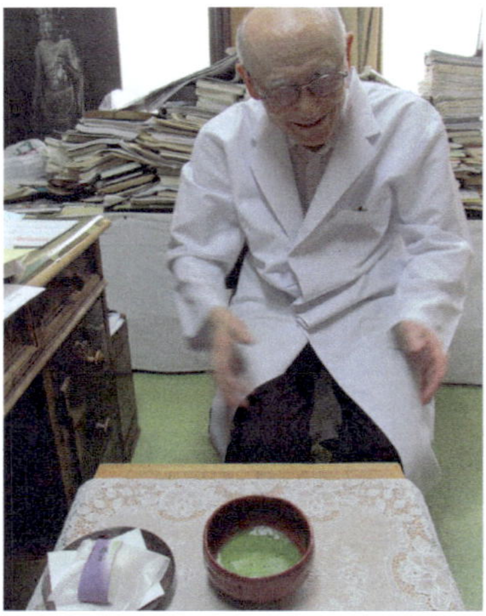

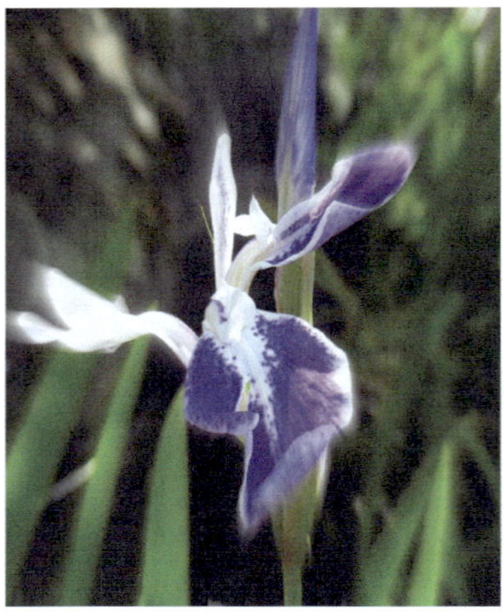

Over a cup of green tea prepared kindly by Dr. Usa in his consulting room. In the early summer morning outside, the eagle-tail irises presented by the Japanese Emperor to Tōfuku-ji temple in the 19th century were in their full bloom (June 2013)

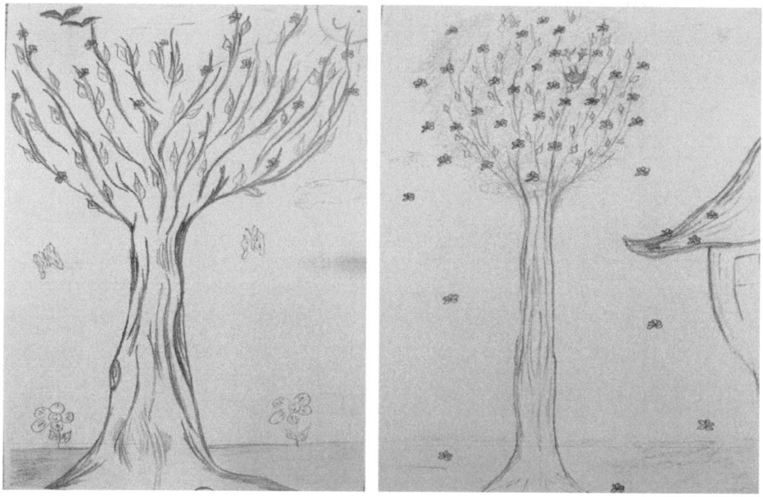

The author's two Baum test drawings on the hospitalization day (May 2013)

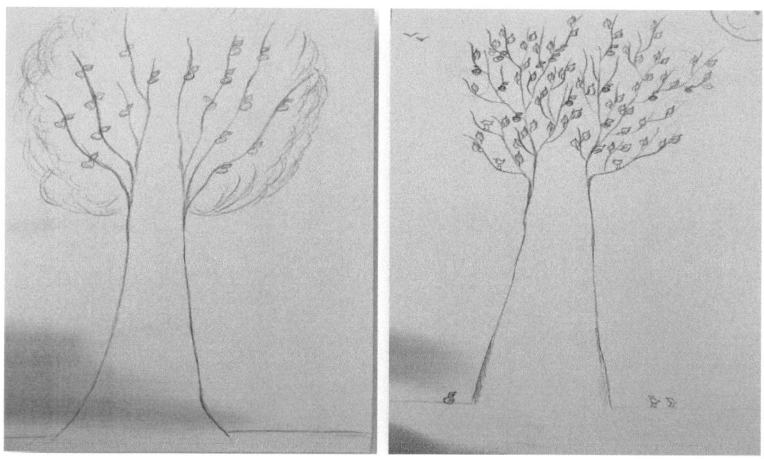

and two weeks later, on the day the author was discharged from the hospital (June 2013)

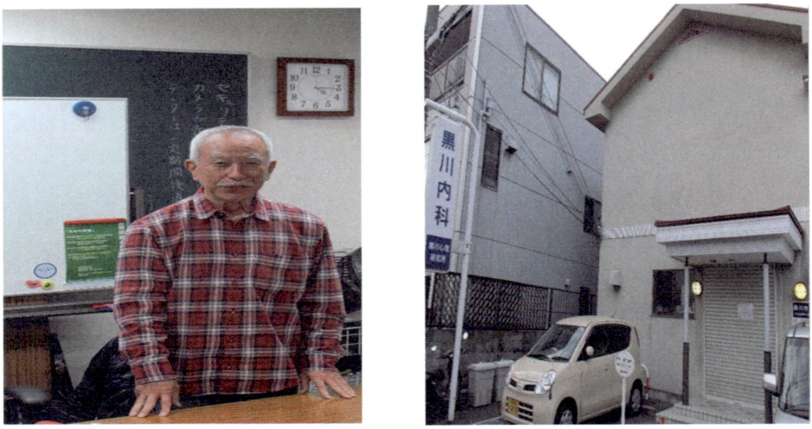

Dr. Nobuo Kurokawa, Director of Kurokawa Clinic of Internal Medicine in Osaka, in his consulting room. Dr. Kurokawa applies outpatient Morita therapy to clients with psychosomatic conditions; on the right: the clinic is located in a two-story house in a silent neighborhood (December 2015)

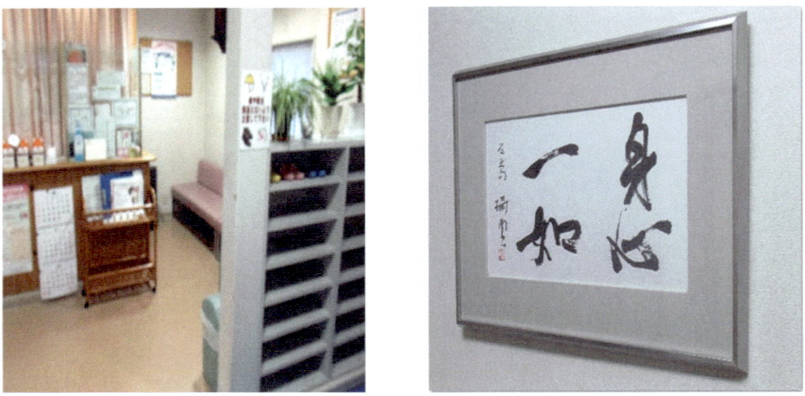

The entrance and the reception desk of Kurokawa Clinic of Internal Medicine. In contrast to many other contemporary hospitals, patients must take off their shoes upon entering and use slippers—a rule which creates a home-like atmosphere; on the right: on one of the corridor walls there is a calligraphy work reading *shinjin-ichinyo* 「身心一如」 ("body-mind oneness"; see footnote 7 in Sect. 4.2) (December 2015)

Appendix II

Naikan Therapy

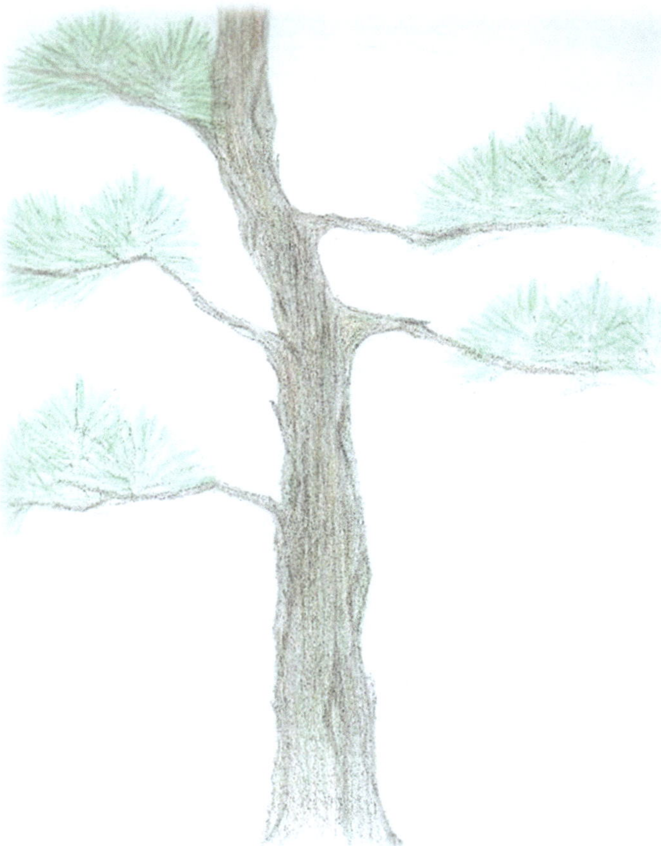

内観療法

V. Chervenkova, *Japanese Psychotherapies*,
DOI 10.1007/978-981-10-3126-7

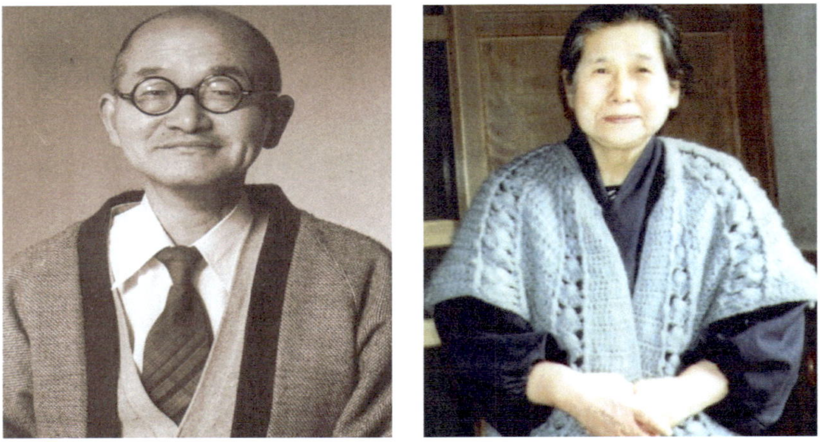

Naikan therapy's founder, Rev. Ishin Yoshimoto (1916–1988), and his wife Kinuko Yoshimoto (1920–2000) (courtesy of Yamato Naikan Training Center). Not only did the spouses commit their whole life to Naikan, but they also raised a big family with two daughters, three sons, and many grandchildren

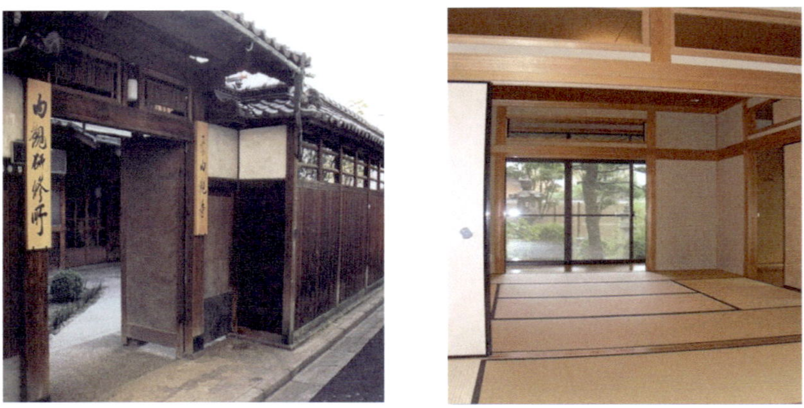

The main entrance to Yamato Naikan Training Center in Yamato-kōriyama, Nara prefecture; on the right: the main training hall with folding screens and *tatami* straw mats, and a beautiful Japanese garden in front of the window. The center was opened in 1953 by Rev. Ishin Yoshimoto and is now headed by his direct disciple, Prof. Teruaki Maeshiro. The center was fully renovated in 2003 (June 2012)

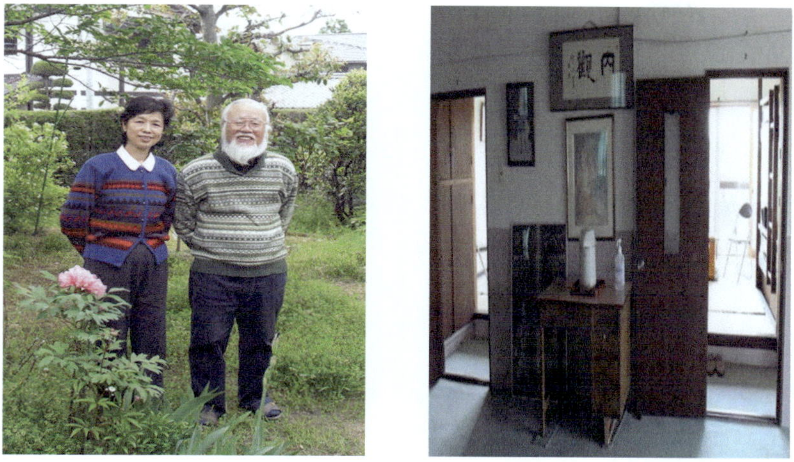

Prof. Yoshihiko Miki and Junko Miki, direct disciples of Rev. Ishin Yoshimoto, in the garden of Nara Naikan Training Center that they operate; on the right: the cener's main corridor with the entrances to the individual rooms. On the wall there is an original calligraphy work by Rev. Ishin Yoshimoto, reading *naikan* (May 2011)

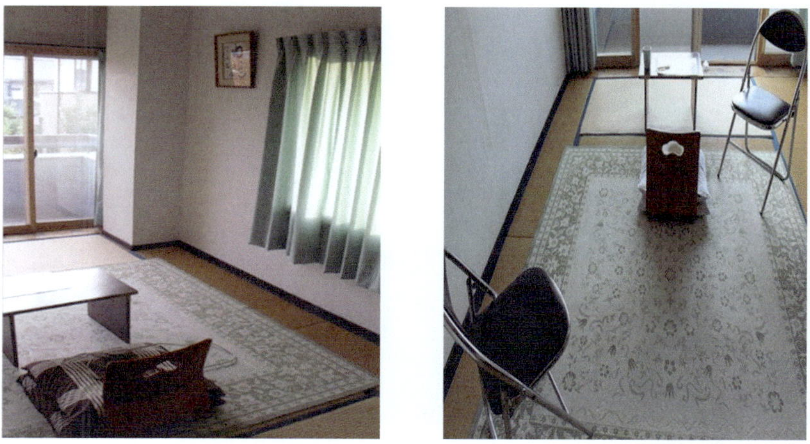

One of the rooms for intensive Naikan at the center. No folding screens are used here and each client is accommodated in a private room. While practicing Naikan, the client sits on a *zabuton* cushion with a backrest, but during the interviews both client and interviewer sit on chairs (May 2011)

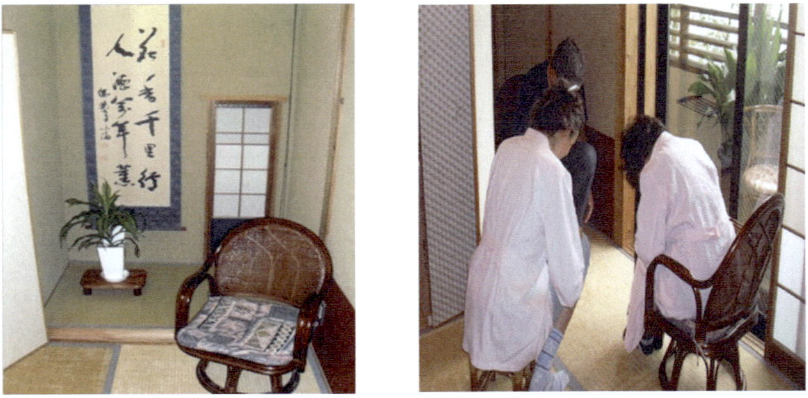

One of the corners with a folding screen for practicing intensive Naikan at Osaka Naikan Training Center. The hanging scroll on the wall reads 「花ノ香千里行人徳万年薫」—"The fragrance of the flowers floats for thousand miles, the man's virtues smell sweet for ten thousand years"; on the right: the center's director Mieko Hariki and a foreign client bowing to each other after a Naikan interview interpreted by the author (November 2011)

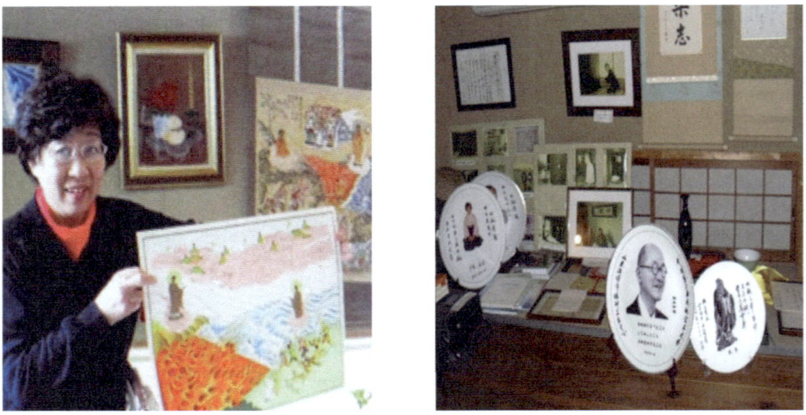

Director Mieko Hariki shows a picture of *Niga-Byakudō* (二河白道, lit. "two rivers and a white road"), an important *Jōdo Shinshū* metaphor referring to two torrential rivers—of water (greed and obsessiveness) and of fire (anger and hatred)—and a white narrow path (thorough self-reflection) between them, which promises to lead the devotees to the Pure Land Paradise. This picture, included in the Mindfulness Sūtra (see Sect. 6.1.6), Ishin Yoshimoto put on the inner side of the folding screens that he used for Naikan;on the right: various paraphernalia of Rev. Ishin Yoshimoto such as photo albums and hanging scrolls are duly kept at Osaka Naikan Training Center. The center is located not far away from the house where once the *Taikan-an* religious group used to come together (October 2012)

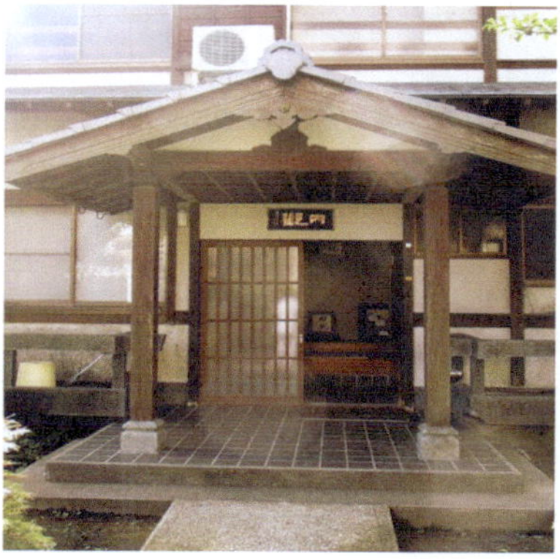

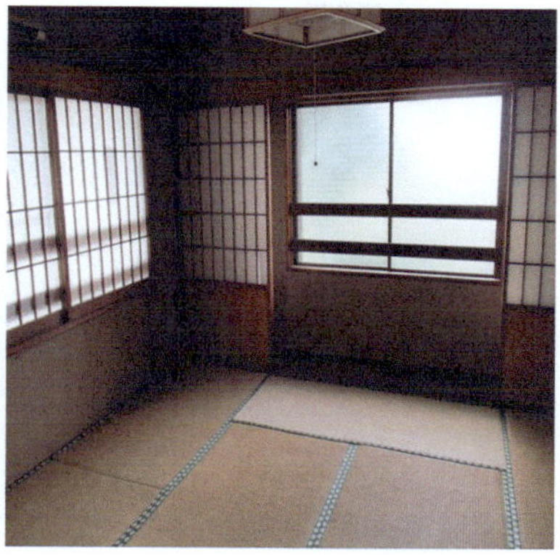

The main entrance to the Naikan training center within Ibusuki Takemoto Hospital in the pastoral hot-spring town of Ibusuki, Kagoshima prefecture. The center, opened in 1975, targets mainly inpatients with alcohol and substance dependence for whom the intensive Naikan practice is part of their treatment plan; on the right: the Naikan room is a Japanese-style one (October 2013)

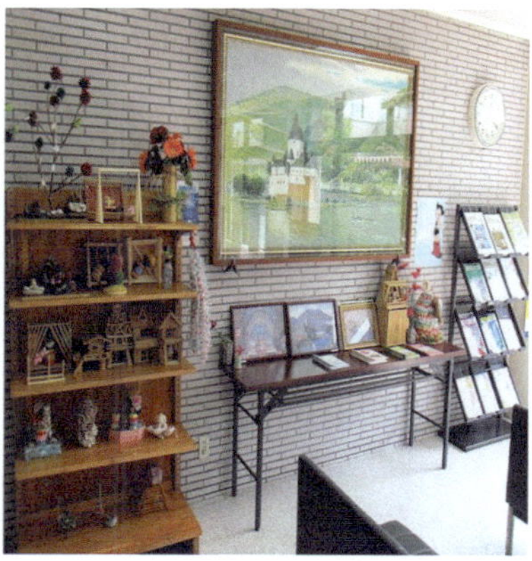

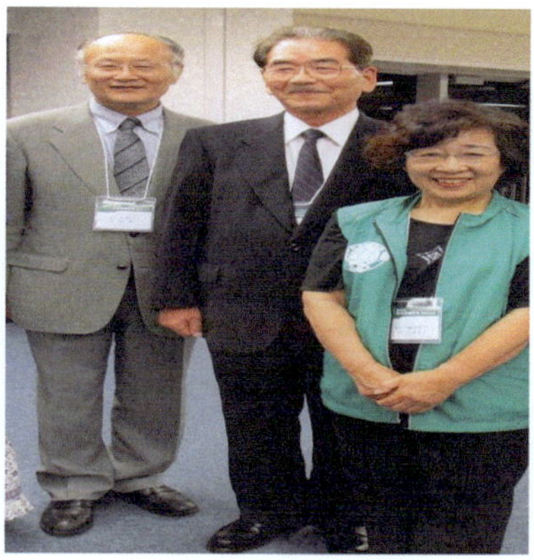

The reception waiting room of the Ibusuki Takemoto Hospital where handiworks by inpatients are displayed. The hospital opened in 1972 to deal primarily with alcohol dependences and psychiatric disorders, and now has a capacity of 211 beds (October 2013); on the right: the hospital director Dr. Takahiro Takemoto (middle) together with Dr. Shō'ichi Ihara of St. Martin Hospital in Kagawa prefecture (left) and Mieko Hariki, head of Osaka Naikan Training Center (right), at the 36th Annual Congress of the Japan Naikan Association in Wakayama (June 2013)

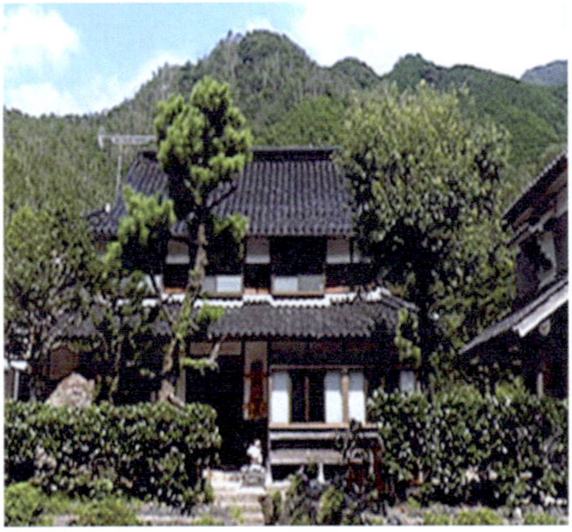

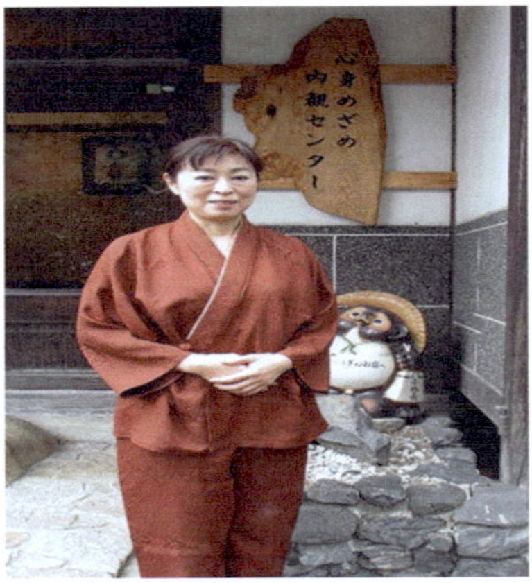

The newest Naikan center in Japan, *Shinshin-Mezame* Naikan Center, opened in June 2014 in Tottori prefecture. Its name means "mind-body awakening" (心身めざめ). The center is accommodated in a traditional Japanese-style house in a rural area endowed with beautiful nature; on the right: the center's director, Rev. Mari Sengoku, Ph.D., in front of the center's entrance (March 2016)

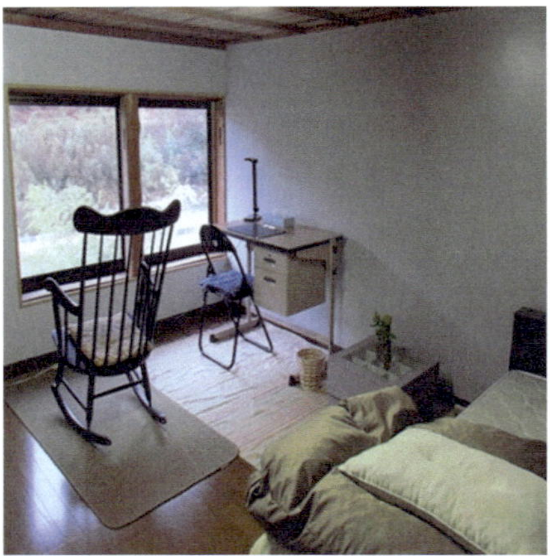

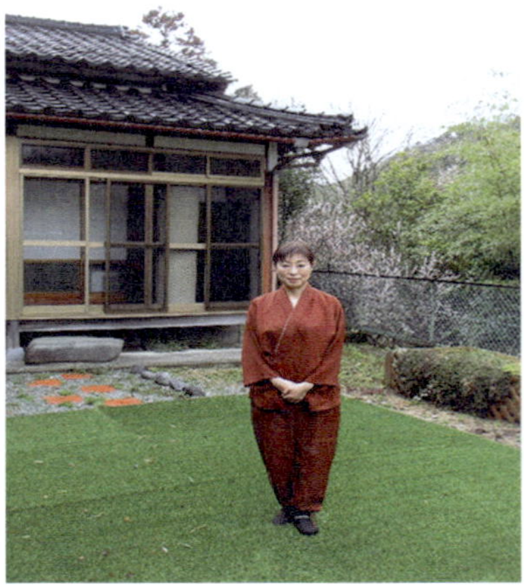

One of the Naikan rooms at the *Shinshin-Mezame* Naikan Center; on the right: together with Naikan therapy, Dr. Sengoku applies to her clients also breathing and meditation techniques at the lawn of the center's backyard. The center accepts also foreign clients, whom Dr. Sengoku interviews in English (March 2016)

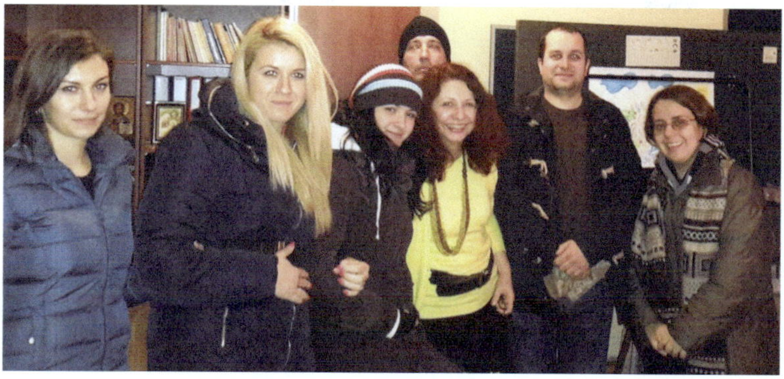

The staff of the "Solidarity" day-care center for rehabilitation of drug, alcohol, and gambling addictions in Sofia (Bulgaria). The first Naikan therapy-related fieldwork research in Bulgaria was carried out among the clients of the center (August 2011/February 2012). The center's director, Dr. Elena Nikolova, smiles in the middle (courtesy of "Solidarity", January 2016)

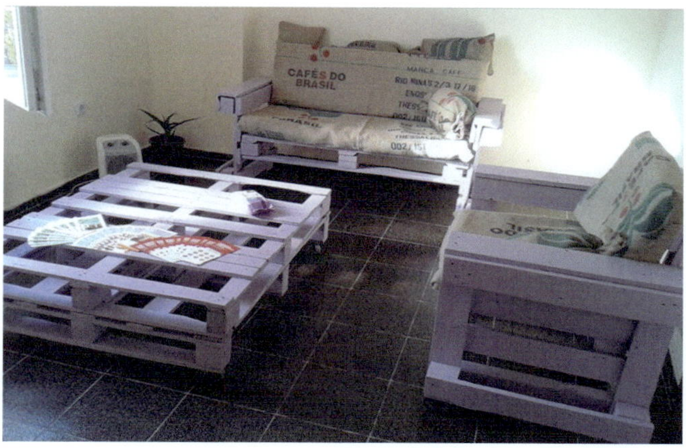

The counseling room at the "Solidarity" day-care center. Its furniture, made of industrial pallets, was created through the joint efforts of the center's staff and clients (courtesy of "Solidarity", January 2016)

Appendix III

Dohsa-hou Therapy

動作法

V. Chervenkova, *Japanese Psychotherapies*,
DOI 10.1007/978-981-10-3126-7

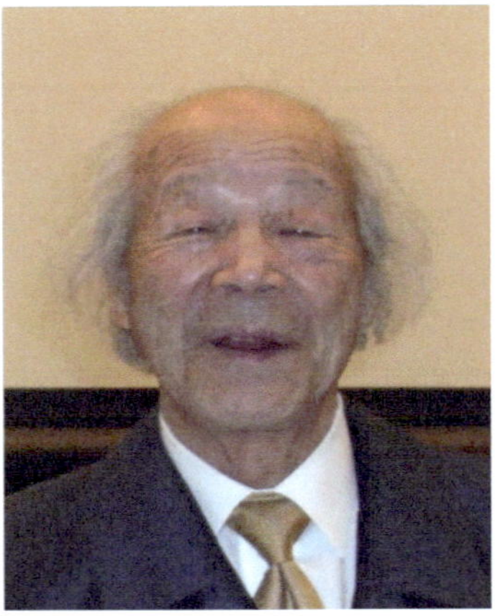

The founder of Dohsa-hou therapy Gosaku Naruse (1924–), Honorary Professor at Kyushu University, at the 36th Annual Congress of Rehabilitation Psychology in Nagoya (December 2010). Notwithstanding his venerable age, Prof. Naruse still keeps on working under a strict daily schedule. The hobbies of his earlier age included skiing, windsurfing, and horse-riding. Known for his curiosity and proactive attitude, which allegedly have contributed to the development of Dohsa-hou, in 2001 Prof. Naruse was conferred the Japanese Imperial decoration Second Class Order of the Sacred Treasure

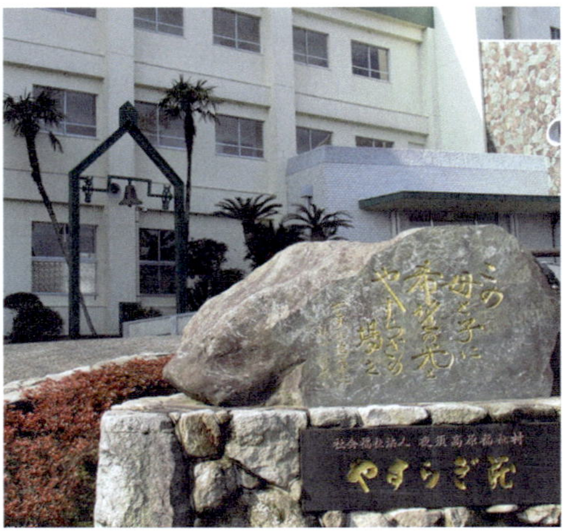

The main entrance to the *Yasuragi-sō* welfare village in Yasu Plateau, Fukuoka prefecture, where the Japanese Association of Rehabilitation Psychology holds Dohsa-hou camps several times a year. The stone-inscribed words read “To the mothers and their children—a place for solace where the light of hope shines” (March 2014)

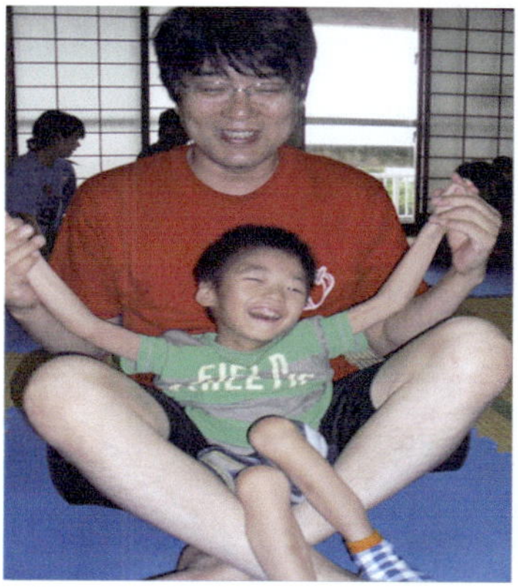

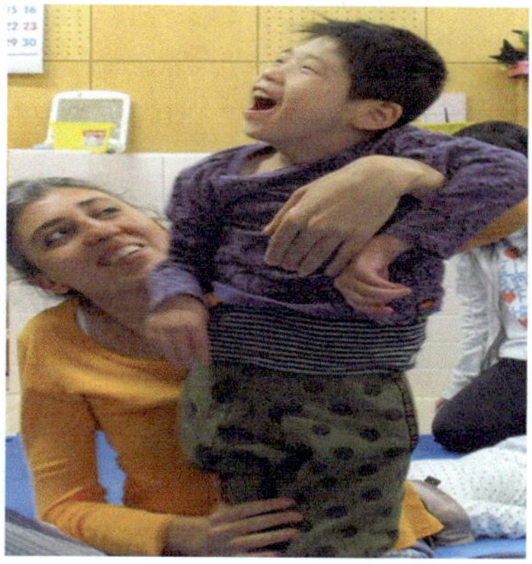

Six-year-old Sei Tanaka, suffering from hydrocephaly, enjoys playful moments with his team supervisor, Prof. Osamu Imura, during the summer Dohsa-hou camp on the island of Ishigaki, Okinawa prefecture (August 2010). Thanks to the camp training, Sei's facial expression and communication skills improved significantly; on the right: with only a little support from the trainer, Sei gladly performs a proper *ritsui* position (November 2013)

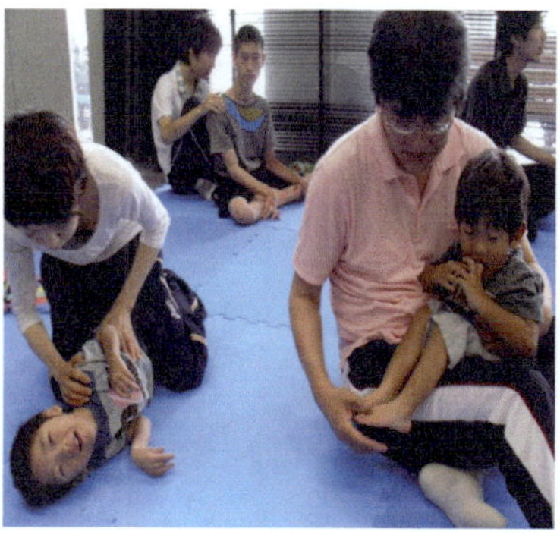

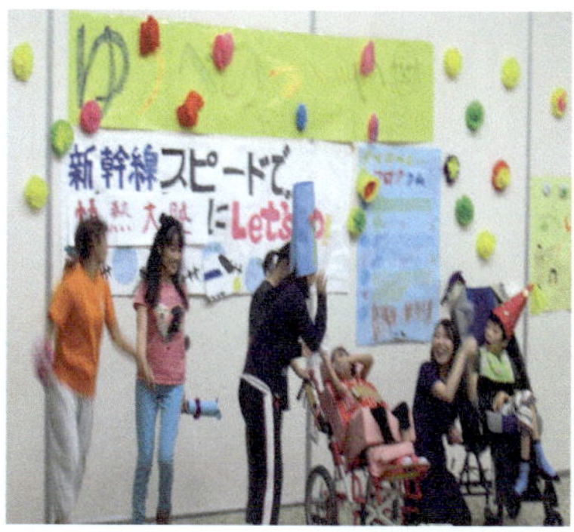

A moment from a therapeutic session with several trainee-trainer pairs during a Dohsa-hou training in Osaka University (July 2010); on the right: a moment from a group therapy session during a summer Dohsa-hou camp in Kyoto (August 2015)

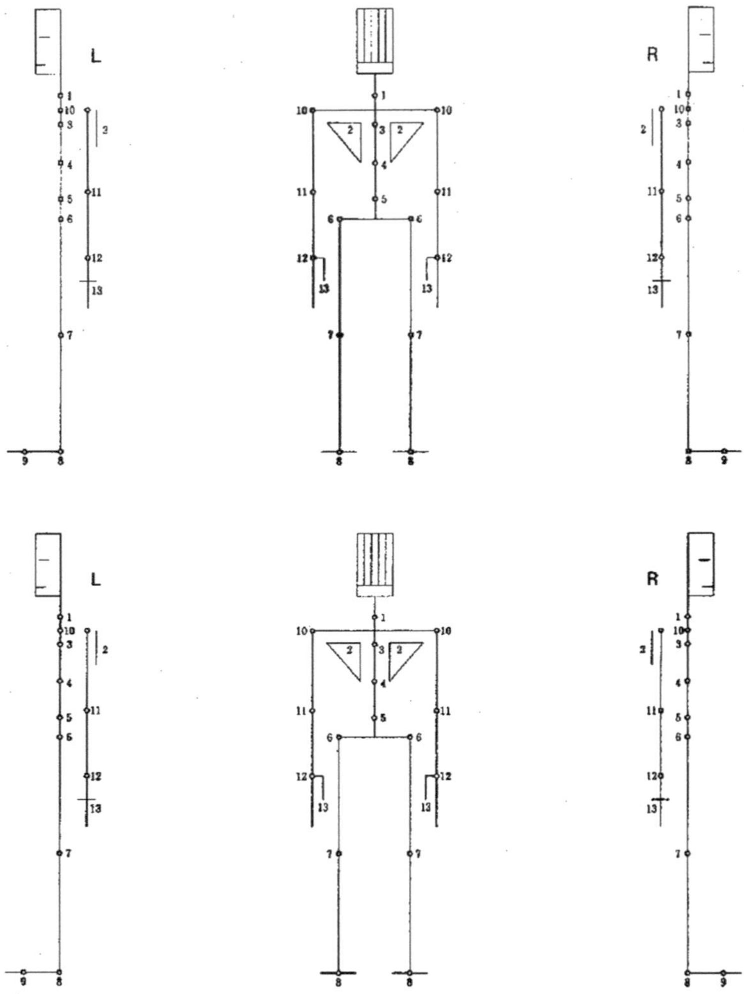

ASSESSMENT

I. Tension

Examine the resistance to examiner's hand. Direction and degree are represented by sign like as follows

i) region : ◯   ii) direction :

II. Joint for test

1. neck	2. scapula	3. breast	4. back	5. waist	6. hip	7. knee
8. ankle	9. toe	10. shoulder	11. elbow	12. wrist	13. hand	

Schema A.1 Schema of body dynamics used in Dohsa-hou assessment (courtesy of Prof. Imura's Laboratory of Clinical Psychology, Osaka University, 2016)

Table A.1 An exemplary schedule for a 4-day/3-night Dohsa-hou camp (courtesy of Prof. Imura's Laboratory of Clinical Psychology, Osaka University, 2016)

Day First		**Day Second**		**Day Third**		**Day Fourth**	
		10:00	Morning greetings	10:00	Morning greetings	10:00	Morning greetings
		10:15	Dohsa-hou session-II	10:15	Dohsa-hou session-V	10:15	Dohsa-hou session-VIII
		11:05	Break	11:15	Break	11:05	Break
		11:15	Training for trainers-II	11:15	Training for trainers-III	11:15	Instructions for parents
		12:05	Break	12:05	Break	11:45	Evaluation of the therapeutic outcomes
12:30	Trainer meeting	12:15	Lunch	12:30	Lunch	12:15	Break
13:00	Orientation for trainees					12:25	Closing ceremony
13:30	Opening ceremony	13:15	Dohsa-hou session-III	13:15	Dohsa-hou session-VI	12:45	End of the camp
14:00	Intake (training for trainers-I)						
		14:05	Break/Nap	14:05	Break/Nap		
14:50	Break	14:15	Group therapy-I	14:15	Group therapy-II		
15:00	Dohsa-hou session-I						
		15:05	Break	15:05	Break		
15:50	Session closing greetings	15:15	Dohsa-hou session-IV	15:15	Dohsa-hou session-VII		
16:05	Break for trainers (supervisor meeting is held at that time)						
		16:05	Session closing greetings	16:05	Party		
16:35	Team meetings						
		16:20	Break for trainers (supervisor meeting is held at that time)				
				17:05	Break for trainers (supervisor meeting is held at that time)		
17:20	General meeting	16:50	Team meetings				
				17:35	Team meetings		
18:05	End	17:35	General meeting				
				18:20	General meeting		
		18:20	End	19:05	End		

Glossary

General terms

Dō **(道)** "path, way"; "doctrine, principle"; the way the Universe functions; the absolute law of life, which cannot be grasped rationally but only as an actual living experience

Dōjō **(道場)** training hall; training establishment

Fumon **(不問)** strategic inattention, disregard of symptoms (lit. "regardless of …")

Gen-fūkei **(原風景)** arche/proto-landscape; the original landscape engraved in one's heart that evokes feelings of nostalgia or déjà-vu

Jibun **(自分)** self, oneself; in person; for one's own part

Jiriki **(自力)** self-power; on one's own; the ability to attain enlightenment through one's own efforts

Kokoro **(心)** heart, mind; center, consciousness; the inner man; mentality

Ma **(間)** interval; in-between; span, time; silence

Mi **(身)** body; oneself, one's character or true mind

Nembutsu **(念仏)** prayer to the Buddha (lit. "I take refuge in Amida Buddha")

Satori **(悟り)** in Zen Buddhism, especially the Rinzai school, refers to enlightenment, awakening; understanding of one's true nature

Shin-fūkei **(心風景)** inner landscape; psychoscape

Shinshin-ichinyo/Shinjin-ichinyo **(心身一如 ・ 身心一如)** body-mind unity; body-mind interconnectedness or interdependence

Morita Therapy

Arugamama **(あるがまま)** the world/reality as it is; frankly, as it is

V. Chervenkova, *Japanese Psychotherapies*,
DOI 10.1007/978-981-10-3126-7

Jijitsu **(事実)** fact, truth; reality

Jun-na kokoro **(純な心)** pure heart

Sei-no-yokubō **(生の欲望)** will to live; vital force

Shinkeishitsu **(神経質)** nervous constitution or temperament

Taitoku **(体得)** to realize, to understand; to learn through one's firsthand experience

Tongo **(頓悟)** abrupt enlightenment, a breakthrough in consciousness; one of the main concepts of the Zen Buddhist Rinzai school

Toraware **(とらわれ)** obsession, mental attachment (lit. "to be biased on; obsessed with")

Zenchi **(全治)** complete cure; total healing

Naikan Therapy

Akunin-shōki **(悪人正機)** a concept by *Jōdo Shinshū*'s founder, Shinran, which suggests that the evil person is the true object of Buddha's compassion and salvation

Byōnin **(病人)** a person that undergoes *mishirabe* (lit. "a sick person")

Jōdo **(浄土)** the Paradise in *Jōdo Shū* and *Jōdo Shinshū* Buddhism (lit. "Pure Land")

Jōdo Shinshū **(浄土真宗)** the True Pure Land school of the Japanese Buddhism, also known as Shin Buddhism. It was founded by monk Shinran, disciple of Hōnen

Jōdo Shū **(浄土宗)** the Pure Land school of the Japanese Buddhism, which was founded by monk Hōnen (1133–1212) in 1175

Jōsan **(定散)** in the *mishirabe* practice this is a person who has learned Buddhism intellectually, but they lack religious experience and their mind is yet attached to mundane matters

Mishirabe **(身調べ)** an austere religious practice heretical to the *Jōdo Shinshū* ranks, considered the predecessor of the Naikan method (lit. "to explore oneself")

Muga **(無我)** selflessness; to "overcome", to "empty" oneself

Mujōkan **(無常観)** awareness of the impermanence of all things

Shinjitsu **(真実)** the one who has attained enlightenment through *mishirabe*

Shinran **(親鸞)** the founder of the *Jōdo Shinshū* school of Japanese Buddhism (born 1173-died 1263). Shinran is known for discarding the monastic vows of celibacy and vegetarianism. In so doing, he emphasized that Buddha Amida's salvation was not reserved for monks and priests only but it was intended for everyone who prayed to Buddha sincerely

Tariki **(他力)** Other-power; the Buddha's salvation power

Zange **(懺悔)** confession, penance

Dohsa-hou Therapy

Agura-zai **(胡坐座位** —"sitting cross-legged on the floor") a task of the *tate-kei* group, *agura-zai* helps the trainer check how flexible the trainee's hip joints are, and if the trainee can keep their back and head upright. The trainer puts their hands on the trainee's shoulders and slightly pushes downward (Ill.1)

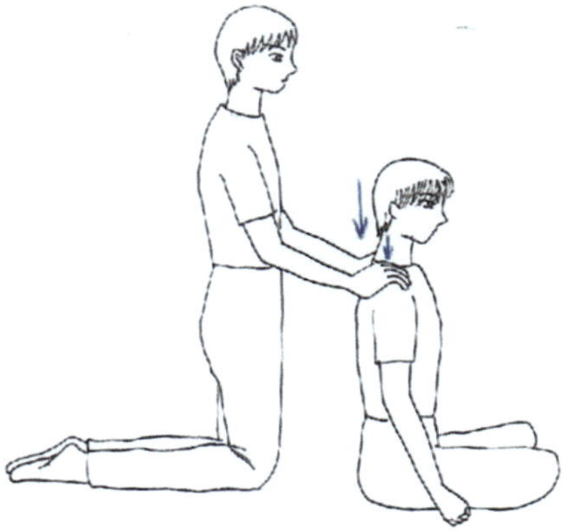

Illustration 1: *Agura-zai*

Hiza-dachi **(膝立ち** —"kneeling") another task of the *tate-kei* group, *hiza-dachi* is important for testing waist flexibility and also for checking the condition of the hip joints and the trainee's ability to stand upright (Ill.2)

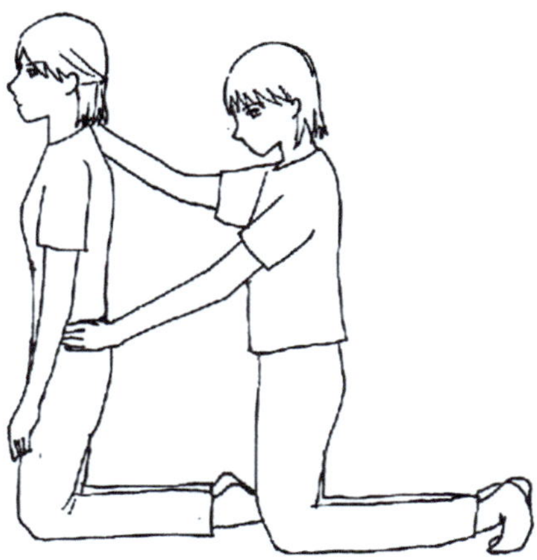

Illustration 2: *Hiza-dachi*

Hokō **(歩行**—"walking") a task of the *tate-kei* group, *hokō* tests the trainee's ability to properly shift their bodyweight from one leg to another while walking

Jiku-zukuri **(軸作り)** "shaping" the body axis applied for the *tate-kei* group of tasks

Karada-de-oboeru **(体で覚える)** to memorize/learn or "remember" through one's body, i.e., through physical practice. This term is somewhat akin to the *taitoku* principle in Morita therapy

Kata (型) figure, form, shape; pattern, type, model

Kukan-no-hineri **(躯幹の捻り**—"twisting of the torso") this task is performed on the floor while the trainee lies on their side. The trainer helps the trainee twist their torso so that the back of their shoulder reaches the floor. It is important that at this point the trainer blocks the trainee's bottom by their knees, while slightly pressing the shoulder to the floor; than the trainer helps the trainee twist their torso in the opposite direction, to the front. This is a key relaxation technique (Ill.3)

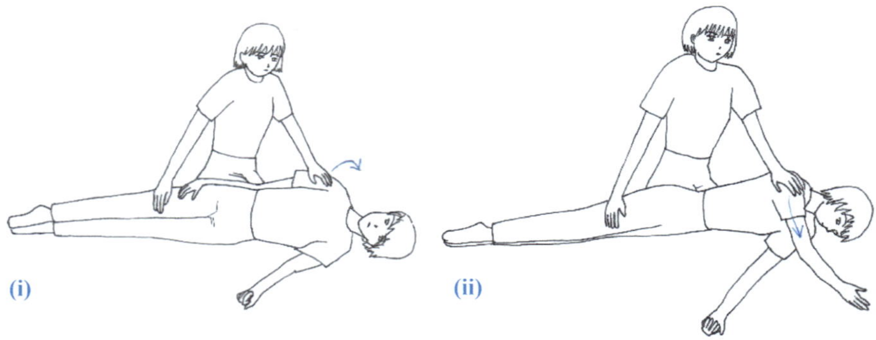

Illustration 3: *Kukan-no-hineri* to the back (i) and to the front (ii)

Ritsui **(立位**—"standing upright") another task of the *tate-kei* group, the simple task of *ritsui* helps the trainer check to which side the trainee's bodyweight tends to shift more, and if they can keep balance and stand upright (Ill.4)

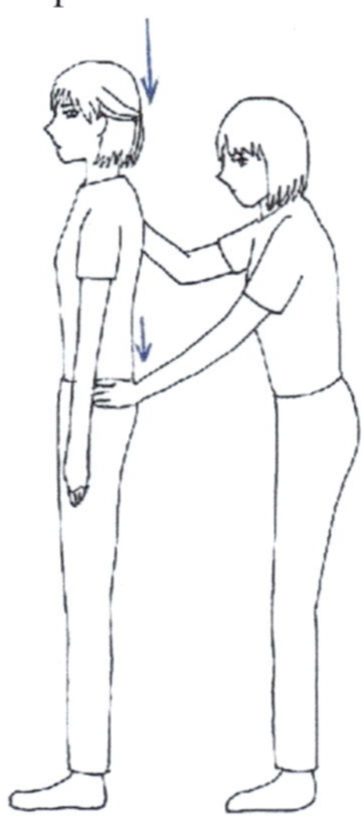

Illustration 4: *Ritsui*

Tate-kei **(**タテ系—"straighten up") this is a general term for all tasks that test the trainee's ability to stand upright and maintain their balance against gravity. These tasks are *agura-zai*, *hiza-dachi*, *ritsui*, and *hokō*

Ude-age **(**腕挙げ—"arm lifting") this task can be performed while the trainee lies on the floor or sits on a chair. The trainer helps the trainee raise their arm while following the imaginary vector of the arm's proper movement. This is one of the main tasks for warming up and for establishing communication between trainer and trainee. *Ude-age* is also applied for the establishment of joint attention, which is especially important in the therapeutic work with children with autism and hyperactivity disorders (Ill.5)

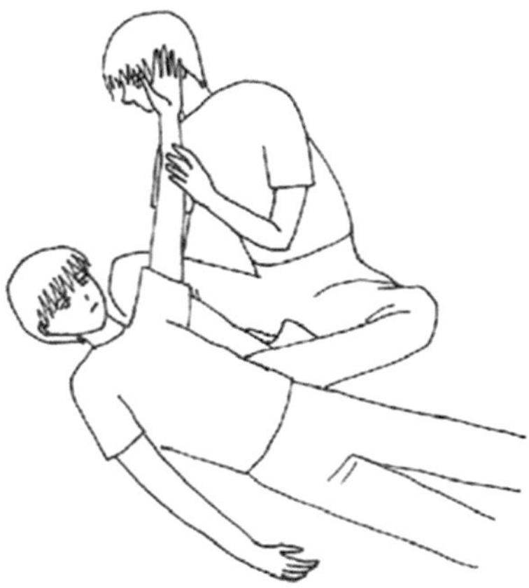

Illustration 5: *Ude-age*

Japanese-Language References

Chapter 1

- 秋田巌(編): 日本の心理療法—思想篇、新曜社、2014
- 小泉晋一: 日本における戦前までの「心理療法」と「精神療法」、日本における臨床心理学の導入と受容過程、日本心理学会第68回大会ワークショップ、 retrieved from http://www.ritsumeihuman.com/uploads/publications/97/9_35.pdf、立命館大学、2004
- 田中淳夫: 森を歩く—森林セラピーへのいざない、暁印刷、2009
- 長山恵一、清水康弘: 内観法—実践の仕組みと理論、日本評論社、2006
- 三木義彦、黒木賢一 (共編): 日本の心理療法—その特質と実際、朱鷺書房、1998
- 森本兼曩、宮崎良文、平野秀樹 (共編) : 森林医学、朝倉書店、2006

Chapter 2

- 秋田巌 (編): 日本の心理療法—思想篇、新曜社、2014

Chapter 3

- 魚住孝至: 道を極める—日本人の心の歴史、放送大学教育振興会、2016
- 内田樹: 日本辺境論、新潮社、2009
- 太田昭彦: 山の神さま･仏さま—面白くてためになる山の神仏の話、ヤマケイ新書、2016
- オギュスタン・ベルク: 空間の日本文化 (訳:宮原信)、筑摩書房、1994
- 門脇佳吉: 道の形而上学—芭蕉・道元・イエス、岩波書店、1990
- 河合隼雄: 中空構造日本の深層、中央公論社、1999
- 神原正明 :日本の美術— 美意識のルーツを探る、勁草書房、2001
- 木村敏: 人と人の間—精神病理学的日本論、弘文堂、1972
- 栗田勇: 日本文化のキーワード—七つのやまと言葉、祥伝社新書、2010
- 鈴木大拙: 東洋的な見方、岩波書店、1997
- 高橋こうじ: 日本の大和言葉を美しく話す— こころが通じる和の表現、東邦出版、2014
- 多田道太郎: 身辺の日本文化、講談社学術文庫、1988
- 中西進:日本人の忘れもの(2)、ウェッジ、2008
- 中野明、大久保喬樹: 日本文化論—名著25冊で読み解く日本人のアイデンティティ、朝日新聞出版、2015
- 長澤規矩也 (編): 新漢和中辞典、三省堂、1967

V. Chervenkova, *Japanese Psychotherapies*,
DOI 10.1007/978-981-10-3126-7

- 芳賀綏: 日本人らしさの構造—言語文化論講義、大修館書店、2004
- 藤田千尋: 森田療法でいわれる不問の意味、 精神療法研究、 第1巻1号、 精神療法研究会、1969
- 安田武: 型の日本文化、朝日新聞社、1984
- 山久瀬洋二: 日本人のこころ—Heart & Soul of the Japanese (対訳ニッポン双書、 transl. Michael A. Cooney)、IBCパブリッシング、2011
- 山崎宏: 日本画と日本建築の時空、青山社、2011
- 吉田裕子: 大和言葉—たしなみ帖、永岡書店、2015

Chapter 4

- 織田尚生: 心理療法と日本人のこころ—神話を生きる、培風館、2005
- 小俣和一郎: 日本における精神病院の起源とその類型(明治維新以前)、第12回世界精神医学会横浜大会シンポジウム、精神経誌、第105巻2号、日本精神神経学会、2003
- 大山正、上村保子: 心理学史、放送大学教育振興会、1998
- 河合隼雄: 心理療法序説 <心理療法>コレクションIV、岩波書店、2009
- 仲紘嗣: 「心身一如」の由来を道元・栄西それぞれの出典と原典から探る、心身医学、第51巻8号、日本心身医学会、2011
- 湯浅康雄: 身体の宇宙性—東洋と西洋、岩波書店、1994

Chapter 5

- 穐山貞登: 創造の心理、誠信書房、1962
- 市川光洋: 外来森田療法—神経症の短期集中治療、白揚社、2008
- 岩田真理: 森田正馬が語る森田療法—「純な心」で生きる、白揚社、2003
- 岩田真理: 流れと動きの森田療法—森田療法の新しい世界、白揚社、2012
- 宇佐玄雄、宇佐晋一: 真実に生きる、三聖病院・三省会、1981
- 宇佐晋一、木下勇作: あるがままの世界—仏教と森田療法、東方出版、1987
- 宇佐晋一、木下勇作: あるがままの世界 (続)—宗教と森田療法の接点、東方出版、1995
- 牛島定信: 森田療法と精神分析の対話—今後の精神療法の方向を探る、東京慈恵会医科大学雑誌、第120巻2号、東京慈恵会医科大学、2005
- 大谷孝行: 森田療法における自然観、富山国際大学人文社会学部紀要、第2巻、富山国際大学、2002
- 大谷孝行: 森田療法における認知的働きかけ—特に言語使用の側面から、富山国際大学現代社会学部紀要、第4巻、富山国際大学、2012
- 大原健士郎: あるがままに生きる—森田療法の心の処方箋、講談社、1997
- 大原健士郎、大原浩一(共編): 森田療法、世界保険通信社、1990
- 岡本重慶: 「禅的森田療法」についての研究—三聖病院の歴史と歩み、総合社会科学研究、第3集2号、総合社会科学会、2010
- 岡本重慶: 波また波—仏教・森田療法・認知行動療法・瞑想、retrieved from kyoto-morita.org、京都森田療法研究所、2012
- 岡本重慶:森田療法の忘れ物—隠れた先哲たちの知恵、retrieved from kyoto-morita.org、京都森田療法研究所、2013
- 岡本重慶: 忘れられた森田療法—生歴史と本質を思い出す、創元社、2015
- 小田晋:東洋の狂気誌、思索社、1990
- 小田晋: 宗教と精神療法—東西文化における並行進化、第15回日本内観学会大会論文集、日本内観学会、1992
- 川原隆造、巽信夫、吉岡伸一 (共編): 東洋思想と精神療法—東西精神文化の邂逅、日本評論社、2004

- 北西憲二: 実践・森田療法、講談社、1999
- 北西憲二: 森田療法 (「個人史と心理療法」)、安田生命社会事業団、2000
- 北西憲二: 森田療法のすべてがわかる本、講談社、2007
- 北西憲二: 森田療法の過去・現在・未来—森田療法の源流から考える、慈恵医大誌 (森田療法センター開設記念論文)、2008
- 北西憲二: 外来精神療法としての森田療法—その理論と技法、精神経誌、第114巻1号、日本精神神経学会、2012
- 北西憲二: はじめての森田療法、講談社現代新書、2016
- 熊野明夫: 森田療法とFrankl の Logotherapie—特に治療環境の相違の意味について、精神療法研究、第1巻2号、精神療法研究会、1969
- 近藤章久: 精神療法におけるアクセプタンス(受け入れ)の意義について、神経質、第3巻1号、神経質研究会、1962
- 桜井図南男: 森田神経質について断想、精神療法研究、第1巻2号、精神療法研究会、1969
- 鈴木知準: ノイローゼの生活指導—森田的性格化の実際、誠信書房、1970
- 鈴木知準: 森田療法を語る、誠信書房、1977
- 中山和彦: 言葉で理解する森田療法—まったく新しい森田療法のかたち、白揚社、2014
- 野村章恒: 森田正馬評伝、白揚社、1974
- 帚木蓬生: 生きる力— 森田正馬の15の提言、朝日新聞出版、2013
- 本多義治、鈴木英鷹、本多秀治、入澤聡:地方都市精神病院における作業療法の草分け (大正初期における七山病院の取り込み)、精神経誌、第111巻9号、日本精神神経学会、2009
- 丸山櫻薫: 森田正馬の人間観、鳴門教育大学大学院、1995
- 三木義彦、黒木賢一 (共編): 日本の心理療法—その特質と実際、朱鷺書房、1998
- 森田正馬: 神経質及神経衰弱症の療法、日本神経医学会、1922
- 森田正馬: 神経質の本能と療法—精神生活の開眼、白揚社、1960
- 森田正馬: 森田正馬全集(編集:高良武久)、第一巻、白揚社、1974
- 渡辺直樹: 森田療法の文化的背景、精神経誌、第105巻5号、日本精神神経学会、2003

Chapter 6

- 五十嵐一夫: 一定案としての内観禅、第14回日本内観学会大会論文集、日本内観学会、1991
- 石井光: 一週間で自己変革— 「内観法」の驚異、講談社Sophia Books、1999
- 石井光: 内観療法(「個人史と心理療法」)、安田生命社事業団、2000
- 石井光: 内観への誘い、西村企画出版、2011
- 市川浩・山崎賞考選委員会: 身体の現象学、河出書房新社、1977
- 市川浩: <身>の構造—身体論を超えて、講談社学術文庫、1993
- 一條信子、川内知子、竹元隆洋: 内観療法による嘔吐発作からの解放—嘔吐症の1女性例、第14回日本内観学会大会論文集、日本内観学会、1991
- 五木寛之: 自力と他力、筑摩書房、2014
- 井原彰一: 精神療法としての内観、第24回内観療法ワ—クショップ–サイコセラピーに果たす内観の役割について(未刊)、2012
- 岩岡正: 内観法の源流をたずねて—吉本伊信の言いたかったこと、倉栄出版、2002
- 宇佐美秀慧: あふれる涙を、ありがとう— 「内観」から「布薩念仏」へ、専光坊、1988
- 奥村二吉、佐藤幸治、山本晴雄(共編): 内観療法、医学書院、1972
- 織田尚生:心理療法と日本人のこころ—神話を生きる、培風館、2005
- カール・ベッカー:死の体験—臨死現象の探求、法藏館、1992
- 金光寿郎:東洋の知恵・内観—こころの洗濯法、光雲社、1985
- 亀井勝一郎: 無常感—日本文化研究 (3)、新潮社、1969
- 河合隼雄: 心理療法序説 <心理療法>コレクションIV、岩波書店、2009
- 川原隆造: 内観療法、新興医学出版社、1996
- 川原隆造(編): 内観療法の臨床—理論とその応用、新興医学出版社、1998

- 川原隆造、 東豊、 三木義彦(共編): 心理療法の本質—内観療法を考える、 日本評論社、1999
- 草薙正夫: 幽玄美の美学、 塙書房、1973
- 草野亮: タナトロジーと内観、内観研究、第7巻、 日本内観学会、2001a
- 草野亮: 内観における「死と再生」 のテーマ—絵画より見た内観者の世界、 日本内観医学会、2001b
- 楠正三: 内観法のしくみ、内観研修所、1980
- 楠正三: 心の探検—内観法、日本内観学会、1983
- 栗田勇: 白隠禅師の読み方—今に甦る「心と体の調和-内観法」 の極意、 祥伝社黄金文庫、2001
- 佐藤幸治(編): 禅的療法・内観法、 文光堂、1972
- 佐藤実枉: 吉本式内観法について、 現代密教、第6号、 智山伝法院、1993
- 清水康弘: 実践内観面接論、内観研究、第5巻、日本内観学会、1999
- 新村拓 (編): 日本医療史、吉川弘文館、2006
- 鈴木大拙: 日本的霊性、岩波文庫、1972
- 千石真理: 内観療法と浄土真宗—アメリカにおける心理療法と仏教の関わり、 内観研究、 第11巻、2005
- 滝野功: 喪の営みとしての内観、第3回日本内観学会大会論文集、日本内観学会 1980
- 竹元隆洋 (編): 瞑想の精神療法 (内観療法の理論と実践)、現代のエスプリ、第202号、至文堂、1984
- 竹元隆洋: 内観法のなりたち、第12回日本内観学会大会論文集、日本内観学会、1989
- 竹元隆洋: 内観と医学、指宿竹元病院内観研修所、1994
- 田中久文: 日本美を哲学する—あはれ・幽玄・さび・いき、青土社、2013
- 田中英: 集中内観の体験に関する臨床心理学的研究—内観療法を分析心理学の観点から理解する試み、大阪大学、2004
- チェルヴェンコヴァ ヴェリザラ: ブルガリア人に対する内観療法の試み—その課題と可能性 ～薬物常用者と健常人に対する記録内観の比較研究～、 内観研究、 第18巻、 日本内観学会、2012
- チェルヴェンコヴァ ヴェリザラ: 本来の自分巡礼—自分自身を集中内観の対象とすることとは、大阪大学教育学年報、第18号、大阪大学、2013
- 長島正博: 原法から見た変法、第14回日本内観学会大会論文集、日本内観学会、1991
- 長島正博: 内観法の立場から、内観研究、第10巻、日本内観学会、2004
- 長島正博、長島美稚子: 内観で<自分>と出会う、春秋社、2001
- 長山恵一 、清水康弘: 内観法—実践の仕組みと理論、日本評論社、2006
- 西牟田久雄: 死の哲学、東京図書出版会、2009
- 日本内観学会 (編): 内観—節—吉本伊信の生涯、日本内観学会、1989
- 野口三千三: 原初生命体としての人間—野口体操の理論、岩波書店、2003
- 波多野二三彦: 内観法はなぜ効くか—自己洞察の科学、信山社、1999
- 服部佐和子: 内観と自己の時間をめぐる—考察、 第34回日本内観学会大会論文集、日本内観学会、2011
- 馬場謙一 、福島章 、小川 捷之 、山中康裕(共編): 日本人の深層分析—母親の深層、有斐閣、1984
- 馬場謙一 、福島章 、小川 捷之 、山中康裕(共編): 日本人の深層分析—日本人の深層、有斐閣、1990
- 稗方富蔵:日本人の美学、早稲田出版、2009
- フランツ リッター: 内観とヨーロッパの心理学、内観研究、第8巻、日本内観学会、2002
- 真栄城輝明: 心理臨床からみた心のふしぎ–内観をめぐる話、朱鷺書房、2001
- 真栄城輝明: 心理療法としての内観、朱鷺書房、2005
- 真栄城輝明: 「身調べ」 の「身」 とは、retrieved from http://yamato-mahoroba.sakura.ne.jp/blog/2010/03/post-62.html、大和まほろばの会 (大和内観研修所)、2010
- 真栄城輝明、 榛木美恵子: 吉本伊信小史[1]、 第17回日本内観学会大会論文集、 日本内観学会、1994

・真栄城輝明、 榛木美恵子: 吉本伊信小史[3]、 第18回日本内観学会大会論文集、 日本内観学会、日本内観学会、 1995
・松下棟治、中村宏子: アルコール症に併発した汎発性脱毛症に対する内観的精神療法と自律訓練の併用について、第15回日本内観学会大会論文集、 日本内観学会、 1992
・三木潤子、三木善彦: 内観志向的カウンセリングと集中内観—5年間の身体の痛みからの解放、内観研究、第15巻、日本内観学会、2009
・三木善彦: 内観療法入門—日本的自己探求の世界、創元社、1976
・三木善彦: 「相手の立場に立つ」 ことの意味、第13回日本内観学会大会論文集、日本内観学会、1990
・三木善彦、黒木賢一 (共編): 日本の心理療法—その特質と実際、朱鷺書房、1998
・三木善彦、真栄城輝明 (共編): 内観療法の現在 (日本文化から生まれた心理療法)、現代のエスプリ、第470号、至文堂、2006
・三木善彦、真栄城輝明、竹元隆洋 (共編): 内観療法、ミネルヴァ書房、2007
・三木善彦、三木潤子: 内観ワーク—心の不安を癒して幸せになる、二見書房、1998
・三木善彦、三木潤子: 摂食障害を悩んでいる若い女性の内観事例研究、大阪大学 (未刊)、2011
・三宅忠六: 内観に救われて— 愛の再体験、 文芸社、 2006
・宮崎忠男: 内観の源法とは何か(下)、 内観ニュース、 第12号、 日本内観学会、 1992
・村瀬孝雄: 内観法研究の基本的問題点、 精神療法研究、 第2巻1号、 精神療法研究会、 1970
・村瀬孝雄: 心理療法と価値: 序論–内観的価値を中心に、 内観研究、 第1巻、日本内観学会、 1995
・村瀬孝雄: 自己の臨床心理学–内観　理論と文化関連性、 誠信書房、 1996
・村松基之介: 禅と内観—不安と葛藤の中を生きるヒント、朱鷺書房、 1991
・村松基之介: 「自己発見の扉」 への招待、第18回日本内観学会大会論文集、日本内観学会、 1995
・本山陽一: 内観の本質—第24回内観学会大会のシンポジストとして田村質問に答えて、 内観研究、 第8巻、 日本内観学会、 2002
・森神逍遥: 侘び然び幽玄のこころ—西洋哲学を超える上位意識、 桜の花出版、 2015
・森川恵昭: 日本美の性格、 朝倉書店、 1984
・安田登: 日本人の身体、 筑摩書房、 2014
・矢田部英正: たたずまいの美学—日本人の身体技法、 中公文庫、 2011
・柳田鶴声: 内観実践論—自己確立の修行法、 いなほ書房、 1995
・柳田鶴声:愛の心理療法・内観—よろこびとやすらぎの世界、いなほ書房、1997
・山久瀬洋二: 日本人のこころ–Heart & Soul of the Japanese (対訳ニッポン双書、 transl. Michael A. Cooney)、 IBCパブリッシング 、 2011
・吉本伊信: 反省(内観)、大和軍需加工(有)、1945
・吉本伊信: 内観法—四十年の歩み、 春秋社、 1965・1989
・吉本伊信: 内観法、 春秋社、 1965・2007
・吉本伊信: 内観療法に至るまで 、 精神療法研究、 第2巻1号、 精神療法研究会、 1970
・吉本伊信: 内観の話、 「やすら樹」 別冊、 自己発見の会、 1977
・吉本伊信: 内観への招待、 朱鷺書房、 1983
・吉本伊信: 信前信後—私の内観体験、 内観研修所、 1985
・吉本伊信: 内観日めくり—吉本伊信の言葉、 自己発見の会、 2004
・吉本清信: 偲び草—内観に捧げた一生、平井眞美館、1989
・吉本正信、本山陽一とのインタビュー、retrieved from https://www.aware-publishing.com/interview-20110612.html、アウェアパブリッシング 、 2011

Chapter 7

- 秋田巌(編): 日本の心理療法—身体篇、新曜社、2017
- 糸永和文: 障害児に対する心理リハビリテーション、 大阪教育大学紀要、 第57巻1号、 大阪教育大学、 2008
- 井村修: 障害児臨床と動作法、 大阪大学小児発達学研究科、大阪大学(未刊)、 2012
- 井村修 、 古川卓: 沖縄県における心理リハビリテーションの発展:琉球大学における地域貢献のひとつのあり方、 琉球大学法文学部紀要人間科学、 第13巻、琉球大学、 2004
- 大野清志、 村田茂 (共編): 動作法ハンドブック—初心者のための技法入門、 慶應義塾大学出版会、 1993
- 河野文光 (監修:成瀬悟策): 動作で「わかる」—心理臨床の援助過程 (動作が変われば「こころ」も「からだ」も変わる)、 禅文化研究所、 2013
- 今野義孝: 発達心理臨床におけるタッチの意義、 教育学部紀要、 第33巻、 文教大学、 1999
- 今野義孝: とけあい動作法—心と身体のつながりを求めて、 学苑社、 2005
- 重橋史朗: 形を整える—「おまかせ脱力」と「形づくり」、 ふぇにっくす、 46号、 総合臨床心理センター、 九州大学、 1994
- 田中康夫 (監修:後藤修司): 東洋医学のきほん、 日本実業出版社、 2009
- 鶴光代: 臨床動作法への招待、 金剛出版、 2007
- 冨永良喜 、 三好敏之 、 中野弘治: からだは語る・からだに語る—阪神淡路大震災: 動作法による被災者の心のケア実践報告、 リハビリテイション心理学研究、 第21巻、日本リハビリテイション心理学会、 1995
- 成瀬悟策: Bobath理論との比較による動作と動作訓練の理論、 教育学部紀要、 第18巻2号、 九州大学、 1974
- 成瀬悟策: イメージの時代、 誠信書房、 1988
- 成瀬悟策 (編):健康とスポーツ臨床動作法、現代のエスプリ、 別冊、 至文堂、 1992
- 成瀬悟策: 姿勢のふしぎ—しなやかな体と心が健康をつくる、 ブルーバックス、 1998
- 成瀬悟策: 動作療法—まったく新しい心理療法の理論と方法、 誠信書房、 2000
- 成瀬悟策: リラクセーション—緊張を自分で弛める法、ブルーバックス、2001
- 成瀬悟策: 動作訓練、 心理リハビリテーション研究所、 2005
- 成瀬悟策: 動作のこころ、 誠信書房、 2007
- 成瀬悟策: からだとこころ—身体性の臨床心理、 誠信書房、 2009
- 成瀬悟策: 動作療法の展開—こころとからだの調和と活かし方、 誠信書房、 2014
- 野口三千三: 野口体操—からだに貞 (き) く、 春秋社、 2002
- 春木豊(編): 身体心理学—姿勢・表情などからの心へのパラダイム、 川島書店、 2002
- 保坂隆 (編): リハビリテーション心理学、現代のエスプリ、 第343号、 至文堂、 1996
- 三木善彦、 黒木賢一 (共編): 日本の心理療法—その特質と実際、 朱鷺書房、 1998
- 良原誠崇: キャンプ療法としての動作法キャンプの心理学的意義、 大阪大学教育学年報、 第15号、大阪大学、 2010

Chapter 9

- 草野亮: アルコール依存症にたいする内観療法—その作用機序について、 第15回日本内観学会大会論文集、 日本内観学会、 1992
- 古賀聡: 心理劇にあるアルコール依存症者の対人関係再構築と将来展望への援助、 心理臨床学研究、 29(2)、 日本心理臨床学会、 2011
- 小林桜児: いわゆる「パーソナリティ障害」症例におけるアルコール・薬物問題をどのように認識し、 対応するか—Khantzianの「自己治療仮説」と「信頼障害」という観点から、 精神医学、 54 (11)、 医学書院、 2012
- 忠井俊明: 逃亡者たち—脱現実と自己愛の病理、 ミネルヴァ書房、 2005

・チェルヴェンコヴァ ヴェリザラ: ブルガリア人に対する内観療法の試み—その課題と可能性 ～薬物常用者と健常人に対する記録内観の比較研究～、内観研究、第18巻、日本内観学会 、2012
・チェルヴェンコヴァ ヴェリザラ: 「父母と話ができるようになった！」 静寂の臨床的側面と治癒力をめぐって 内観療法に関するブルガリア薬物依存症者との集団面接、内観研究、第19巻、日本内観学会、2013
・辻田奈保子、 森下文、 真栄城輝明: 「内観研究」 の動向分析—日本内観学会大会の一般演題を中心に、内観研究、第17巻、日本内観学会、2011
・三木善彦、三木潤子: 内観ワーク—心の不安を癒して幸せになる、二見書房、1998
・吉本伊信: 内観法、 春秋社、 1965・2007

Chapter 10

・市川光洋: 外来森田療法—神経症の短期集中治療、白揚社、 2008
・井手雅弘、 大林正博: 心療内科入門—臨床に役に立つ、NCコミュニケーションズ、 2003
・宇佐玄雄、 宇佐晋一: 真実に生きる、 三聖病院・三省会、 1981
・宇佐晋一: 歴史を超える森田療法、精神経誌、第105巻5号、日本精神神経学会、2003
・宇佐晋一: 禅的森田療法(付: 入院日記)、三省会、2004
・宇佐晋一、木下勇作: あるがままの世界—仏教と森田療法、東方出版、1987
・宇佐晋一、木下勇作: あるがままの世界(続)—宗教と森田療法の接点、東方出版、1995
・宇佐晋一、高林昭二: 禅•森田療法•京都—宇佐玄雄博士生誕百年記念講演集、三省会、1987
・岡本重慶: 「 禅的森田療法」 についての研究—三聖病院の歴史と歩み、 総合社会科学研究、 第3集2号、 総合社会科学会、 2010
・中山和彦: 言葉で理解する森田療法—まったく新しい森田療法のかたち、 白揚社、 2014
・星野良一: 浜松医大の入院森田療法 ・ 外来の森田療法—わかりやすい森田療法に取り込んだ20年、 メンタルニュース、 No.33、 (公財) メンタルヘルス岡本記念財団、 2015

Chapter 11

・岡本五十雄: ゆらぐこころ—日本人の障害と疾病の受容と克服、 医歯薬出版株式会社、 2004
・北西憲二: 実践・森田療法、 講談社、 1999
・長山恵一、 清水康弘: 内観法—実践の仕組みと理論、 日本評論社、 2006

Name Index

V. Chervenkova, *Japanese Psychotherapies*,
DOI 10.1007/978-981-10-3126-7

Subject Index

V. Chervenkova, *Japanese Psychotherapies*,
DOI 10.1007/978-981-10-3126-7

MIX
Papier aus verantwortungsvollen Quellen
Paper from responsible sources
FSC® C105338

If you have any concerns about our products,
you can contact us on
ProductSafety@springernature.com

In case Publisher is established outside the EU,
the EU authorized representative is:
Springer Nature Customer Service Center GmbH
Europaplatz 3, 69115 Heidelberg, Germany

Printed by Libri Plureos GmbH
in Hamburg, Germany